SURGERY - PROCEDURES, COMPLICATIONS, AND RESULTS

SPONTANEOUS SUBARACHNOID HAEMORRHAGE

WELL-KNOWN AND NEW APPROACHES

SURGERY - PROCEDURES, COMPLICATIONS, AND RESULTS

Additional books in this series can be found on Nova's website under the Series tab.

Additional e-books in this series can be found on Nova's website under the e-book tab.

SURGERY - PROCEDURES, COMPLICATIONS, AND RESULTS

SPONTANEOUS SUBARACHNOID HAEMORRHAGE

WELL-KNOWN AND NEW APPROACHES

THOMAS KAPAPA AND RALPH KÖNIG
EDITORS

New York

Library of Congress Cataloging-in-Publication Data

ISBN: 978-1-63485-270-8
Library of Congress Control Number: 2016939085

Published by Nova Science Publishers, Inc. † New York

CONTENTS

PREFACE

Johann Wolfgang von Goethe once wrote: "Certain books seem to be written, not that we might learn from them, but in order that we might see how much the author knows." This is not the intention here. This book is far more in keeping with the writings of Thomas Aquinas: "Wonder is the desire for knowledge."

In retrospect, the various advances in the treatment of spontaneous subarachnoid haemorrhage reflect the changes that have taken place not only in neurosurgery but in medicine and medical technology as a whole. The treatment of aneurysms has progressed from surgical ligation of the carrier vessel to the use of complex radiological endovascular and neurosurgical revascularisation methods. The most significant steps in this journey were not taken until recent decades tightly interwoven with the work of our partners especially in Neuroradiology. The improved diagnostics contributed significantly to the development of the surgical treatment of aneurysms. Yet it also has triggered the shift from open operation to endovascular treatment. A development not at its end, encompassing the great danger of dissociation between treatment and patient care – just as the handling of patients with subarachnoid haemorrhage has become a multidisciplinary field. An achievement that - while not denying the significance and the pivotal role of the individual neurosurgeon - shifts the focus onto the well-being of the patient. More and more studies are demonstrating that surgery is not the first, let alone the only possible treatment. Consequently, the number of those mastering this art with both virtuosity and versatility is dwindling. The number of vascular neurosurgeons is declining with the number of procedures that have to be performed on the vascular system supplying the brain. It would appear that many surgical procedures will also be replaced by endovascular therapies in the future.

Yet the treatment of spontaneous subarachnoid haemorrhage implies far more than merely the occlusion of an aneurysm. Neuro*surgical* skills still are needed as far as the treatment of intracerebral haemorrhage, impaired CSF circulation and, in particular, complex aneurysm constellations are concerned not to mention options for intensive care. It is only this additional knowledge of the pathological condition that will fully complete the spectrum of treatment. This book has been written with this in mind: to generate enthusiasm for this neurosurgical condition and ignite the spark of wonder that leads to the desire for deeper knowledge and expertise. It has been written for budding neurosurgeons and those with an interest in this pathological condition. Young (and old) doctors involved in treating these conditions should have a thorough understanding of what lies behind the (surgical) procedures. This well-structured, compact book offers in depth information on the pathological condition and hopefully will inspire further reading. By providing a comprehensive view on all aspects of the illness from the origin to long term outcomes of our patients to all involved in their therapy this book unites the players in the game despite the proceeding sub-specialization in many areas of medicine.

Prof. Dr. med. Christian Rainer Wirtz
University of Ulm
Germany

In: Spontaneous Subarachnoid Haemorrhage
Editors: Thomas Kapapa and Ralph König
ISBN: 978-1-63485-270-8

Chapter 1

History of Subarachnoid Haemorrhage

Dieter H. Woischneck
Neurosurgical Department, Hospital Landshut, Landshut, Germany

Abstract

The modern definition of an "aneurysm" as being the "dilatation of a weakened artery" originated in 1728 (Lancisis). Cerebral aneurysms were further described by Morgagni (1761) and Biumi (1778) in the 18th century. Beadles (1907) noticed that cerebral aneurysms could in almost all cases only be diagnosed post-mortem. Air encephalography also did nothing to increase diagnostic confidence: the invention of cerebral angiography would be the answer in 1926 (E. Monitz). Seldinger's catheter method pushed the technology further in1953. In 1911, Cushing developed a clip for securely occluding inaccessible tumour vessels. McKenzie modified this silver clip and in 1937 Walter Dandy was the first surgeon to treat an intracranial aneurysm with a clip. The first embolisation treatments of intracranial malformations thus resulted in the 1960s and 70s. As a result of international norms the further developments were standardised.

Keywords: history, intracranial aneurysm, subarachnoid hemorraghe, surgical equipment, interventional radiography

Cerebral aneurysms were first described by Morgagni (1761) and Biumi (1778) in the 18th century. The authors had by that time already surmised that subarachnoid haemorrhage was the result of perforated blood vessels. Evidence for this affliction came in 1859: during post-mortem examinations of young men after their sudden deaths, Sir William Gull found haemorrhages in the meshes of the pia mater that had developed as a result of a ruptured aneurysm. However, despite studying these developments methodically the classic triad of symptoms eluded him. The solution was found by Charles Symonds in 1823/24. At the beginning of the 20th century, there then developed a great source of frustration: Beadles (1907) noticed that cerebral aneurysms could in almost all cases only be diagnosed post-mortem. At this stage, surgeons performing craniotomy were by chance confronted with intracranial aneurysms, especially when treating sellar masses. This is evidenced by a report from Sir Victor Horsley of an incidental finding of an aneurysm in the optic nerve, which he treated with bilateral ligation of the cervical portion of the carotid artery. As the former foremost expert in pituitary gland surgery, Harvey Cushing came across numerous such cases, opening up the sacs (aneurysms) and filling them with muscle tissue. Air encephalography also did nothing to increase diagnostic confidence: the invention of cerebral angiography would be the answer.

About the Invention and Establishment of Cerebral Angiography

In 1926 the Portuguese neurologist Egas Moniz carried out initial experiments into cerebral angiography on dogs, using lithium and strontium bromide as contrast media. When first used in humans this method was by no means successful, causing some patients to die. Surgical exposure of the carotid artery with subsequent direct puncture was carried out for the first time on Patient 6. The examination was technically successful but this patient also died from complications. Cerebral angiography was first survived by a patient on 28 June 1927. The method was published in 1927, and a monograph by the inventor with 180 cases appeared in 1931. Sodium iodide was replaced as a contrast medium in 1931 by Thorotrast. In 1934, Moniz described the four angiographic phases. In 1933, Lima and Caldas published the first results of serial angiography. The angiographic findings for intracranial tumours (Lima) and cerebrovascular aneurysms (Cairns, Dott and Jefferson) were presented at a meeting of the British Society of Neurological Surgeons in 1935.

By the mid-30s, Bergstrand, Olivecrona and Tönnis were presenting angiographic images of arteriovenous malformations. In 1936, percutaneous carotid angiography was described by Lomann and Myerson and disseminated by Shimidzu. In 1940, Takahashi published a study on percutaneous vertebral artery puncture. In Europe, angiography was universally accepted relatively quickly, while in the USA the method was initially received with much scepticism due to issues with the employed contrast agents. This situation was improved through the introduction of tri-iodinated contrast media, leading to widespread use of the method from 1945 onwards. In 1944 Dandy pronounced ambivalent: "There is no doubt whatever of the excellent demonstrations of aneurysms by this method; it is unquestionably the most important, if not the only function that this procedure serves." Even pioneers did not seem to be able to predict the future.

Seldinger's catheter method pushed the technology further (1953). The first embolisation treatments of intracranial malformations thus resulted in the 1960s and 70s. In 1973, computer tomography (CT) was also introduced as a cerebral diagnostic method. First attempts at CT-DSA by Oldendorf (1978) passed off initially without repercussions, and the method became established by the beginning of the 80s.

The History of Surgery on Cerebral Aneurysms

As is often the case, it was in ancient times, around 2725 BC, that Imhotep became somewhat well-known: for arterial aneurysm. There was no further mention until Galen (200

AD). The modern definition of an "aneurysm" as being the "dilatation of a weakened artery" originated in 1728 (Lancisis). The attempt to treat aneurysms through ligation of the proximal artery also dates from this period. In 1760, Jean-Louis Petit reported an aneurysm of the carotid bifurcation that spontaneously healed as a result of thrombosis. These observations led John Hunter, in around 1800, to systematically treat aneurysms by afferent artery ligation with the aim of inducing thrombosis. The method is named "Hunterian Ligation" in his honour. In 1885, Sir Victor Horsley used this principle to treat an aneurysm of the intracranial carotid artery, discovered by chance during a craniotomy, with ligation of the extracranial internal carotid artery. However, the outcomes of incidental findings in the era of carotid ligation that was now beginning were poor. In 1931, Normann Dott was the first surgeon in history to attack a suspected aneurysm after SAH in a planned and targeted way using frontal craniotomy. He had found an aneurysm of the internal carotid artery that he covered with muscle tissue. In the 1930s Harvey Cushing, in particular, attempted to strengthen the wall of the aneurysm ("wrapping") by removing muscle tissue from the leg. The Silverstone clamp, with which the carotid artery could be gradually closed at the neck, provided an interlude. The aim was to achieve collateral circulation via the circle of Willis prior to final vascular occlusion and thus prevent ischaemic complications of the carotid ligature.

Running parallel to these attempts was the development of aneurysm clips. Initially, it was once again Norman Dott who attempted to ligate intracranial aneurysms through a surgical suture at the neck. This method was favoured time and again up until the late 60s (Brake and Anmacher, 1969). In 1911, Cushing developed a clip for securely occluding inaccessible tumour vessels. McKenzie modified this silver clip and in 1937 Walter Dandy was the first surgeon to treat an intracranial aneurysm with a clip: he treated a 43-year-old, alcoholic man with oculomotor nerve palsy for internal carotid artery aneurysm. The surgical procedure went well, as Cushing reported, even through the brain atrophy. The patient did not have an angiogram prior to surgery. The door was therefore open to the development of ever more specialised clips.

The Development of Aneurysm Clips

The development of clips has repeatedly been referred to as an evolution. The literature certainly gives the impression of a teleological development, which is not exactly evolution. In 1840, in France, the toolmaker Joseph Charrière devised vascular clips that intersected, opened in response to pressure and closed as the pressure decreased. This principle was adopted in the emerging field of neurosurgery: Olivecrona had the idea of attaching further posterior winged blades to the so-called Dandy clip so that the clip could be opened and repositioned. Schwartz developed miniaturised spring forceps as clips. Mayfield continued to develop Schwartz's inventions in the 1950s by adding a grooved clip surface, kinked introducer and continuing miniaturisation. Together with Kees, an engineer, Mayfield developed a whole range of individual clips. He persuaded seven volunteers to undergo a temporal craniotomy procedure so that he could test his clips in vivo. As far as we know from what has been written, there were no deaths. In subsequent years, many details and specifications concerning the clips were presented: The Drake clip had fenestrations for efferent vessels. Mayfield devised clips with arms that did not intersect when closed so that they would not act like scissors. McFadden devised round clip arms with blunt tips. Heifetz attempted specifically to devise a clip with an additional spring for secure closure. The next generation of clips was then made to the specifications of microneurosurgery (Yasargil, Sugita, Spetzler). Clips were also developed that permit examinations with magnetic resonance imaging.

The success story of clips has also had its darker sides: new developments were often made by companies that had no knowledge of biocompatibility or metallurgy. There were catastrophic results due to clips rusting in the body or lethal complications from magnetic resonance imaging. That improved with the introduction of national standards.

The Investigation of Cerebral Vasospasm

Sir William Gull, who, as already mentioned, was one of the first physicians to attribute SAH to a ruptured aneurysm, was also the first to describe secondary deterioration as a result of cerebral infarctions: 150 years ago, he reported the case of a young woman who fell into a coma five days after suffering SAH, developed wide and fixed pupils, and subsequently died. The post-mortem examination uncovered a ruptured aneurysm of the middle cerebral artery, a blood clot around the vessel and focal softening in the cortex.

The Existence of Cerebral Vasospasm

Physiologists gathered the next findings en route to the discovery of vasospasm: in 1925, Florey described cerebral vasospasms in cats, caused by mechanical and electrical stimulation of the cerebral vessels. In 1944, Zucker found evidence of spasmogenic substances in the serum of laboratory animals. In 1949, Jackson injected blood into the cisterna magna of dogs and assumed that the resulting vasospasm was caused by the components of the red blood cells. The clinical breakthrough in defining "spasm" was made in 1951 by Ecker and Riemenschneider: they detected a spasm in humans using angiography, which was at its strongest at the site of the largest collection of blood, i.e., near the aneurysm. They described the time limitation, reporting that no spasms occurred after day 26 post SAH. This dependence on time led to the realisation by Allcock and Drake in 1965 that the spasm was particularly frequent and pronounced in the first three days after SAH and that the timing of surgery should account for the frequency of the spasm. During this period, Kennedy was the first to develop the theory that a surgical reduction of the SAH volume could lead to spasm prophylaxis. In the 1970s, the existence of cerebral vasospasm and its basic clinical features were recognised, and research into prophylaxis and treatment began:

About the Prophylaxis and Treatment of Cerebral Vasospasm

As early as the 1960s, there were initial clinical recommendations to avoid an excessive drop in blood pressure, even after SAH, in order to improve cerebral perfusion. In 1972, Wise recommended a systolic pressure of 150-170, and a diastolic pressure of 85-100 mm Hg. In the next few years, however, consideration was given to increasing the central venous pressure so as to improve the neurological outcome. The administration of whole blood, plasma or albumin was recommended. Triple-H therapy was in its infancy. In 1979, Allen described the positive effect of calcium antagonists on a vasospasm induced in an experiment on dogs. Allen was also the initiator of nimodipine tests. From then on, treatment of vasospasm played a very influential role in the development of intensive therapy (and vice versa). Questions related to the ventilation strategy and the use or otherwise of invasive neuromonitoring continue to dominate discussions to this day and run parallel to the other major issue of neurosurgical intensive care - neurotraumatology.

In the late 1970s, Weir, Suzuki and Hashimoto established a link between surgical timing and spasm prophylaxis, which is acknowledged today: operations in the first few days after SAH have been found to deliver a better outcome, as the spasm was not yet formed – they are now also regarded as a means of preventing and treating spasms:

Surgical Timing Over the Decades

Until well into the 1950s, the management of ruptured aneurysms was based on case-by-case decisions and personal opinions: in 1951, Slosberg observed that the surgical occlusion of ruptured aneurysms was about as effective as reducing blood pressure with drugs. In 1963, Merritt wrote that ruptured aneurysms should only be approached when operating on space-occupying haematomas. Among the first to recommend surgery, at least for patients in good condition, were Hunt and Hess in 1968. Consequently, they developed a scale for assessing patients after SAH which would make the decision to operate easier. Throughout the 1970s, it was then recognised that after a period of bed rest, drug treatment and stabilisation, better long-term outcomes were achieved with, rather than without surgery. The high rate of later second bleeds could thus be reduced.

In the 1980s, a number of pioneers in aneurysm surgery (Dott, Drake, Yasargil) were still recommending surgery after stabilising the patient, with clipping proving to be significantly better than the wait-and-see attitude alone. However, many patients died while waiting for surgery – not only due to the vasospasm as first described in 1951, but also because of recurring haemorrhages. The improved outcomes of aneurysm surgery were therefore the result of a bias, since the patients with worse baseline conditions or complications were not included in the statistics reported by the surgeons. That was the dichotomy of the 80s: Kasel and Drake complained that although the surgical outcomes had improved, the management outcomes in terms of SAH symptoms had not. Suzuki, Yoshimoto and Norden achieved good surgical outcomes even with early surgery. The International Cooperative Study on the Timing of Aneurysm Surgery recommended early surgery in patients in good condition. It certainly would not have done any harm. In the 90s, early surgery was carried out in patients whose baseline status was poor. Some of the trailblazers of cerebral aneurysm surgery were poor statisticians and fell short with a view to the overall patient population. Retrospectively, this blinkered view of surgical outcomes alone has hampered the advancement of aneurysm treatment. The next expansion of the therapeutic spectrum is also attributable to neurosurgery:

The Development of Interventional Neuroradiology

The neurosurgeon Luessenhop carried out the first attempts at embolisation on malformations in Washington in 1960. Lehmann used an adhesive substance (cyanoacrylate) for the first time in 1967. In 1973, Djindjian described the embolisation of extracranial tumours and vascular malformations. The rapid technological advancement in X-ray diagnostics was the driving force for interventional neuroradiologists: the ability to visualise the smallest of blood vessels using digital subtraction angiography, "online" imaging in two planes and the development of the flow- or guidewire-directed microcatheter. The wheel of time is turning very quickly in this medical field: 20 years ago interventional procedures were a rarity, 10 years ago detachable coils did not exist, and five years ago today's stents were a distant reality. The two trailblazers of this technology and their background are presented below:

Fedor Andreevich Serbinenko (1928 – 2002) was a pioneer of embolisation treatment. After completing his studies, Serbinenko joined the N.N. Burdenko Neurosurgery Institute in Moscow in 1954, which was being established at that time as a neurocentre. Supported by the then luminaries of Russian neurosurgery (Shlykov, Salazzkin), he focused his attention on percutaneous angiography. In 1959, during the May Day celebrations in Red Square, he observed how children were playing with helium-filled balloons and trying to steer them like kites on long strings. And so the idea of endovascular balloon embolisation was born. In 1964, his first attempt at balloon occlusion of an intracranial vessel was successful, and in 1969 or 1970 the first permanent occlusion in the case of a malformation was achieved. By 1962, 162 embolisations had taken place, with a valve being developed to prevent spontaneous emptying. Later, Serbinenko worked with Alexander Luria to carry out psychological tests after experimental vascular occlusion. Despite Cold War restrictions, the techniques became more widespread and continued to be developed elsewhere, particularly as doctors from abroad were invited to visit the institute in Moscow. There was one overriding goal: greater individual adaptation to the aneurysm with the embolic agent than with the balloon. It is at this point that the second greatest pioneer in the field appeared: the neurosurgeon Guido Guglielmi, born in Rome in 1948. He took Mullen's idea from the 1960s of using electrolysis to detaching a metallic coil from the catheter, developing it further. Because of its elasticity (memory effect), the coil assumes its original shape and so several coils can be packed into the aneurysm. Stasis and thrombosis occur in the aneurysm as an immediate effect. Epithelialisation to achieve an intact vascular wall is the long-term effect. Guglielmi began his work in Rome in 1976. In 1983, he began working with Fernando Vinuela in London. After many years of correspondence, Vinuela invited him to the UCLA in Los Angeles in 1989, where the GDC (Guglielmi Detachable Coil) was ultimately developed. Guglielmi is now back at work in Rome.

With the dual approach of surgery and embolisation, an interest developed in obtaining more detailed information on a patient's progress in order to achieve a better prediction. The search began for criteria as to which patient would benefit more from which treatment. Attempts then began to describe treatment outcomes on an individual level:

THE EXPLORATION OF HEALTH-RELATED QUALITY OF LIFE

Whilst until the 1990s the treatment outcome of SAH was given as mortality or, more specifically, was categorised according to the Glasgow Outcome Score, since the start of the new millennium many working groups have been exploring health-related quality of life. The quality-of-life research that has now been ongoing for 15 years pursues two goals: 1) The search for sophisticated predictors with which treatment can be optimised individually (intervention yes or no, operation or coiling, expansion or reduction of intensive therapy) and 2) an estimation of the extent to which rehabilitation is feasible. At the beginning of the 2000s, quality-of-life scales from internal medicine or neurotraumatology were used one-for-one to this end in SAH research. In the last few years, there have been attempts to develop specific tools for measuring the symptoms. What complicates matters is that a lot of statistical data on SAH is subsumed in health and disease registries under the keyword "stroke", leading to a loss of information on the particular features of the clinical condition. In rehabilitation research, scales are also traditionally used for SAH patients which originate from stroke research and are presumably inadequate.

CONCLUSION

The first modern descriptions of SAH as a pathological condition and cerebrovascular aneurysms were formulated by the neurologists of the 19th century. With the development of neurosurgery in the first half of the 20th century, SAH became a preserve of this new discipline. Hence, therapies were introduced that had been developed from neurosurgery and subsequently opened out into their own disciplines – special intensive therapy and interventional neuroradiology are perfect examples. Neurosurgeons have relinquished their powers at the expense of more individualised treatment. Despite all the medical and technological advances, the clinical experience endemic to neurology and neurosurgery must not be overlooked.

REFERENCES

Heros RC, Morcos JJ. Cerebrovascular surgery: past, present, and future. *Neurosurgery.* 2000; 47: 1007-1033.

Louw D.F., Louis D.F., Asfora W.T., Sutherland G.R. A brief history of aneurysm clips. *Neurosurgical Focus.* 2001; 11: 1-4.

Polevaya N.V., Kalani M.Y., Steinberg G.K., Tse V.C. The transition from hunterian ligation to intracranial aneurysm clips: a historical perspective. *Neurosurgical Focus.* 2006; 20: E3.

Prestigiacomo C.J. Historical perspectives: the microsurgical and endovascular treatment of aneurysms. *Neurosurgery.* 2006; 59: 39-4.

Rahimi S.Y., Brown J.H., Macomson S.D., Jensen M.A., Alleyne C.H. Jr. Evolution of the treatment of cerebral vasospasm. *Neurosurgical Focus.* 2006; 20: E4.

Stein S.C. Brief history of surgical timing: surgery for ruptured intracranial aneurysms. *Neurosurgical Focus.* 2001; 11: E3.

Teitelbaum G.P, Larsen D.W., Zelman V. Lywsachev A.FG., Likhterman L.B. A tribute to Dr. Fedor A. Serbinenko, founder of endovascular neurosurgery. *Neurosurgery* 2000; 46: 462-469.

In: Spontaneous Subarachnoid Haemorrhage
Editors: Thomas Kapapa and Ralph König

ISBN: 978-1-63485-270-8

Chapter 2

ARTERIAL AND VENOUS VASCULARISATION OF THE BRAIN

Horst Claassen
Institute of Anatomy and Cell Biology,
Martin Luther University Halle-Wittenberg
Halle (Saale), Germany

ABSTRACT

This chapter has been written especially for neurosurgeons currently in training. To begin with, a description is provided of the cerebral arteries and veins as well as their relevant ramifications. The symptoms of ischaemia will also be mentioned. Thereafter, the neighbouring structures of the cerebral arteries will be described specifically in relation to the surgical treatment of aneurysms. Current textbooks on the subject of anatomy provide functional descriptions of structures often to the detriment of topography, or the two topics are covered together without making any identifiable distinction. In the surgical treatment of aneurysms in particular, it is important to be aware of and possibly avoid damaging the tracts and structures in the immediate vicinity.

Keywords: cerebral arteries; cerebral veins; aneurysms; functional anatomy; topographical anatomy

1. INTRODUCTION

Life-threatening subarachnoid haemorrhage is often the result of a ruptured aneurysm. This type of aneurysm often develops at the bifurcations of the cerebral arteries. Aneurysms, or arterial outpouchings, usually develop due to a congenital structural abnormality of the arterial walls, particularly of the tunica media, or due to the excessive pressure arising from hypertension (Drenckhahn 2004; Bähr and Frotscher 2014). The arteries most commonly affected by such outpouchings are the anterior communicating artery, followed by the internal carotid artery (Paulsen and Waschke 2010). Post-mortem examinations have revealed the following incidence of aneurysms with advancing age: 4.1% at 20-29 years of age, 11% at 30-49, 8.4% at 50-69, and 20% over the age of 90.

As a preventative measure, aneurysms can be secured with a clip. Otherwise they have to be occluded with a clip if acute subarachnoid haemorrhage occurs. Alternatively, endovascular catheter treatment can be undertaken, by inserting platinum-coated metal coils. This causes a thrombus to form in the saccular bulge of the aneurysm, thereby preventing rupture of the bulging arterial wall. This novel concept is called endovascular coiling. In all cases it is essential to consider the surrounding anatomic structures when performing surgery.

2. Arterial Blood Supply to the Brain

The brain is supplied by two arterial territories, namely the internal carotid artery and the vertebral artery (Figure 1). Corrosion casts of the cerebral arteries illustrate this quite clearly (Tillmann 1997). The cerebral part of the internal carotid artery divides into the anterior and middle cerebral arteries. The intracranial part of the vertebral artery first gives rise to the posterior spinal artery, then the posterior inferior cerebellar artery, and finally the anterior spinal artery. The vertebral arteries then join from both sides to form the basilar artery, from which in each case two further cerebellar arteries emerge: the anterior inferior arteries and the superior cerebellar arteries. Having emitted the superior cerebellar arteries, the basilar artery branches off into the two posterior cerebral arteries.

The posterior communicating artery, which is the penultimate branch of the internal carotid artery, usually anastomoses with the posterior cerebral artery to connect the anterior carotid territory with the posterior vertebral territory. The two anterior cerebral arteries are likewise joined together by a connecting artery, namely the anterior communicating artery. The resulting structure is a closed arterial loop, known as the *circle of Willis,* which encircles the optic chiasm, infundibulum and mamillary bodies (Figure 1). Out of 1,000 brains, however, the circle of Willis as described in textbooks is found only in 53.8% (Leonhardt 1988). Variations appear in 46.2%, often involving the communicating arteries, with the posterior communicating arteries differing more frequently than the anterior communicating artery.

Below is a description of the branches of the major cerebral arteries and the territories they supply, based largely on the observations of Töndury et al. (1987) presented in the Textbook and Atlas of Human Anatomy by Rauber/Kopsch (*Lehrbuch und Atlas der Anatomie des Menschen* Volume III, 1987). The three cerebral arteries are in each case divided into segments, as is customary in neurosurgery. Corning (1923) distinguished between two types of branches in the case of cerebral arteries: 1. The cortical branches which supply blood to the grey matter of the cerebral and cerebellar cortex, and partly ensure perfusion of the semioval centre. 2. The basal branches are small branches that enter the brain vertically and perfuse the "central grey matter", i.e., the basal ganglia, internal capsule, thalamus, cranial nerve nuclei as well as parts of the semioval centre. An analysis of the structure of the cerebral arteries, including phylogenetic aspects, has been provided by Lasjaunias and colleagues (2001). Yasargil (1969) describes the fine structure of the cerebral arteries. Based on his observations, the middle layers of the intracranial arteries contain far fewer collagen fibres than the extracranial arteries. This is possibly a factor that predisposes to aneurysms.

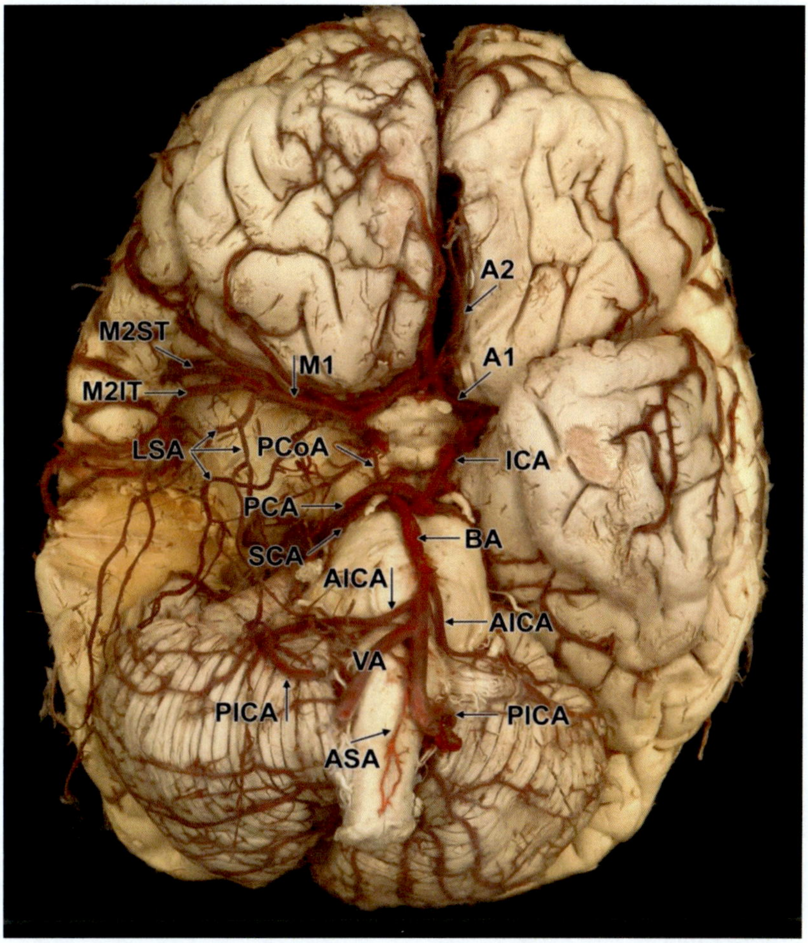

Figure 1. Injected specimen showing the arteries of the brain – basal aspect. The blood is supplied to the brain by the internal carotid artery (ICA) and vertebral artery (VA). The two circulations are connected by the posterior communicating arteries (PCOA). The resulting structure is the circle of Willis, which surrounds the optic chiasm, infundibulum and mamillary bodies. The anterior half of the right temporal lobe has been removed from the specimen. The lenticulostriate arteries (LSA), which supply the basal ganglia and internal capsule, are therefore exposed. Note that the lenticulostriate arteries, due to the special preparation technique, hang down from the M1 segment of the middle cerebral artery. These arteries would normally permeate the cerebral matter and ascend toward their supply territories in a formation similar to an onion skin. Also note the ascending posterior inferior cerebellar artery (PICA) on the right, versus the descending posterior inferior cerebellar artery (PICA) on the left. The following major arteries and arterial branches are visible: A1 – A2 = segments of the anterior cerebral artery, AICA = anterior inferior cerebellar artery, ASA = anterior spinal artery, BA = basilar artery, ICA = internal carotid artery, LSA = lenticulostriate artery, M1 – M2 = segments of middle cerebral artery, M2ST = middle cerebral artery of superior trunk, M2IT = middle cerebral artery of inferior trunk, PCA = posterior cerebral artery, PCoA = posterior communicating artery, PICA = posterior inferior cerebellar artery, SCA = superior cerebellar artery, VA = vertebral artery. Image of a wet specimen (1933, Trautmann preparative technique) in a jar (W/D/H 21 x 10 x 26 cm) from the Meckel Collections of the Institute of Anatomy and Cell Biology of Martin Luther University Halle-Wittenberg.

2.1. Branches of the Internal Carotid Artery

The *internal carotid artery* supplies the cerebrum, pituitary gland, orbital content, forehead, as well as the mucous membranes of the frontal sinus cavity, ethmoidal sinuses and anterior nasal cavity. It runs parallel to the pharynx as far as the base of the skull and passes through the carotid canal of the petrosal bone, entering the middle cranial fossa at the pyramidal apex. The artery then traverses the carotid sulcus on both sides of the body of the sphenoid bone and passes through the cavernous sinus. After penetrating the dura mater anteriorly at the sella turcica, it branches off on reaching the subarachnoid space. Next to the sella turcica, the artery curves to form an S shape which is referred to as the "carotid siphon" (Sobotta/Becher 1973). As it carries on, the artery is divided into the following segments:

Cervical Part

At the neck, the interior carotid artery initially lies posterior and lateral to the external carotid artery, but then winds in a more medial direction on its ascent. Immediately before it enters the carotid canal, the artery forms a medial convexity.

Petrous Part

At its petrous part, the interior carotid artery ramifies to supply the tympanic cavity (caroticotympanic arteries). The artery of the pterygoid canal also emerges here, and is anastomosed with the artery of the same name arising from the maxillary artery.

Cavernous Part

At this point the internal carotid artery is surrounded by the venous blood of the cavernous sinus. It releases the following branches:

- Tentorial basal branch
- Tentorial marginal branch
- Meningeal branch to the dura mater of the anterior cranial fossa
- Cavernous branch
- Inferior hypophysial artery
- Branch to trigeminal ganglion
- Branches to cranial nerves IV and V

Cerebral Part

The cerebral part, as it is called, is reached on penetration of the dura mater. It is here where the following arteries emerge, the supply territories of which are described below: superior hypophysial artery, clivus branches, ophthalmic artery, posterior communicating artery, anterior choroidal artery, anterior cerebral artery, middle cerebral artery.

- The superior hypophysial artery leads to the pituitary stalk and the basal hypothalamus.
- The clival branches supply the meninges at the clivus.
- The ophthalmic artery supplies the tear ducts, the eye and the choroid, the ciliary body and iris, as well as the eyelids.

- The posterior communicating artery anastomoses with the posterior cerebral artery and forms part of the cerebral arterial circle (of Willis). The branches of the following are emitted: optic chiasm, oculomotor nerve, thalamus, hypothalamus, tail of caudate nucleus.
- Anterior choroidal artery, runs beneath the optic tract past the lateral geniculate body, arriving at the choroid line through the choroidal fissure of the inferior horn of the lateral ventricle. In vertebrates, this artery once played a pivotal role due to its vast vascular territory. The anterior choroidal artery in humans also has numerous branches, the failure of which, if diagnosable, is not without its problems.

The *anterior choroidal artery* is the final branch of the internal carotid artery before it divides into the anterior and middle cerebral artery. It covers an expansive territory, including parts of the choroid plexus of the lateral ventricle and the third ventricle, the basal ganglia, internal capsule, parts of the diencephalon with the junction boxes for the auditory and optic tracts, as well as portions of the mesencephalon. Damage to the anterior choroidal artery will lead to motor, sensory and visual deficits (Deller 2015). Branches of the anterior choroidal artery:

- Choroidal branches to lateral ventricle, forming the choroid plexus in the inferior horn of the lateral ventricle.
- Choroidal branches to third ventricle, supplying the choroid plexus of the third ventricle.
- Branches to anterior perforated substance, passing through the anterior perforated substance to the genu of the internal capsule.
- Branches to optic tract.
- Branches to lateral geniculate body, the fourth synapse in the visual pathway.
- Branches to internal capsule, leading to the posterior limb of the internal capsule where the pyramidal, optic and auditory pathways, amongst others, are located.
- Branches to globus pallidus, a basal ganglion that is responsible, amongst others, for "more mobility".
- Branches to tail of caudate nucleus, a basal ganglion.
- Branches to tuber cinereum.
- Branches to hypothalamic nuclei.
- Branches to substantia nigra, a brainstem nucleus that degenerates in the presence of Parkinson's disease.
- Branches to red nucleus, which plays a central role in extrapyramidal motor function.
- Branches to amygdaloid body, a basal ganglion.
- Anterior cerebral artery = *anterior terminal branch* of the internal carotid artery.
- Middle cerebral artery = *lateral terminal branch* of and continuation of the internal carotid artery.

2.1.1. Anterior Cerebral Artery

A distinction is made between two segments (Figure 1, 2): the precommunicating part (Pars praecommunicalis, or A1 segment) at the base of the brain, and the postcommunicating part (Pars postcommunicalis, or A2 segment) emerging behind the anterior communicating artery.

2.1.1.1. Precommunicating Part (A1 Segment)

- Short central arteries (lateral group): 8-12 branches permeate the medial anterior perforated substance and supply the anterior hypothalamus, column of fornix, anterior commissure, head of caudate nucleus, globus pallidus and anterior limb of the internal capsule.
- Long central artery (recurrent artery of Heubner): this artery leads back to the lateral anterior perforated substance. It supplies the head of the caudate nucleus, the anterior third of the lentiform nucleus, and anterior limb of the internal capsule. *Clinical features:* Long central artery dysfunction can result in aphasia, hemiparesis and paralysis of the muscles of the face and tongue. The artery should be spared when clipping aneurysms (Lang and Wachsmuth 1979).

2.1.1.2. Anterior Communicating Artery

- Short central arteries (anterior group): the anterior group of these arteries form 6-7 narrow ramifications that perfuse the optic chiasm.

2.1.1.3. Postcommunicating Part (A2 Segment)

The postcommunicating part winds around the genu of the corpus callosum, ramifying onto the medial frontal lobe and the cingulate gyrus. Above the corpus callosum, the A2 segment divides into the pericallosal and callosomarginal arteries (Figure 2).

- Pericallosal artery (Figure 2): supplies the corpus callosum and anastomoses at the splenium of the corpus callosum with the posterior cerebral artery.
- Callosomarginal artery (Figure 2): passes over the cingulate gyrus in the cingulate sulcus, ramfiying onto the medial surface of the hemisphere.

The cortical branches of the A2 segment not only supply the medial surface of the hemisphere, but also a narrow strip on the lateral surface of the cortex. Close to the superior margin of the cerebral hemisphere, the branches of the A2 segment anastomose with the middle cerebral artery. *Clinical features:* Owing to the described anastomotic processes, both anterior cerebral arteries can, if necessary, be occluded distal to the anterior communicating artery.

2.1.2. Middle Cerebral Artery

The middle cerebral artery (Figure 1) is divided into two segments: the sphenoid part (M1 segment) running parallel to the lesser wing of the sphenoid, and the insular part (M2 segment) ascending in the lateral sulcus. In rare cases, the middle cerebral artery may be duplicated. Adachi (1928) observed a duplicated middle cerebral artery five times (3%) in 166 hemispheres of donated Japanese bodies.

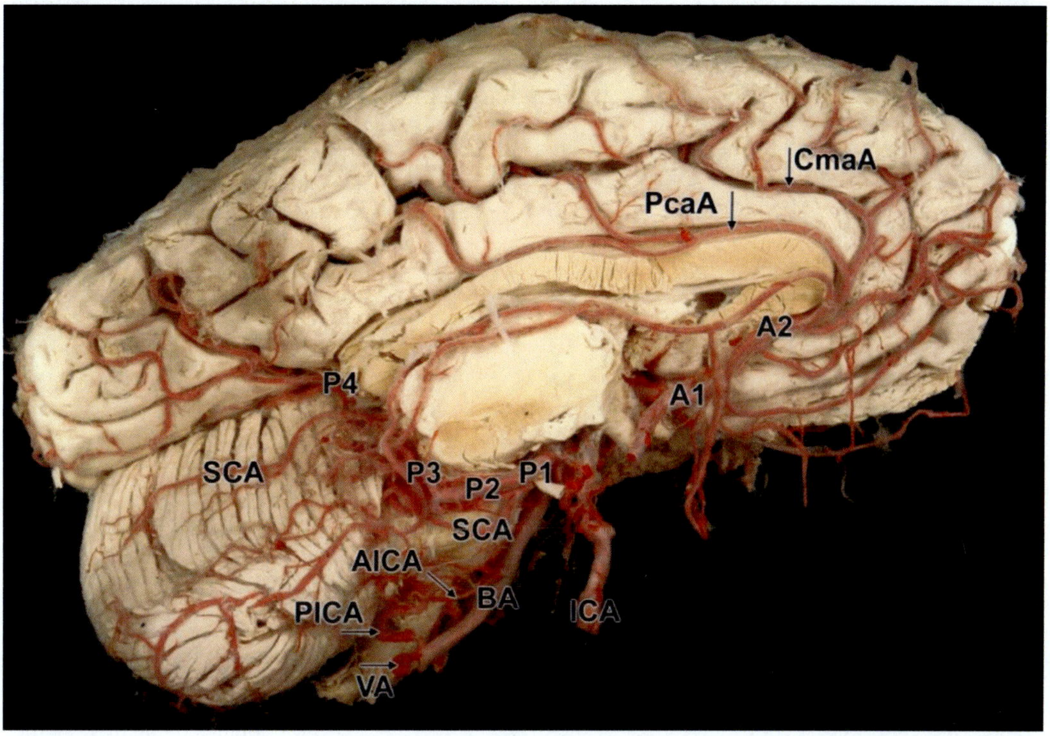

Figure 2. Injected specimen of the arteries of the brain – medial section. Caudally, the stumps of the internal carotid artery (ICA) and vertebral artery (VA) are visible. The brain is supplied with blood by these two arteries and their ramifications. Note how the supply territories of the anterior cerebral artery (A1 – A2) and posterior cerebral artery (P1 – P4) are connected by the pericallosal artery (PcaA). The following major arteries and arterial branches are identifiable: A1 – A1 = segments of the anterior cerebral artery, AICA = anterior inferior cerebellar artery, SCA = superior cerebellar artery, BA = basilar artery, CmaA = callosomarginal artery, ICA = internal carotid artery, P1 – P4 = segments of the posterior cerebral artery, PcaA = pericallosal artery, PICA = posterior inferior cerebellar artery, VA = vertebral artery. Image of a wet specimen (1957, Trautmann preparative technique) in a jar (W/D/H 22 x 10 x 25 cm) from the Meckel Collections of the Institute of Anatomy and Cell Biology of Martin Luther University Halle-Wittenberg.

2.1.2.1. Sphenoid Part (M1 Segment)

- Anterolateral central arteries (lenticulostriate arteries, Figure 2): these arteries infiltrate the lateral half of the anterior perforated substance, ascending cranially and supplying the putamen, internal capsule, as well as the head and body of the caudate nucleus. *Clinical features:* One branch ascending at the outer aspect of the putamen is referred to as the “artery of cerebral haemorrhage”.

2.1.2.2. Insular Part (M2 Segment)

The M2 segment bifurcates at the limen insulae, or insular threshold, into a superior and inferior trunk (Figure 3).

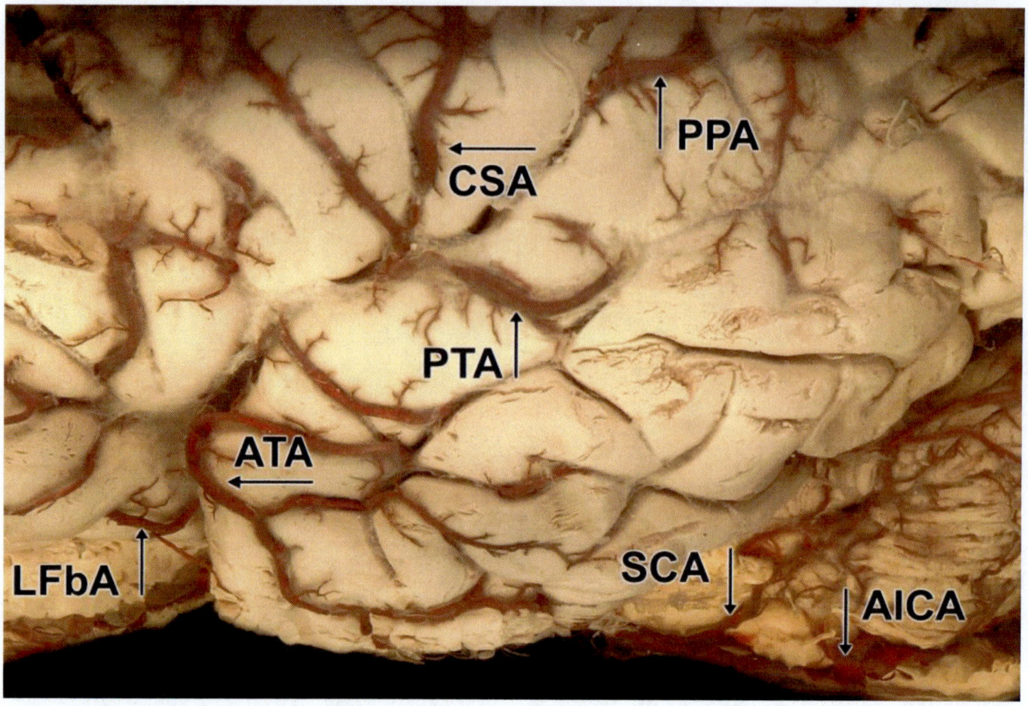

Figure 3. Injected specimen of the arteries of the brain – lateral view. The branches of the M2 segment of the middle cerebral artery are visible. The M2 segment passes through the Sylvian fissure. The branches of the M2 segment supply, among others, the motor speech centre (Broca's area), the sensorimotor cortex, the primary auditory centre, and the sensory speech centre (Wernicke's area). The following major arteries and arterial branches are visible: AICA = anterior inferior cerebellar artery, ATA = anterior temporal artery, CSA = central sulcal artery, LFbA = lateral frontobasal artery, PTA = posterior temporal artery, SCA = superior cerebellar artery, PPA = posterior parietal (supramarginal) artery. Image of a wet specimen (1957, Trautmann preparative technique) in a jar (W/D/H 22 x 10 x 25 cm) from the Meckel Collections of the Institute of Anatomy and Cell Biology of Martin Luther University Halle-Wittenberg.

- Superior trunk: The arteries of the precentral sulcus, central sulcus (Figure 3) and postcentral sulcus are ramifications of the superior trunk, perfusing the convolutions of the sensorimotor cortex. Further branches supply Broca's area, the motor centre for speech. The supramarginal arteries (Figure 3) and angular gyri lead to Wernicke's area.
- Inferior trunk: The branches of the inferior trunk supply the lateral gyri of the temporal lobe and the primary auditory centre in Heschl's convolutions. The terminal branch of the M2 segment is the posterior temporal artery (Figure 3), which perfuses the majority of Wernicke's area. *Clinical features:* The middle cerebral artery is the largest branch and the continuation of the internal carotid artery. Hence, embolisms from the distal territory of the internal carotid artery are often deposited in the middle cerebral artery (Clara 1959). Occlusion of the posterior temporal artery can affect the sensory speech centre. This artery is therefore also referred to as the "artery of Wernicke's aphasia".

2.2. Branches of the Vertebral Artery

The **vertebral artery** (Figure 1, 2) travels through the foramen of the transverse process of the cervical spine to the atlas, entering the skull through the foramen magnum. Its branches supply blood to the brain stem, cerebellum, the auditory and vestibular system, as well as, via the posterior cerebral artery, the occipital lobe of the telencephalon with visual centre.

2.2.1. Posterior Spinal Artery

The posterior spinal artery is the first intracranial branch of the vertebral artery. It supplies the core areas of the spinobulbar tract.

2.2.2. Posterior Inferior Cerebellar Artery

The posterior inferior cerebellar artery (Figures 1, 2) is the largest branch of the vertebral artery. It supplies the majority of the inferior aspect of the cerebellar hemisphere, the inferior portion of the vermis and core areas of the medulla oblongata. The terminal segment emits the choroidal branch to the fourth ventricle for the choroid plexus of the fourth ventricle.

- Arteries of posterolateral sulcus: the arteries of this lateral vascular system supply parts of the medulla oblongata with the trigeminal nerve nucleus (V) as well as the solitary, ambiguus and dorsal nuclei of the vagus nerve (X) and hypoglossal nucleus. *Clinical features:* A deficit in the lateral vascular system will lead to the development of Wallenberg's syndrome, which is characterised by dysphonia (nerve X), dysphagia (IX), gustatory anaesthesia (VII, IX, X), sensory disorders in the face (V), vertigo and nystagmus (medial longitudinal fasciculus).

2.2.3. Anterior Spinal Artery

The anterior spinal artery (Figure 1) emerges shortly before the confluence of the two vertebral arteries that forms the basilar artery. The pyramidal arteries arising from the anterior spinal artery perfuse the medullary pyramids.

2.2.4. Basilar Artery

At the lower aspect of the pons, the basilar artery (Figures 1, 2) bifurcates, giving way to the anterior inferior cerebellar arteries. Once the superior cerebellar arteries have been discharged at the upper aspect of the pons, the artery divides into a pair of posterior cerebral arteries. The following arteries also emerge:

- Artery of the anterior median fissure: The anterior segment of the pyramidal tract in the lower ventral medulla oblongata is supplied by this artery.
- Medial medullary branches of the anterior median fissure artery: perfusion of the area of the medial longitudinal fasciculus and tectospinal tract in the upper ventral portion of the medulla oblongata.
- Median pontine branches: enter the pons and supply the area of the medial longitudinal fasciculus, tectospinal tract, medial and lateral lemniscus pathways as well as trigeminal lemniscus.

- Short pontine branches: travel into the region of the pontine nuclei and corticospinal tract.
- Labyrinthine artery (though only in 15%; see below).

2.2.5. Anterior Inferior Cerebellar Artery

The anterior inferior cerebellar artery (Figures 1, 2) perfuses the flocculonodular lobe of the cerebellum, and emits a branch to supply the choroid plexus of the fourth ventricle.

- Labyrinthine artery: the artery supplying the auditory and vestibular system is in 85% of cases a branch of the anterior inferior cerebellar artery. Only in 15% of cases does this artery originate from the basilar artery.
- Long pontine branches: lead to the superior cerebellar peduncle as well as to the area of the anterior spinocerebellar tract and the motor nucleus of trigeminal nerve V in the pons.

2.2.6. Superior Cerebellar Artery

The superior cerebellar artery (Figures 1-3) is the largest of the three cerebellar arteries. It supplies the entire superior surface of the cerebellar hemisphere and superior aspect of the vermis. The artery anastomoses with the branches of the inferior cerebellar arteries, and with the posterior cerebral artery in the area of the quadrigeminal bodies.

2.2.7. Posterior Cerebral Artery

The posterior cerebral artery (Figures 1, 2) is divided into four segments. The precommunicating part (P1) is located in front of the posterior communicating artery, with the postcommunicating part (P2) behind. The P2 segment extends as far as the origin of the posterior inferior temporal branch. The quadrigeminal part (P3) begins here, ascending to the quadrigeminal bodies. The terminal part (P4), which winds its way towards the occipital pole, begins at the level of the quadrigeminal bodies.

2.2.7.1. Precommunicating Part (P1 Segment)

- Interpeduncular perforating arteries (posterolateral central arteries): these arteries supply the posterior limb of the internal capsule, the thalamus and hypothalamus, as well as the territories of Perlia's nucleus (oculomotor nerve, III), Edinger-Westphal nucleus and medial longitudinal fasciculus in the mesencephalon. *Clinical features:* A deficit in this arterial segment is described as a peduncular syndrome: homolateral paresis of the eye muscles, contralateral hemianaesthesia, impaired coordination of the eye movements.

2.2.7.2. Postcommunicating Part (P2 Segment)

- Short circumferential arteries: responsible for supplying the red nucleus and substantia nigra.
- Quadrigeminal artery: supplies the quadrigeminal bodies.
- Thalamogeniculate artery: supplies the posterolateral portion of the thalamus.

- Anterior and posterior inferior temporal branches: supply the basal gyri of the temporal lobe. At the hippocampal sulcus, the branches of these arteries form a T-shape bifurcation, thus supplying the hippocampus and dentate gyrus with tiny branches that form an arcade-like pattern. *Clinical features:* Given the vascular architecture, the CA1 region (cornu ammonis 1, Sommer sector) is more susceptible to ischaemia than CA2/CA3 (cornu ammonis 2/3, Spielmeyer sector).

2.2.7.3. Quadrigeminal Part (P3 Segment)

- Lateral and medial posterior choroidal arteries: perfuse the choroid plexus of the third ventricle.

2.2.7.4. Terminal Part (P4 Segment)

- Lateral occipital artery: this artery contributes to the perfusion of the basal surface of the occipital lobe and posterior segments of the temporal lobe.
- Medial occipital artery: the parieto-occipital branch of this artery leads to the superior aspect of the cuneus belonging to the occipital lobe, and the calcarine branch to the pole of the occipital lobe. The visual cortex is perfused in 42% of cases exclusively by the parieto-occipital branch, in 23% by the calcarine branch, and in 31% by both.

3. Aneurysms and Neighbouring Structures of the Intracranial Arteries

3.1. Internal Carotid Artery

Aneurysms of the internal carotid artery (Figures 1, 2) can occur where the artery passes through the cavernous sinus (cavernous part of internal carotid artery) (Duus 1993). The artery curves at this point to form an S shape (carotid siphon) and is surrounded by venous blood. In the immediate vicinity, the following nerves, listed in caudal to cranial order, traverse the sinus wall: maxillary, ophthalmic, trochlear and oculomotor nerves (Sobotta/Becher 1983; Leonhardt 1988). The abducens nerve passes immediately below the artery. A caudally positioned aneurysm will exert pressure on cranial nerves V1, V2, IV and VI. Paraesthesias in the upper and mid face, as well as abducens nerve palsy, can develop as a result. An orally located aneurysm will more likely affect the oculomotor nerve. This can be manifested as a cranial and lateral shift in the position of the eyeball as well as double vision. In addition, the parasympathetic fibres of cranial nerve III may be affected. The pupils will then dilate (mydriasis). An arteriovenous fistula will result from a ruptured aneurysm. In this case, arterial blood will spread via the sphenoparietal and superior petrosal sinuses to more distant sinus cavities.

Aneurysms develop more frequently in the cerebral part of the internal carotid artery, known as the supraclinoid segment (30% according to Bähr and Froscher 2014). These arterial bulges are found near to the ophthalmic or posterior communicating artery (ophthalmic and posterior communicating aneurysm). Given the proximity to the anterior clinoid process and to the cavernous sinus, it is difficult to operate on such aneurysms (Kyoshima et al. 2006). Secondary involvement of the optic nerve, optic chiasm, or optic tract in the aneurysmal process is possible. If the decussating fibres of the optic chiasm are affected, the nasal fields of the retina, which represent the temporal fields of vision, can be impaired (heteronymous hemianopsia). The field of vision is thus laterally disturbed on both sides. Unilateral impairment of an optic tract will lead to homonymous hemianopsia, causing dysfunction in one temporal and one nasal field of vision.

3.2. Anterior Cerebral Artery

Aneurysms of the anterior cerebral artery (Figures 1, 2) affect the anterior communicating artery in 40%-45% of cases (anterior aneurysm). This artery forms the border between the A1 and A2 segments. An anterior aneurysm is located in front of the optic chiasm. It usually projects superiorly or anteriorly, and less often inferiorly or posteriorly (Sanches-Mejia et al. 2006). Sections of the rhinencephalon such as the olfactory tract and anterior perforated substance are in close proximity. Basal sections of the frontal lobe, such as the rectal gyrus and orbital gyri, likewise border the anterior communicating artery. When operating on this area, it is important to spare the short central arteries and long central artery (both from the A1 segment), which supply the basal ganglia and the internal capsule. Furthermore, the short central arteries (from the anterior communicating artery) supply the optic chiasm. Subarachnoid haemorrhage resulting from a ruptured anterior aneurysm can spread ventrally into the pericallosal cistern and dorsally into the chiasmatic cistern via the cistern of lamina terminalis, which is traversed by the anterior cerebral artery.

3.3. Middle Cerebral Artery

In approx. 20% of cases aneurysms of the middle cerebral artery (Figures 1-3) affect the beginning of the M2 segment (MCA aneurysms according to Bähr and Frotscher 2014). Here, the artery divides into a superior and an inferior trunk. The MCA aneurysm, measuring 2-14 mm, is larger than other types of aneurysm (Rinne et al. 2006). Due to subarachnoid haemorrhage, a ruptured MCA aneurysm more often results in death than other types of ruptured aneurysms. The bleeding may be associated with intraventricular haemorrhage. The inferior horn of the lateral ventricle is affected in such cases. MCA aneurysm is related to the parahippocampal gyrus, as part of the limbic system, and to the amygdala, a basal ganglion. Aneurysmal subarachnoid haemorrhage will spread in the cistern of the lateral fissure, since the M2 segment of the artery passes through the Sylvian fissure (Figure 3). Consideration must therefore be given to the proximity of important telencephalic centres, such as the motor speech centre (Broca's area) in the inferior frontal gyrus, the primary auditory centre in the Heschl convolutions of the superior temporal gyrus, and the sensory speech centre (Wernicke's area) in the supramarginal and angular gyri. On surgical intervention, care must also be taken not to interfere with the branches of the M2 segment that supply the motor and premotor cortex as well as the sensory cortex. Ultimately, the artery does not only bifurcate, namely into the superior and the inferior trunks (Figure 1), but multiple divisions also occur

(Lang and Wachsmuth 1979). If MCA aneurysms are to be occluded, it is important to know about a potential bi-, tri- quad- or pentafurcation so that branches concealed by the side of the aneurysm facing away from the surgeon are not also occluded.

3.4. Posterior Cerebral Artery

Aneurysms of the posterior cerebral artery (Figures 1, 2) are rare and usually affect the postcommunicating P2 segment. This type of aneurysm is found near the oculomotor nerve. Also in close proximity are the cerebral crura of the mesencephalon and parahippocampal gyrus, as part of the limbic system. A subarachnoid haemorrhage will spread into the ambient cistern, which is traversed by the superior cerebellar artery (Figure 2) and the trochlear nerve. Trochlear nerve palsy causes the eyeball to deviate inward and downward.

3.5. Basilar Artery

Basilar artery aneurysms (Figures 1, 2) occur at a rate of 10% (Bähr and Frotscher 2014) in the so-called basilar tip (basilar tip aneurysms), at the upper margin of the pons. The basilar artery divides at this point into the two superior cerebellar arteries and the two posterior cerebral arteries. Immediately ventral to this aneurysm are the mamillary bodies, infundibulum and floor of the hypothalamus. Dorsolaterally, the aneurysm meets with the oculomotor nerve and the fine arteries of the P1 segment (Figure 2) of the posterior cerebral artery that supply the internal capsule and thalamus. A haemorrhage will also spread into the ambient cistern via the interpeduncular cistern. Liliequist's membrane, which extends between the two temporal lobes, prevents the haemorrhage from crossing into the chiasmatic cistern. A basilar tip aneurysm is a space-occupying process in the region of the tentorial incisure (Lang 1985). Compression of the oculomotor nerve is therefore to be expected. The aneurysm can moreover displace the cerebral aqueduct dorsally, and the posterior wall of the third ventricle superiorly (Lang 1985). Intraoperative complications can entail unintentional injury to the fine arteries of the P1 segment of the posterior cerebral artery (Hernesniemi et al. 2006). Damage to one of the small-calibre interpeduncular perforating arteries running through the posterior perforated substance alone can have drastic consequences for the patient (Lawton 2011).

Aneurysms occur less often at the junction of the middle to lower third of the artery, roughly at the level of the origin of the anterior inferior cerebellar artery (1%-2%, according to Bähr and Frotscher 2014), than at the basilar tip (Figure 1). The abducens nerve is found dorsal, and the trigeminal nerve lateral to such aneurysms. Any haemorrhage will spread via the medial pontine cistern into the pontocerebellar cistern, located in the cerebellopontine angle, through which the facial and vestibulocochlear nerves pass. The lateral aperture of the fourth ventricle (Luschka) discharges into the pontocerebellar cistern; adhesion can occur in the event of bleeding. Internal hydrocephalus can result.

Basilar artery aneurysms are difficult to treat surgically on account of the fact that the neighbouring structures of this artery, namely the brain stem, territory of the clivus and tentorial incisure, are very hard to reach from lateral access points in the middle or posterior cranial fossa (Pernkopf 1957). Pterional (where the frontal bone, parietal bone, squamous bone and greater wing of the sphenoid bone converge), subtemporal and suboccipital approaches are suggested (Hernesniemi et al. 2006). Using modern surgical techniques, such as endovascular coiling of the aneurysm as mentioned at the start, treatment outcomes have improved.

3.6. Anterior Inferior Cerebellar Artery

Aneurysms of the anterior inferior cerebellar artery (Figures 1-3) are rare and are usually found close to the origin of the basilar artery. The abducens nerve is located near to such an aneurysm. The artery runs through the pontocerebellar cistern together with the facial and vestibulocochlear nerves, as well as the labyrinthine artery. The foramen of Luschka also passes into this cistern. Hence, a subarachnoid haemorrhage would also prevent CSF from exiting the lateral aperture of the fourth ventricle (foramen of Luschka). Internal hydrocephalus would be the result.

3.7. Posterior Inferior Cerebellar Artery

Aneurysms of the posterior inferior cerebellar artery (Figures 1, 2) are also rare. They mostly develop where the given artery emerges from the vertebral artery (Figure 1). A distinction is made between the descending and the ascending posterior inferior cerebellar artery (Figure 1). In both cases, the aneurysm is located near the inferior olive and is linked with cranial nerves IX, X, XI and XII (Pernkopf 1957). A subarachnoid haemorrhage will spread into the lateral cerebellomedullary cistern, on the posterolateral aspect of the medulla oblongata. Corresponding membranes separating the adjacent cisterns probably prevent the haemorrhage from infiltrating the pontocerebellar and cerebellomedullary cisterns. During surgical treatment of an aneurysm of the posterior inferior cerebellar artery, occlusion of the small arteries involved in supplying the caudal cranial nerves can occur (Bertalanffy et al. 2006). Wallenberg's syndrome would be the result.

4. Venous Drainage of the Brain

The description of the major cerebral veins and their branches is provided, as with the arteries, on the basis of the relevant chapter by Töndury et al. in the Textbook and Atlas of Human Anatomy by Rauber/Kopsch (1987). With thin walls and no valves, the cerebral veins drain into the dural venous sinuses. They are distributed independently of the arteries and can be divided into two main groups: 1) Superficial cerebral veins: The superficial cerebral veins transport the blood of the cerebral cortex to the superior sagittal sinus and basal sinus. 2) Deep cerebral veins: The deep cerebral veins transport blood from the medulla, basal ganglia and diencephalon to the great cerebral vein (or vein of Galen).

4.1. Superficial Cerebral Veins

The venous blood in the upper half of the outer surface of the cerebral hemispheres flows through the ascending, i.e., superior cerebral veins, into the superior sagittal sinus, and that in the lower half through the descending, i.e., inferior cerebral veins, into the transverse and sphenoparietal sinus. The superficial middle cerebral vein transports venous blood from both territories to the sphenoparietal sinus. Ultimately, the superficial cerebral veins also include the veins of the medial and basal aspects of the cerebral hemisphere.

4.1.1. Superior Cerebral Veins

These are 6-12 ascending veins that can be divided into four groups: frontal, frontoparietal, parietal and occipital veins. The frontal veins drain the blood from the gyri of the frontal lobe. The triad of frontoparietal veins (veins of Rolando) is made up of the precentral, central and postcentral veins. These veins lead into the sulci of the same names and transport the blood away from the precentral and postcentral gyri. The parietal and superior veins transport blood from the parietal lobe and the upper occipital lobe. Characteristically, the frontal veins drain in the direction of the blood flow, whereas the parietal and occipital veins drain in the opposite direction to the flow of the venous blood into the superior sagittal sinus.

4.1.2. Inferior Cerebral Veins

These comprise the inferior temporal and inferior occipital veins, which transport venous blood from the temporal lobe and from the lower occipital lobe down to the transverse sinus. The superficial middle cerebral vein, moreover, which descends through the lateral sulcus to the sphenoparietal sinus, carries blood out of the supramarginal and angular gyri.

The superficial cerebral veins on the outer aspect of the cerebral hemisphere are connected via two important anastomoses: 1. Superior anastomotic vein (vein of Trolard): This vein is formed from the postcentral vein and the superficial middle cerebral vein. It links the superior sagittal sinus to the sphenoparietal sinus. 2. Inferior anastomotic vein (vein of Labbé): This vein facilitates the anastomosis of the largest inferior temporal vein with the superficial middle cerebral vein. Via the vein of Trolard, the superior sagittal sinus is joined with the transverse sinus.

4.1.3. Veins of the Medial Surface

The frontopolar, medial anterior and posterior frontal, paracentral, precuneal veins, and the medial occipital veins drain blood from the territories of the frontal, parietal and occipital lobe belonging to the medial surface. The anterior cerebral (anterior limbic) vein and the dorsal (posterior limbic) vein of corpus callosum transport blood out of the corpus callosum and cingulate gyrus.

4.1.4. Veins of the Basal Surface

The anterior cerebral vein takes the same course as the artery of the same name. The deep middle cerebral artery is found deep in the lateral sulcus under the middle cerebral artery. The basal vein (of Rosenthal) emerges in the territory of the anterior perforated substance from the confluence of the anterior cerebral and deep middle cerebral veins. The vein travels dorsally along the optic tract, ascending to the quadrigeminal bodies, and discharges into the great cerebral vein (of Galen).

The anterior cerebral veins, the anterior communicating vein, the basal segments of the basal veins and the interpeduncular veins with posterior communicating vein form a cerebral venous circle (also referred to as Trolard's hexagon) beneath the cerebral arterial circle (Figure 1).

4.2. Deep Cerebral Veins

The deep cerebral veins, i.e., the septum pellucidum, thalamostriate and superior choroid veins, drain the blood from the basal ganglia, internal capsule, semioval centre of the white matter and the choroid plexus of the lateral ventricle and third ventricle. They merge at the posterior margin of the interventricular foramen in the anterior venous confluence with the internal cerebral vein.

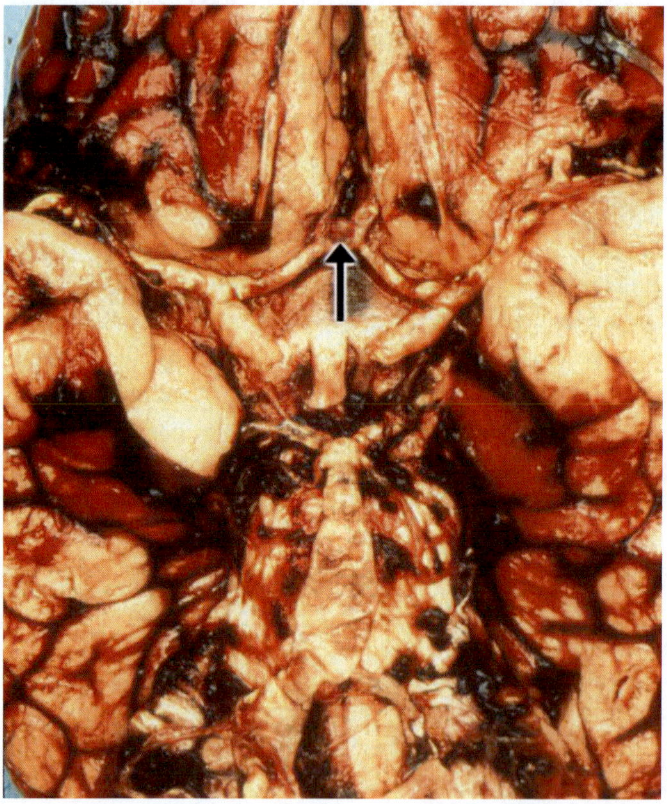

Figure 4. Aneurysm of the anterior communicating artery (anterior aneurysm). In 40%-45% of cases, the anterior communicating artery is affected. This artery forms the border between the A1 and A2 segments of the anterior cerebral artery. In this case the aneurysm (arrow) projects caudally, which tends to be rare. The aneurysm has ruptured. The subarachnoid haemorrhage has spread into the lamina terminalis cistern and, in particular, into the Sylvian, ambient and pontocerebellar cisterns. Image of an original specimen from a donated body, used in the Neuroanatomy Course at the Institute of Anatomy of Christian Albrechts University Kiel.

The vein of septum pellucidum transports blood from the genu of the corpus callosum, the head of the caudate nucleus and from the white matter of the frontal lobe. Unlike the name suggests, the thalamostriate vein does not drain blood from the thalamus, but rather from the striate body, the internal capsule and the white matter of the frontal and parietal lobe. The superior choroid vein removes blood from the hippocampus, fornix and corpus callosum.

The subependymal veins of the posterior and inferior horns drain blood from the white matter of the parietal and occipital lobe, and the temporal lobe and hippocampus, respectively, transporting it to the basal vein.

The internal cerebral vein takes venous blood from the thalamus, fornix, hippocampus, pineal body and quadrigeminal bodies. The largest thalamic vein, namely the superior thalamic vein, leads vertically into the middle of the internal cerebral artery. The interior cerebral veins on both sides unite via the pineal body to from the great cerebral vein (of Galen).

The great cerebral vein (of Galen) discharges into the right sinus immediately behind the confluence of the inferior sagittal sinus. It incorporates the caudally ascending basal vein (of Rosenthal) and the medial superior cerebellar vein. Furthermore, numerous smaller veins arrive at the great cerebral vein from the territories of the cuneus of the occipital lobe, epithalamus and quadrigeminal bodies.

4.3. Veins of the Cerebellum and Brain Stem

The cerebellar veins follow a similar pattern to the cerebral arteries, though they are independent of the latter. Their larger branches cross furrows and convolutions in a sagittal, and only rarely transverse direction. A differentiation is made between one medial and two lateral groups of veins. The medial veins drain blood from the vermis; the lateral veins remove blood from the cerebellar hemispheres.

The medial superior cerebellar vein carries blood from the upper part of the cerebellar vermis to the great cerebral vein; the medial inferior cerebellar vein transports blood from the inferior vermis to the transverse sinus. The lateral superior cerebellar vein carries the blood of the upper half of the hemisphere to the transverse sinus or straight sinus. The lateral inferior cerebellar vein drains blood from the lower half of the hemisphere, transporting it to the transverse sinus.

The superior petrosal (or Dandy's) vein ascends from the cerebellopontine angle along the trigeminal nerve to the superior petrosal sinus. It removes only a small amount of blood from the cerebellum, since it mainly drains the pons and medulla oblongata. However, this vein can also substitute the lateral superior and inferior cerebellar veins, among others. In this particular case, the superior petrosal vein drains almost the entire cerebellar hemisphere.

The veins of the brain stem are the continuation of the spinal veins, linking them to the basal cerebral veins. Caudally they create a longitudinal and transverse system in a similar way to the spinal veins. Topographically, the veins of the medulla oblongata and pons, like the cerebellar veins, are part of the infratentorial system.

Clinical features: The cerebral veins have specific source territories in which venous stasis can develop in the event of cerebral vein or sinus thrombosis, ultimately resulting in haemorrhagic infarcts in the cortex or medulla, as well as accompanying oedema. Cerebral venous and sinus thromboses are caused not only by thrombi rising from the pelvic and leg veins, but also by cardiovascular disorders, trauma, tumours, and inflammatory processes in the brain, skull and paranasal sinuses.

Thrombosis leads to an increase in intracranial pressure, and in extreme cases to compression of the tentorium. The consequences are headaches, nausea, vomiting, disorders of consciousness and, depending on the localisation of the pathological process, motor and sensory deficits. Thrombosis of the superior cerebral veins can result in a haemorrhagic infarct, mostly accompanied by contralateral hemiparesis or hemiplegia. Thrombosis of the inferior cerebral veins leads to an infarct in the region of the temporal or basal occipital lobe. The resulting symptoms are aphasia or contralateral homonymous hemianopsia. Thrombosis of the deep cerebral veins causes clouding of consciousness that progresses rapidly and can result in coma.

5. Relevance of Cerebral Veins and Dural Venous Sinuses to Surgical Aneurysm Repair

5.1. Superficial Cerebral Veins

When taking a lateral approach, such as for middle cerebral artery aneurysms, attention must be paid to the veins of the Sylvian fissure. The superficial middle cerebral vein courses over the surface together with the branches of the M2 segment of the middle cerebral artery (Figure 3). The deep middle cerebral vein can be found deep in the lateral fissure. At the base of the brain it enters the basal vein (of Rosenthal) along with the anterior cerebral vein. The superficial veins that drain the Sylvian fissure are referred to as "guardians" (Lawton 2011). This structure can vary, draining superiorly, anteriorly or posteriorly (Lawton 2011). In case of superior drainage, the venous blood flows into the frontoparietal veins, the superior anastomotic vein (vein of Trolard), and the superior sagittal sinus. In case of anterior drainage, the blood is discharged into the sphenoparietal, cavernous, superior petrosal and inferior petrosal sinuses. Finally, if the blood is drained posteriorly, it is transported into the inferior temporal veins, inferior anastomotic vein (vein of Labbé), and the transverse sinus.

5.2. Veins of the Cerebellum and Brain Stem

If taking a posterolateral approach through the asterion (junction of the lambdoid, parietomastoid and occipitomastoid sutures), the proximity of the transverse and sigmoid sinuses must first be taken into consideration. The medial inferior and lateral superior cerebellar veins drain the blood from the cerebellar vermis and hemispheres into the transverse sinus. The superior petrosal vein transports blood from the pons and medulla oblongata to the superior petrosal sinus.

ACKNOWLEDGEMENTS

I wish to thank Professor Dr. sc. med. R. Schultka, Director of the Meckel Anatomical Collections at the Institute of Anatomy and Cell Biology of Martin Luther University Halle-Wittenberg, for kindly loaning the injected specimens of the cerebral arteries for imaging purposes. I also thank Mr. G. Bothe, photographer at the Institute of Forensic Medicine of Martin Luther University Halle-Wittenberg for the excellent images and expert labelling of the collected specimens.

REFERENCES

Adachi B (1928): Das Arteriensystem der Japaner. Band I: A. pulmonalis, Aorta bis Arcus volaris profundus. Maruzen, Kyoto, S. 113.

Bähr M, Frotscher M (2014): Neurologisch-topische Diagnostik. 10. Auflage. Thieme, Stuttgart und New York, S. 521-527.

Bertalanffy H, Benes L, Heinze S, Tirakotai W, Sure U (2006): Surgical management of aneurysms of the vertebral and posterior inferior cerebellar artery complex. In: Schmidek HH, Roberts DW (Eds.), Schmidek and Sweet's Operative Neurosurgical Techniques, Section XIII: Management of Intracranial Aneurysms. 5th Edition, Saunders, Elsevier, pp 1209-1223.

Clara M (1959): Das Nervensystem des Menschen. 3. neubearbeitete Auflage. Johann Ambrosius Barth, Leipzig, S. 716.

Corning HK (1946): Lehrbuch der topographischen Anatomie. 23. Auflage. Springer, Berlin, S 36-42.

Deller T (2015): Hirngefäße. In: Waschke J, Böckers TM, Paulsen F (Hrsg.), Anatomie – Das Lehrbuch – Sobotta. 1. Auflage. Elsevier, Urban and Fischer, München, S. 623-644.

Drenckhahn (2004): Blutgefäße des Zentralnervensystems. In: Drenckhahn D (Hrsg.) Benninghoff/Drenckhahn, Anatomie, Band 2. 16. Auflage. Elsevier, Urban and Fischer, München, S. 621-648.

Duus P (1995): *Neurologisch-topische Diagnostik. 6.* Auflage. Thieme, Stuttgart und New York, S. 121, 439-441.

Herneshiemi J, Karatas A, Niemelä M, Ishii K, Peerless SJ, Drake CG (2006): Surgical techniques of terminal basilar and posterior cerebral artery aneurysms. In: Schmidek HH, Roberts DW (Eds.), Schmidek and Sweet's Operative Neurosurgical Techniques, Section XIII: Management of Intracranial Aneurysms. 5th Edition, Saunders, Elsevier, pp 1177-1191.

Kyoshima K, Shibuya M, Kobayashi S (2006): Surgical management of paraclinoid aneurysms. In: Schmidek HH, Roberts DW (Eds.), *Schmidek and Sweet's Operative Neurosurgical Techniques, Section XIII: Management of Intracranial Aneurysms.* 5th Edition, Saunders, Elsevier, pp 1099-1114.

Lang J und Wachsmuth W (1979): Lanz Wachsmuth, Praktische Anatomie, Kopf – Teil 1B: Gehirn- und Augenschädel. Springer, Berlin, Heidelberg und New York, S. 38-48, 123, 181-189.

Lang J (1985): Lanz Wachsmuth, Praktische Anatomie, Kopf – Teil A: Übergeordnete Systeme, Sonderausgabe 2004 der 1985 erschienenen 1. Auflage. Springer, Berlin, Heidelberg, New York et al., S. 438-439.

Lasjaunias P, Berenstein A, ter Brugge KG (2001): *Surgical Neuroangiography.* Vol. 1: Clinical vascular anatomy and variations. Second edition. Springer, Berlin und Heidelberg.

Lawton MT (2011): *Seven Aneurysms. Tenets and Techniques for Clipping.* Thieme, Stuttgart und New York.

Leonhardt H (1988): Kopf – Hals. In: Leonhardt H, Tillmann B, Zilles K (Hrsg.), Rauber/Kopsch, Anatomie des Menschen, Lehrbuch und Atlas, Band IV, Topographie der Organsysteme, Systematik der peripheren Leitungsbahnen. Thieme, Stuttgart und New York, S. 21-183.

Paulsen F, Waschke J (2010): Sobotta – Atlas der Anatomie des Menschen. Kopf, Hals und Neuroanatomie. 23. Auflage. Elsevier, Urban and Fischer, München, S. 266-269.

Pernkopf E (1957): Topographische Anatomie des Menschen. IV. Band, 1. Hälfte: Topographische und stratigraphische Anatomie des Kopfes. Urban and Schwarzenberg, München, Berlin und Wien. S. 193-227.

Rinne J, Ishii K, Shen H, Kivisaari R, Hernesniemi J (2006): Surgical Management of Aneurysms of the Middle Cerebral Artery. In: Schmidek HH, Roberts DW (Eds.), Schmidek and Sweet's Operative Neurosurgical Techniques, Section XIII: Management of Intracranial Aneurysms. 5th Edition, Saunders, Elsevier, pp 1144-1166.

Sanchez-Mejia RO, Quinones-Hinojosa A, Jun P, Lawton MT (2006): Microsurgical Management of Anterior Communicating Artery Aneurysms. In: Schmidek HH, Roberts DW (Eds.), Schmidek and Sweet's Operative Neurosurgical Techniques, Section XIII: Management of Intracranial Aneurysms. 5th Edition, Saunders, Elsevier, pp 1131-1143.

Sobotta/Becher (1973): Atlas der Anatomie des Menschen, Band 3. Ferner H, Staubesandt J (Hrsg.). 17. Auflage. Urban and Schwarzenberg, München, Berlin und Wien, S. 66-67.

Tillmann B (1997): Farbatlas der Anatomie. Zahnmedizin – Humanmedizin. Thieme, Stuttgart und New York, S. 240.

Töndury G, Kubik S, Krisch B (1987): Hirnhäute und Hirngefäße. In: Leonhardt H, Töndury G, Zilles K (Hrsg.), Anatomie des Menschen, Lehrbuch und Atlas, Band III, Nervensystem, Sinnesorgane Thieme, Stuttgart und New York, S. 175-233.

Yasargil MG (1969): Microsurgery applied to neurosurgery. *Chapter 4: Reconstructive and constructive surgery of the cerebral arteries in man.* Thieme, Stuttgart, New York und London, pp 82-95.

In: Spontaneous Subarachnoid Haemorrhage
Editors: Thomas Kapapa and Ralph König
ISBN: 978-1-63485-270-8

Chapter 3

Neuropathology of Subarachnoid Haemorrhage

Angelika Scheuerle
Section Neuropathology, University Ulm, Günzburg, Germany

Abstract

The resulting damages from subarachnoid haemorrhage has a complex pathogenesis encompassing various systems which nevertheless overlap when active simultaneously, consecutively or at staggered intervals. The precise interplay of different factors that lead to alternately pronounced, permanent damage to the central nervous system has not yet been completely and conclusively explained. However, the underlying mechanisms that are activated as a result of bleeding into the subarachnoid space from a blood vessel are presented.

Keywords: subarachnoid haemorrhage, pathogenesis, histology, aneurysm, early and delayed injury

The subarachnoid space is formed by a loosely arranged layer of cells in the pia mater lying next to the glia limitans which is divided by a basal membrane. The outer layer forms densely structured, flat to cuboidal arachnoid cells that are joined with each other by tight junctions. The arachnoid cells have projections which make contact with the pia mater and therefore permeate the space like a spider's web. Individual fibroblasts and collagen fibres, as well as medium-sized blood vessels are also found which, like the intracerebral vessels, have a blood-CSF barrier. The subarachnoid space contains cerebrospinal fluid (CSF) which is transported via the arachnoid villi (arachnoid granulations). If blood penetrates the subarachnoid space, an increase in intracranial pressure, initial vasoparalysis, and impaired CSF drainage will result depending on the extent and magnitude, which will reflect the size of the defect in the vessel. To maintain the cerebral blood flow, the blood pressure will increase along with vasodilation. This leads to an increase in the cerebral blood volume and further increase in intracranial pressure, even global cerebral ischaemia, since the intracranial pressure will exceed the arterial perfusion pressure. This can be seen in the form of apoptosis but also necroses, both in animal experiments and in post-mortem examinations on humans, whereby apoptosis was not only detected in brain cells but also in vascular wall cells. Vascular wall damage causes a disturbance in the blood-brain barrier with subsequent cerebral oedema and a further increase in intracranial pressure. The death receptor, TNF-alpha, p53, and the Caspase cascade appear to play a crucial role in cell death induced by SAH.

If the acute phase of bleeding is survived, haematoma then develops with lysis of erythrocytes, precipitation of fibrin and infiltration of fibroblasts and sprouting of capillaries, from which granulation tissue forms. These organisational processes explain the course of temporal changes which are reflected in the (CSF "cancel") histological findings. These initially exhibit fresh blood with perfectly preserved erythrocytes, granulocytes and leukocytes in the same ratio as in a patient's peripheral blood count. After approx. 12 hours, the erythrocyte boundaries are more indistinct (blurred), and reactive pleocytosis begins. Oxyhaemoglobin and initial erythrophages emerge on the first day post haemorrhage. The breakdown of haemoglobin begins three to four days later with evidence of siderophages. As a result, haematoidin crystals may be visible if there is more pronounced haemorrhaging.

During haemoglobin release and haemoglobin breakdown, oxygen radicals develop, which activate adhesion molecules that attract macrophages and neutrophils. The potent vasoconstrictor leads to the increased detection of TNF-alpha during this phase. Erythrocyte breakdown products in the subarachnoid space can trigger so-called spreading depressions that are linked with the delayed onset of cerebral ischaemia which ensues 5-14 days after the haemorrhage. The slow spread of neuronal ("and glial" cancel) depolarisation detectable on electrophysiological testing can lead to cerebral ischaemia as a result of vasoconstrictive activity.

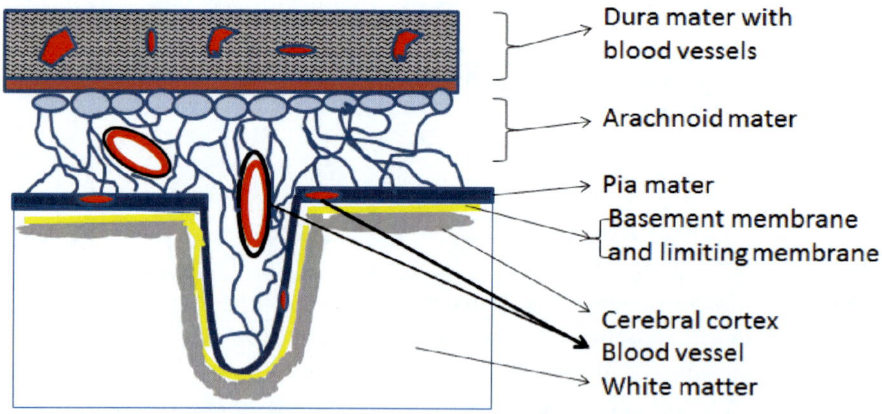

Figure 1. Structure of the subarachnoid space. From the outside inward, the dura mater is identifiable from the firm collagen/fibre-rich connective tissue with embedded blood vessels. Next is the arachnoid mater with dura-facing neurothelium (arachnoidal cells), from where delicate trabeculae traverse the subarachnoid space like a spider's web to reach the pia mater, a delicate layer of vascularised connective tissue.

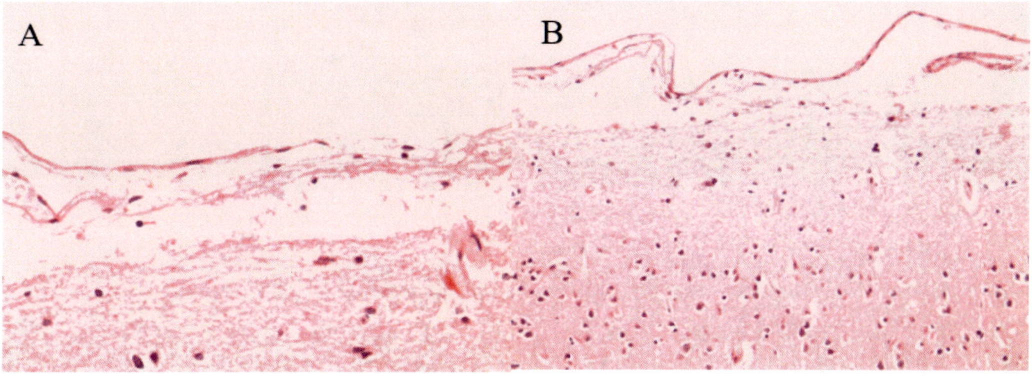

Figure 2. A) Delicate arachnoid mater with narrow, elongated, flat arachnoid cells and embedded blood vessel. B) An adjacent, external band of cortex.

CAUSES OF SAH

Aside from trauma, a ruptured aneurysm (85%) is the main cause of SAH. An aneurysm is the bulging of an arterial wall, the exact origin of which is not yet fully understood. As they are extremely rare in newborn babies and children with no apparent cause (trauma, infections, connective tissue diseases), it is assumed that the change in the vascular wall is acquired. Genetic factors are postulated, since apart from a familial predisposition aneurysms occur increasingly with congenital connective tissue diseases (polycystic kidney disease, Ehler-Danlos syndrome type IV, etc.). Forbes (1930) [1], and later Stehbens (1989) [2], have suggested that a defect appears in the muscle layer at the onset of an aneurysm. Other authors favour the theory that so-called intimal cushions reduced the elasticity locally. This causes increased pressure on the immediately adjacent wall, possibly leading to structural changes in the aneurysm. Calouhi et al. [3] see increasing evidence for an inflammatory event in the pathogenesis of a cerebral aneurysm. Back in 2010, Y. Kanematsu et al. [4] reported that macrophages and cytokines originating from the macrophages assume a key role in haemodynamic blebs. They are particularly effective during the constant remodelling of the wall following haemodynamic stress. It cannot yet be fully understood why some aneurysms rupture, while other aneurysms do not rupture throughout a person's life. Usually, the rupture is assumed to have an inflammatory origin. The risk of rupture grows with the size of the aneurysm, the location of the aneurysm in the posterior circulation, hypertension, alcohol and cocaine abuse.

Histologically, the aneurysm is characterised by the loss of the internal elastic lamina and a thinning or even missing middle coat in the arterial wall, resulting in the wall usually only consisting of collagen fibres, isolated smooth muscle cells and possibly individual elastic fibres. Ruptures usually occur at the dome of the aneurysm where blood and fibrin are deposited. Some fresh and partially organised thrombi are observed in the lumen. Arteriosclerotic changes can take place at the margins of usually fusiform aneurysms.

Aneurysms caused by inflammation are rare and usually accompanied by infectious endocarditis (bacterial or mycotic). Histologically, the bulge in the wall is accompanied by pronounced inflammatory cell infiltrates (granulocytes, lymphocytes).

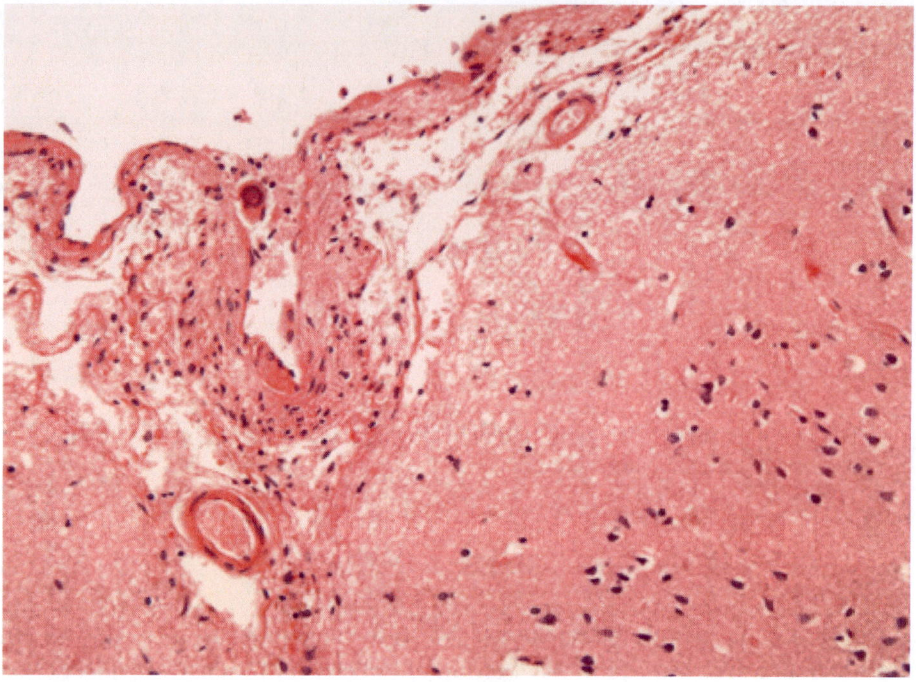

Figure 3. The arachnoid mater follows the invaginated sulcus of the superficial cortex, where it is somewhat fibrosed and the embedded blood vessels are more clearly visible. A small calcified psammoma body can be seen.

Morphologically, arterial dissection reveals a tear in the intima and/or media with subsequent bleeding into the arterial wall which, as well as being caused by trauma, can also be precipitated by amyloid angiopathy. Occasionally, especially in older people and sometimes due to genetic predisposition, deposits of amyloid are found in the walls of the small and medium-sized, mostly arterial blood vessels of the cortex and the leptomeninges. They can be accompanied by Alzheimer's type dementia.

Non-aneurysmal perimesencephalic haemorrhage corresponds to bleeding into the basal interpedicular cisterns, anterior to the midbrain. It can occur in combination but also with no evidence of an aneurysm, and is more frequent in hypertensive patients. The patients have an excellent prognosis and require only a short period of convalescence. In particular, no cerebral ischaemia develops.

Other rare causes of subarachnoid haemorrhage are arteriovenous malformations of the cerebral cortex which usually lead to an intracerebral haemorrhage and in >5% can bleed primarily into the subarachnoid space. Small aneurysmal bulges of delicate afferent and efferent arterial branches have been identified as a cause of haemorrhage. Cavernomas also more likely lead to intracerebral haemorrhage than to subarachnoid haemorrhage.

SAH develops in 30% of children and most adults with sickle cell disease (Cary et al., 1990) [5]. Other rare causes are venous thrombi, vasculitis, severe stenosis, coagulation disorders, inflammations as well as primary and secondary leptomeningeal tumours.

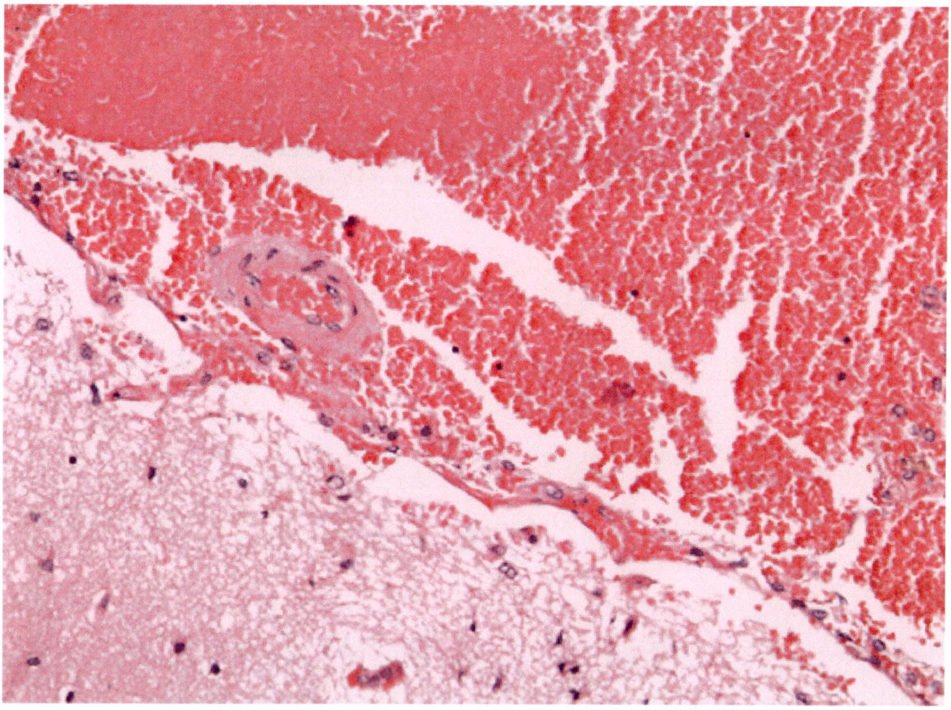

Figure 4. Recent subarachnoid haemorrhage with well-preserved erythrocytes and individual white blood cells, embedded subarachnoid arterial branch and basal outer cortex are also depicted.

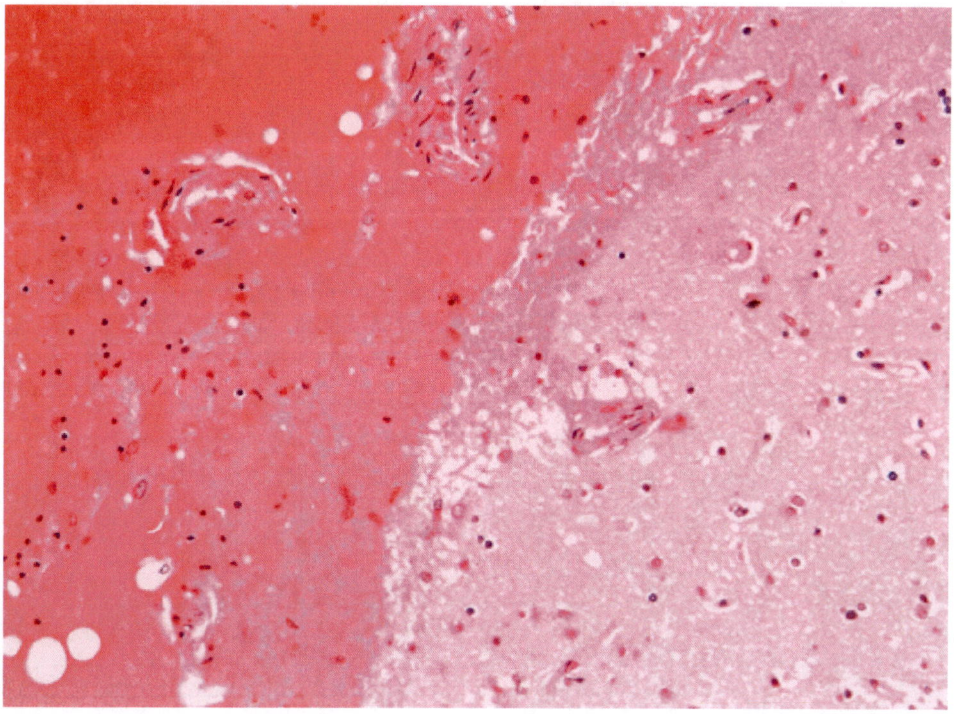

Figure 5. Less recent subarachnoid haemorrhage (approx. 1 day) with depleted erythrocytes that now have blurry contours.

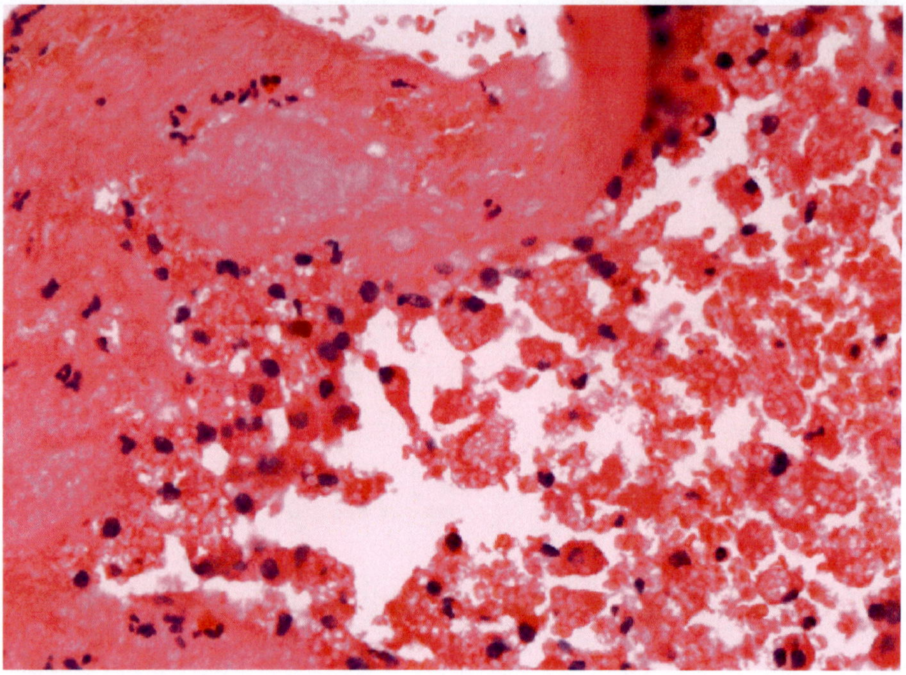

Figure 6. Incipient signs of organisation of a haemorrhage with erythrophages.

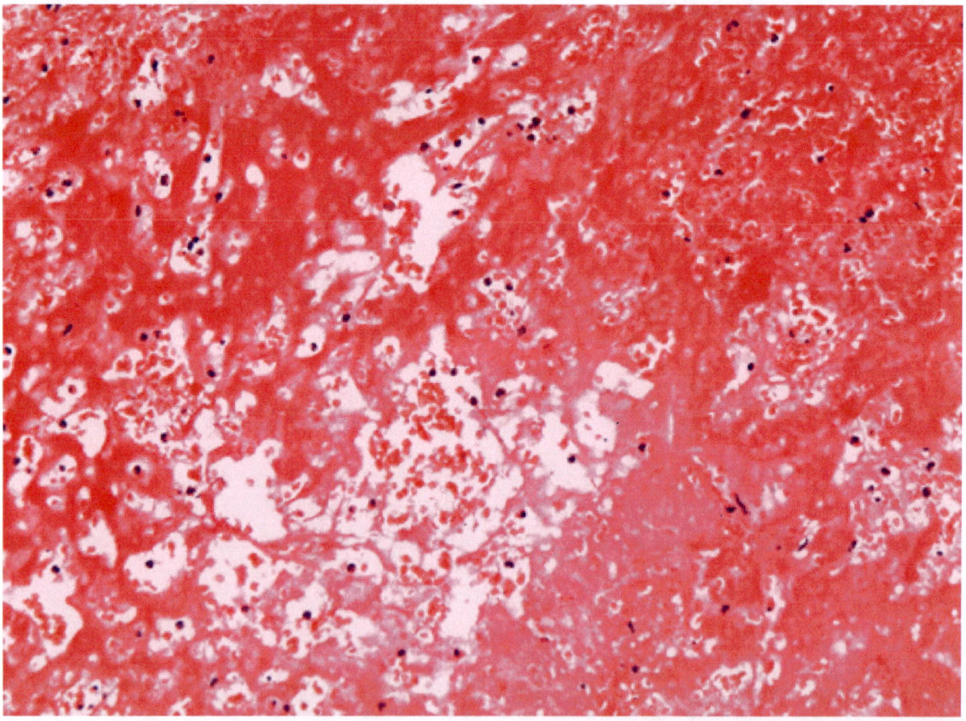

Figure 7. Approx. 1-2 day-old blood with fibrin precipitations, but still loosely distributed leukocytes and interspersed, still well-preserved erythrocytes.

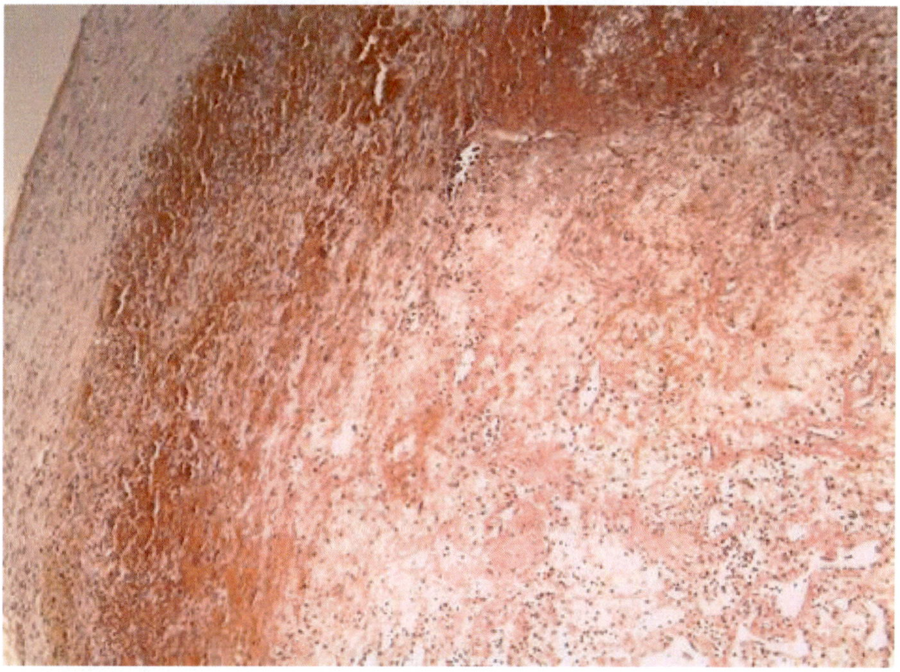

Figure 8. Aneurysm: Partially thrombosed aneurysm (VEG). To the left: sections of the fibrous aneurysm wall with adjacent fresh blood and well-preserved erythrocytes. To the right: advancing hypervascular granulation tissue, corresponding to organised thrombus (VEG staining).

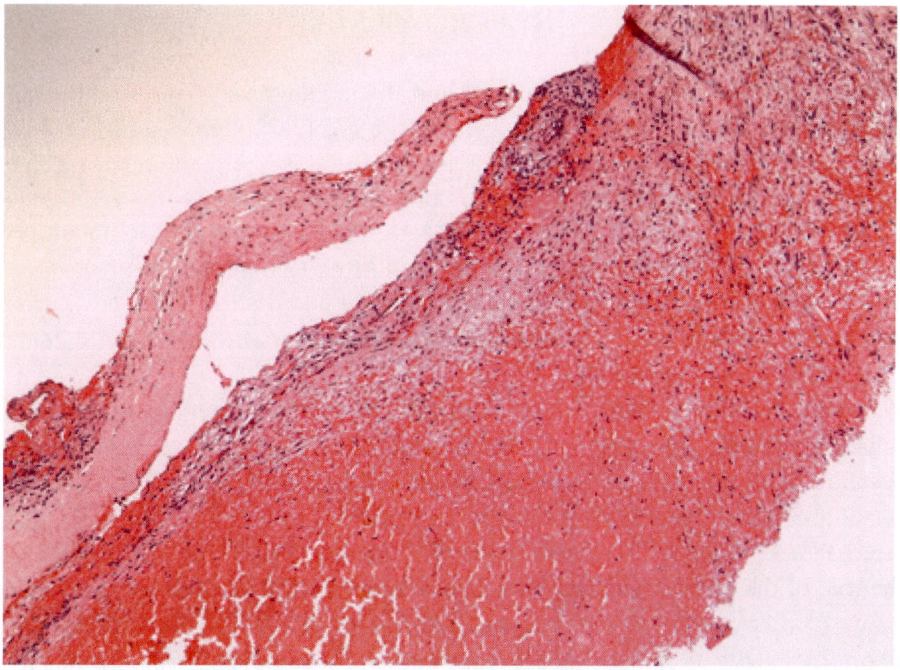

Figure 9. Rupture site of an aneurysm HE: Significantly narrowed aneurysm wall, consisting of rather hypocellular fibrous connective tissue (bottom left). Mononuclear round cells (top centre) at the rupture site. Top right: organised thrombus with fibroblasts and isolated vascular fissures.

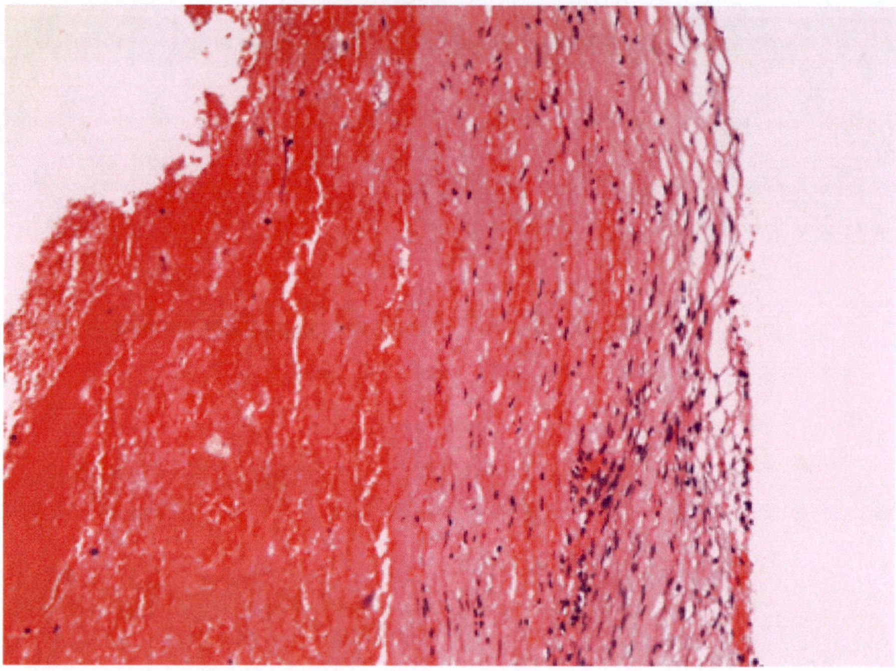

Figure 10. The fibrous wall segments adjacent to the aneurysm rupture site with fresh intramural haemorrhages (right). Left: lumen of the aneurysm sac filled with fresh blood.

References

[1] van Gijn J, Rinkel GJ. Subarachnoid haemorrhage: diagnosis, causes and management. *Brain: a journal of neurology.* 2001 Feb;124(Pt 2):249-78. PubMed PMID: 11157554.

[2] Sabri M, Lass E, Macdonald RL. Early brain injury: a common mechanism in subarachnoid hemorrhage and global cerebral ischemia. *Stroke research and treatment.* 2013;2013:394036. PubMed PMID: 23533958. Pubmed Central PMCID: 3603523.

[3] Cahill J, Calvert JW, Zhang JH. Mechanisms of early brain injury after subarachnoid hemorrhage. *Journal of cerebral blood flow and metabolism: Official journal of the International Society of Cerebral Blood Flow and Metabolism.* 2006 Nov;26(11):1341-53. PubMed PMID: 16482081.

[4] Dreier JP, Woitzik J, Fabricius M, Bhatia R, Major S, Drenckhahn C, et al. Delayed ischaemic neurological deficits after subarachnoid haemorrhage are associated with clusters of spreading depolarizations. *Brain: a journal of neurology.* 2006 Dec;129(Pt 12):3224-37. PubMed PMID: 17067993.

[5] Ostergaard L, Aamand R, Karabegovic S, Tietze A, Blicher JU, Mikkelsen IK, et al. The role of the microcirculation in delayed cerebral ischemia and chronic degenerative changes after subarachnoid hemorrhage. *Journal of cerebral blood flow and metabolism: Official journal of the International Society of Cerebral Blood Flow and Metabolism.* 2013 Dec;33(12):1825-37. PubMed PMID: 24064495. Pubmed Central PMCID: 3851911.

In: Spontaneous Subarachnoid Haemorrhage
Editors: Thomas Kapapa and Ralph König ISBN: 978-1-63485-270-8

Chapter 4

Epidemiology and Risk Factors

Stefan Röhrer
Department of Neurosurgery, University of Ulm, Ulm, Germany

Abstract

The incidence of aneurysmal subarachnoid hemmorrhage is different in miscellaneous countries or regions. Exact global figures are not available. Reasons might be variable medical infrastructure in different countries such as availability of diagnostic methods. Subarachnoid hemorrhage thus could go undiagnosed and a patient may die without prior diagnosis. The common age for subarachnoid hemorrhage is between 40 and 60 years, and women are more affected. Additionally differences between races have been detected in terms of the occurrence of subarachnoid hemorrhage. So black people are statistically more affected. The risk factors for occur of subarachnoid hemorrhage can be separate in modifiable and non-modifiable factors. Examples for modifiable factors are smoking, arterial hypertension and excess alcohol consumption. Familial disposition or genetic diseases are non-modifiable factors.

Keywords: subarachnoid hemorrhage, epidemiology, cerebral aneurysm

Epidemiology of Aneurysmal Subarachnoid Haemorrhage

In the literature the incidence of aneurysmal subarachnoid haemorrhage (SAH) in Western countries is quoted as being 6-10 cases per 100,000 inhabitants a year [1, 2]. In some countries, such as Japan or Finland for example, the occurrence of SAH of unknown cause is significantly higher, reaching annual rates of up to 23 out of 100,000 inhabitants [1, 3]. Exact global figures are not available, as the care structure in the various countries does differ significantly. Not everywhere is a standard or emergency CT imaging method available for diagnosing SAH. SAH thus could go undiagnosed and a patient may die without prior diagnosis. An example of this would be Africa. In principle, an aneurysmal SAH can occur at any age, but tends to be more common in people between 40 and 60 years of age [4, 5].

Gender-specific comparison reveals that the ratio between women and men is 3:2 [1]. The risk of SAH was thereby found to be lower in women who do not give birth to their first child until after the age of 23, or who have had hormone replacement therapy but have never taken oral contraception [17].

Furthermore, differences between races have been identified in terms of the occurrence of SAH. Hence, the risk of spontaneous SAH has been found to be 2.1 times higher in black versus white people [6].

Intracranial aneurysms in children are very rare and constitute 1%-5% of all detected aneurysms [14, 15]. A ruptured aneurysm with consecutive aneurysmal SAH causes haemorrhagic stroke in 10%-15% of paediatric patients [16].

Risk Factors for Aneurysmal Subarachnoid Haemorrhage

When it comes to the risk factors for aneurysmal SAH, a distinction is made between modifiable and non-modifiable factors.

The modifiable and treatable factors which increase the risk of SAH include smoking (1.9%), arterial hypertension (2.8%) and excess alcohol consumption (4.7%) [3]. The risk of spontaneous SAH is also increased by taking oral contraceptives [7]. As patients with these risk factors are increasingly affected by SAH, acquired damage of the internal elastic lamina appears to be the cause of aneurysm formation.

Predictor for ruptured aneurysm	*Points*
Hypertension	
No	0
Yes	1
Population	
North America, Europe	0
Japan	3
Finland	5
Age	
<70 years old	0
>70 years old	1
Aneurysm size	
< 7.0 mm	0
7.0-9.9 mm	3
10.0-19.9 mm	6
>20 mm	10
History of SAH from another aneurysm	
No	0
Yes	1
Location of aneurysm	
Internal carotid artery	0
Middle cerebral arteries	2
Anterior cerebral arteries/posterior cerebral arteries	3

Figure 1. PHASES Score.

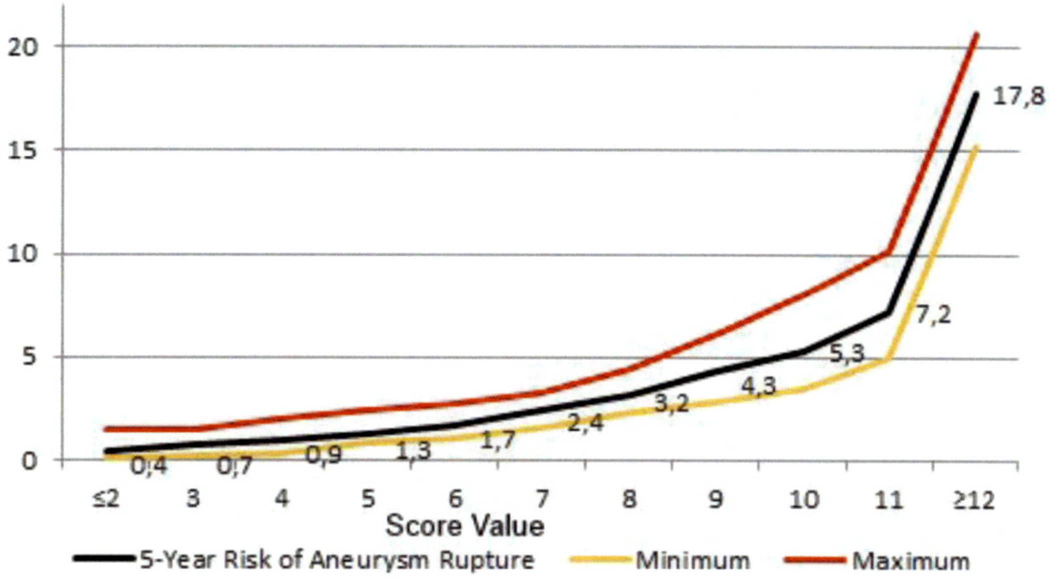

Probability of ruptured aneurysm (%)
Risk score

Figure 2. Five-year risk of a cerebral aneurysm rupturing according to the PHASES Score.

The non-modifiable factors include familial disposition, with 5%-20% of all patients having a positive family history of aneurysmal haemorrhage [8]. In particular, first-degree relatives of patients with aneurysmal SAH are found to have a 3-7 times higher risk of also experiencing such a haemorrhage. In contrast, the risk returns to normal in the second generation [9]. There are genetic factors, moreover, that are responsible for the development of aneurysmal SAH. Connective tissue diseases and polycystic kidney disease would be worth mentioning here [10]. In the case of the latter, mutations can be found on chromosomes 4 or 16, depending on the type. In contrast, Ehlers-Danlos syndrome and Marfan syndrome, which are often mentioned in relation to SAH, are only very rarely noted to be associated with a haemorrhage [11] and, in the case of Marfan Syndrome, studies have not established any relevant link [12].

In order to ascertain the five-year risk of a rupture in incidental cerebral aneurysms, the PHASES Score (following Chapter) was developed. To determine the risk of rupture, this score includes age, arterial hypertension, size and location of the aneurysm, previous history of SAH and the geographic location of the patient [13].

References

[1] Linn F. H. H., Rinkel G. J., Algra A. et al. 1996. Incidence of subarachnoid hemorrhage. Role of region, year and CT scanning: A meta-analysis. *Stroke*, 27: 625-629.

[2] Broderick J. P., Brott T. G., Tomsick T. et al. 1993. Intracerebral hemorrhage more than twice as common as subarachnoid hemorrhage. *J Neurosurg*, 78: 188-191.
[3] Teunissen L. L., Rinkel G. J. E., Algra A., van Gijn J. 1996. Risk factors for subarachnoid hemorrhage: A systematic review. *Stroke*, 27: 544-549.
[4] Longstreth W. T. Jr., Nelson L. M., Koepsell T. D., van Belle G. 1993. Clinical course of spontaneous subarachnoid hemorrhage: a population-based study in King County, Washington. *Neurology*, 43: 712-718.
[5] Lanzino G., Kassel N. F., Germanson T. P., Kongable G. L., Truskowski L. L., Torner J. C. et al. 1996. Age and outcome after aneurysmal subarachnoid hemorrhage: why do older patients fare worse? *J Neurosurg*, 85: 410-418.
[6] Broderick J. P., Brott T. G., Tomsick T., Huster G., Miller R. 1992. The risk of subarachnoid and intracerebral hemorrhages in blacks as compared with whites. *N Engl J Med*, 326: 733-736.
[7] Johnston S. C., Colford J. M. Jr., Gress D. R. 1998. Oral contraceptives and the risk of subarachnoid hemorrhage: a meta-analysis. *Neurology*, 51: 441-418.
[8] Schievink W. I. 1997. Genetics of intracranial aneurysms (Review). *Neurosurgery*, 40: 651-662.
[9] Bromberg J. E. C., Rinkel G. J. E., Algra A., Greebe P., van Duyn C. M., Hasan D. et al. 1995. Subarachnoid haemorrhage in first and second degree relatives of patients with subarachnoid haemorrhage. *BMJ*, 311:288-289.
[10] Schievink W. I., Michels V. V., Piepgras D. G., Wiebers D. O. 1992. Saccular intracranial aneurysms in autosomal dominant polycystic kidney disease. *J Am Soc Nephrol*. 3: 88-95.
[11] Schievink W. I., Michels V. V., Piepgras D. G. 1994. Neurovascular manifestations of heritable connective tissue disorders. A review. *Stroke*, 25: 889-903.
[12] Van den Berg J. S., Limburg M., Hennekam R. C. 1996. Is Marfan syndrome associated with symptomatic intracranial aneurysms? *Stroke*, 27: 10-12.
[13] Gravin J. P. et al. 2014. Development of the PHASES score for prediction of risk of rupture of intracranial aneurysms: a pooled analysis of six prospective cohort studies. *The Lancet Neurology*, 13: 59-66.
[14] Herman J. M., Rekate H. L., Spetzler R. F. 1991. Pediatric intracranial aneurysms: simple and complex cases. *Pediatr Neurosurg*, 17: 66-72.
[15] Krishna H., Wani A. A., Behari S., Banerji D., Chhabra D. K., Jain V. K. 2005. Intracranial aneurysms in patients 18 years of age and under, are they different from aneurysms in adult population? *Acta Neurochir*, 147: 469-467.
[16] Jordan L. C., Johnston S. C., Wu Y. W., Sidney S., Fullerton H. J. 2009. The importance of cerebral aneurysms in childhood hemorrhagic stroke: a population-based study. *Stroke*, 49: 400-405.
[17] Mhurchu Cliona, Anderson Craig, Jamrozik Konrad, Hankey Graeme, Dunbabin David. 2011. Hormonal factors and risk of aneurysmal subarachnoid hemorrhage: an international population-based, case-control study. *Stroke*, 32: 606-612.

In: Spontaneous Subarachnoid Haemorrhage
Editors: Thomas Kapapa and Ralph König

ISBN: 978-1-63485-270-8

Chapter 5

RISK FACTORS: FORMATION, GROWTH, RUPTURE

Karl-Michael Schebesch and Petra Schödel
Department of Neurosurgery, University of Regensburg,
Regensburg, Germany

ABSTRACT

Aneurysms have a pathology that is certainly multifactorial and probably an expression of genetic predisposition. Their incidence is increased in the event of a family history, and they usually occur in considerable numbers with certain genetic diseases. Arterial hypertension, diabetes mellitus, smoking, drug abuse and connective tissue diseases with tunica media insufficiency are suspected risk factors for aneurysm formation. A distinction must be made between the factors that promote the development of cerebral aneurysms and those that cause them to rupture and lead to the occurrence of subarachnoid haemorrhage. In addition to age and sex, size, morphology, positive history of a previous ruptured aneurysm, as well as a positive family history are other significant contributory risk factors for a rupture.

FORMATION

Recent autopsy studies, along with radiological screening, have demonstrated that the prevalence of cerebral aneurysms is in some instances much higher than previously assumed [1, 2]. Aneurysms have a pathology that is certainly multifactorial and probably an expression of genetic predisposition [3, 4]. Their incidence is increased in the event of a family history, and they usually occur in considerable numbers with certain genetic diseases (polycystic kidneys, Marfan syndrome, Ehler's Danlos syndrome) [1, 5, 6]. The following factors are suspected to contribute to the development and growth of cerebral aneurysms: arterial hypertension, diabetes mellitus, smoking, drug abuse and connective tissue diseases with tunica media insufficiency [4, 5, 7].

Elaborate computer-based simulation studies, as well as physical wind tunnel experiments, have to date produced valuable yet inconsistent results which when combined, however, suggest that considerable influence is exerted by the properties of the vessel walls – such as shear stress in the vascular walls, the angle of the exiting vessels and the surrounding pressure. Pathohistological studies of aneurysm-carrying vessels have also demonstrated that a sometimes pronounced inflammatory reaction takes place in the vascular wall, accompanied by an influx of T cells and macrophages. It is therefore presumed that the localised weakening of the vessel wall, together with the flow characteristics of the blood, could result in the formation of cerebral aneurysms [8-10].

Table 1. Phases Score: Predicted risk of rupture in percent within the next 5 years. ICA = Internal Carotid Artery, MCA = Middle Cerebral Artery, ACA = Anterior cerebral Artery, postCirc = posterior circulation including the posterior communicating artery, y = years, SAH = Subarachnoid Haemorrhage

Population in North America and Europe, excluding Finland																
	No hypertension, no history of SAH				Hypertension, no history of SAH				Hypertension and history of SAH							
Size, Age ≥ 70y	ICA	MCA	ACA	postCirc	ICA	MCA	ACA	postCirc	ICA	MCA	ACA	postCirc				
≥ 20 mm	7	13	>15	>15	10	>15	>15	>15	14	>15	>15	>15				
10-19.9 mm	2	4	6	7	3	5	8	9	4	7	11	13				
7-9.9 mm	1	1	3	3	1	2	3	4	2	3	5	6				
<7 mm	0	1	1	1	0	1	1	2	1	1	2	3				
Size, Age <70y	ICA	MCA	ACA	postCirc	ICA	MCA	ACA	postCirc	ICA	MCA	ACA	postCirc				
≥ 20 mm	5	9	15	>15	7	12	>15	>15	10	>15	>15	>15				
10-19.9 mm	1	2	4	5	2	3	6	7	3	5	8	9				
7-9.9 mm	1	1	2	2	1	1	2	3	1	2	3	4				
<7 mm	0	0	1	1	0	1	1	1	0	1	2	2				
Size, Age ≥ 70y	ICA	MCA	ACA	postCirc	ICA	MCA	ACA	postCirc	ICA	MCA	ACA	postCirc				
≥ 20 mm	>15	>15	>15	>15	>15	>15	>15	>15	>15	>15	>15	>15				
10-19.9 mm	5	10	>15	>15	7	13	>15	>15	10	>15	>15	>15				
7-9.9 mm	2	4	7	8	3	5	9	11	4	8	13	15				
<7 mm	1	2	3	4	1	2	4	5	2	3	6	7				
Size, Age <70y	ICA	MCA	ACA	postCirc	ICA	MCA	ACA	postCirc	ICA	MCA	ACA	postCirc				
≥ 20 mm	13	>15	>15	>15	>15	>15	>15	>15	>15	>15	>15	>15				
10-19.9 mm	4	7	11	13	5	9	15	>15	7	13	>15	>15				
7-9.9 mm	2	3	5	6	2	4	6	8	3	5	9	11				
<7 mm	1	1	2	3	1	2	3	3	1	2	4	5				

GROWTH AND RUPTURE

A distinction must be made between the factors that promote the development of cerebral aneurysms (see above) and those that cause them to rupture and lead to the occurrence of subarachnoid haemorrhage (SAH). As a condition, SAH peaks between the ages of 50 and 70 years, and affects women approx. 1.6 times more often than men. In addition to age and sex, however, there are other significant contributory factors, of which the following have been frequently identified: size (craniocaudal diameter or largest diameter) depending on anatomic position (e.g., >5 mm ACOM, >7 mm ICA/MCA/PCOM), morphology (irregular, fusiform, blebs, blisters), positive history of a previous ruptured aneurysm, as well as a positive family history [7, 11-13].

The role of environmental factors such as the weather is not clear, whereas ethnicity has been confirmed as a definite and highly significant factor. Hence, the incidence of aneurysmal SAH in Asia, but also in Finland, is approximately three times higher than in Central and Western Europe [7, 11-13].

A practical risk stratification method for use in patients with cerebral aneurysm is the PHASES score, which accounts for the aforementioned variables and permits estimation of the haemorrhagic risk [14].

Mycotic aneurysms (following cerebral infections), dissecting aneurysms (usually caused by trauma) and giant aneurysms (>24.9 mm) are rare cerebral aneurysmal malformations. These three entities are to be viewed as having a distinct pathophysiology in terms of development and risk of rupture, and according to a number of authors are to be strictly separated from conventional cerebral aneurysms [6, 7, 12, 13].

REFERENCES

[1] Agarwal N, Gala NB, Choudhry OJ, Assina R, Prestigiacomo CJ, Duffis EJ, et al. Prevalence of asymptomatic incidental aneurysms: a review of 2,685 computed tomographic angiograms. *World neurosurgery.* 2014 Dec;82(6):1086-90. PubMed PMID: 23336985.

[2] Mostafazadeh B, Farzaneh Sheikh E, Afsharian Shishvan T, Seraji FN, Salmasian H. The incidence of berry aneurysm in the Iranian population: an autopsy study. *Turkish neurosurgery.* 2008 Jul;18(3):228-31. PubMed PMID: 18814108.

[3] Farlow JL, Lin H, Sauerbeck L, Lai D, Koller DL, Pugh E, et al. Lessons learned from whole exome sequencing in multiplex families affected by a complex genetic disorder, intracranial aneurysm. PloS one. 2015;10(3):e0121104. PubMed PMID: 25803036. *Pubmed Central* PMCID: 4372548.

[4] Sam C, Li FF, Liu SL. Inherited neurovascular diseases affecting cerebral blood vessels and smooth muscle. *Metabolic brain disease.* 2015 Apr 21. PubMed PMID: 25893882.

[5] Weir B. Unruptured intracranial aneurysms: a review. *Journal of neurosurgery.* 2002 Jan;96(1):3-42. PubMed PMID: 11794601.

[6] Wiebers DO, Whisnant JP, Huston J, 3rd, Meissner I, Brown RD, Jr., Piepgras DG, et al. Unruptured intracranial aneurysms: natural history, clinical outcome, and risks of surgical and endovascular treatment. *Lancet.* 2003 Jul 12;362(9378):103-10. PubMed PMID: 12867109.

[7] Suarez JI, Tarr RW, Selman WR. Aneurysmal subarachnoid hemorrhage. *The New England journal of medicine.* 2006 Jan 26;354(4):387-96. PubMed PMID: 16436770.

[8] Doenitz C, Schebesch KM, Zoephel R, Brawanski A. A mechanism for the rapid development of intracranial aneurysms: a case study. *Neurosurgery.* 2010 Nov;67(5):1213-21; discussion 21. PubMed PMID: 20948398.

[9] Hasan DM, Hindman BJ, Todd MM. Pressure Changes Within the Sac of Human Cerebral Aneurysms in Response to Artificially Induced Transient Increases in Systemic Blood Pressure. *Hypertension.* 2015 Aug;66(2):324-31. PubMed PMID: 26056344.

[10] Poelma C, Watton PN, Ventikos Y. Transitional flow in aneurysms and the computation of haemodynamic parameters. *Journal of the Royal Society, Interface / the Royal Society.* 2015 Apr 6;12(105). PubMed PMID: 25694540. Pubmed Central PMCID: 4387528.

[11] Bederson JB, Connolly ES, Jr., Batjer HH, Dacey RG, Dion JE, Diringer MN, et al. Guidelines for the management of aneurysmal subarachnoid hemorrhage: a statement for healthcare professionals from a special writing group of the Stroke Council, American Heart Association. *Stroke; a journal of cerebral circulation.* 2009 Mar; 40(3):994-1025. PubMed PMID: 19164800.

[12] Diringer MN. Management of aneurysmal subarachnoid hemorrhage. Critical care medicine. 2009 Feb;37(2):432-40. PubMed PMID: 19114880. Pubmed Central PMCID: 2820121.

[13] van Gijn J, Rinkel GJ. Subarachnoid haemorrhage: diagnosis, causes and management. *Brain: A journal of neurology.* 2001 Feb;124(Pt 2):249-78. PubMed PMID: 11157554.

[14] Greving JP, Wermer MJ, Brown RD, Jr., Morita A, Juvela S, Yonekura M, et al. Development of the PHASES score for prediction of risk of rupture of intracranial aneurysms: a pooled analysis of six prospective cohort studies. *The Lancet Neurology.* 2014 Jan;13(1):59-66. PubMed PMID: 24290159.

In: Spontaneous Subarachnoid Haemorrhage
Editors: Thomas Kapapa and Ralph König
ISBN: 978-1-63485-270-8

Chapter 6

SCALES

Petra Schödel and Karl-Michael Schebesch
Department of Neurosurgery,
University of Regensburg, Regensburg, Germany

ABSTRACT

There is a variety of scales that have been established specifically for grading Subarachnnoid Haemorrhage. Initial assessment of the level of consciousness is made by the Glasgow Coma Scale. The scales most commonly used for grading SAH are those by Hunt and Hess and the World Federation of Neurological Surgeons. Imaging-based classification systems are represented by the Fisher Rating Scale and Modified Fisher Rating Scale. Volume and distribution of the blood in the initial computed tomography are rated. To describe the outcome objectively, the Glasgow Outcome Score is often used.

The severity and the prognosis of subarachnoid haemorrhage are determined using a variety of scales that have been established specifically for grading SAH [1].

An initial preclinical assessment of the level of consciousness is made using the Glasgow Coma Scale (GCS, see Table 1) [2]. This scale was developed in 1974 by neurosurgeons Graham Teasdale and Bryan Jennett as a means of generally estimating the depth of unconsciousness, and has since become established in emergency medicine worldwide. Owing to its routine use, it is not only neurosurgeons that have become highly proficient in its application. The initially measured GCS score is integrated into other scores specific to SAH. Furthermore, by regularly measuring the GCS it is easy to detect a change in the level of consciousness, such as during the vasospastic phase.

The scales most commonly used for grading SAH are those by Hunt and Hess (HH, see Table 2) and the "World Federation of Neurological Surgeons" (WFNS, Table 3) [3, 4].

Table 1. Glasgow Coma Scale

Glasgow Coma Scale (GCS)		
Eye opening	Spontaneous	4
	In response to voice	3
	In response to painful stimulus	2
	No response	1
Verbal response	Oriented	5
	Confused	4
	Inappropriate words	3
	Incomprehensible sounds	2
	None	1
Motor response	Obeys commands	6
	Localised defence	5
	Withdrawal	4
	Flexion	3
	Extension	2
	None	1
Total (GCS score)		3-15

Table 2. Hunt and Hess Scale

Hunt and Hess grading		
Grade	*Consciousness*	*Clinical severity*
0	Awake	Asymptomatic, incidental
I	Awake	Asymptomatic, mild headache, discrete nuchal rigidity
Ia	Awake	Fixed neurological deficit with no further evidence of SAH
II	Awake	Severe headaches, nuchal rigidity, cranial nerve deficits, no further focal neurological deficit
III	Somnolent	Confusion, slight focal neurological deficit
IV	Soporific	Moderate to severe hemiparesis, onset of decerebrate rigidity, vegetative disorders
V	Deep coma	Signs of decerebrate rigidity

Table 3. World Federation of Neurological Surgeons Grading System (WFNS Scale)

World Federation of Neurological Surgeons Grading System		
Grade	*GCS*	*Motor deficit (hemiparesis, aphasia)*
I	15	No
II	13-14	No
III	13-14	Yes
IV	7-12	Yes/No
V	3-6	Yes/No

Hunt and Hess developed their classification system in 1968 based on 275 SAH patients, in whom they identified a correlation between the initial neurological condition and the severity of the disease course. The patients are stratified on the basis of their initial neurological symptoms, from asymptomatic, mild headache (HH I) to deep coma (HH V). Significant pre-existing conditions, as well as any vasospasm already detectable on an angiogram, will lead to the patient being placed in the next highest HH category. The higher the Hunt and Hess score, the greater the probability of death and a poor neurological outcome, therefore. The original publication describes an increase in the mortality rate from 11% at grade HH I to 100% at HH V. Modern, rapid diagnostic tests and critical care have vastly improved the prognosis of patients whose baseline neurological condition is poor. A recent publication reports a good outcome in 26% of SAH cases rated WFNS V (see below) compared to a mortality rate of 30% in the past [5]. The Hunt and Hess Scale was modified in 1974 with the addition of grades HH 0 (unruptured aneurysm) and HH Ia (no meningeal reaction, but fixed neurological deficit, e.g., oculomotor nerve palsy) [6].

Table 4. Fisher Rating Scale

Fisher grading	
Group	*Evidence of blood on CCT*
1	No evidence of blood
2	Diffuse distribution of blood or evidence of blood in the subarachnoid space, including interhemispheric fissure, insular cisterns or ambient cisterns less than 1 mm thick
3	Localised blood clot and/or evidence of blood in the subarachnoid space more than 1 mm thick
4	Intracerebral or intraventricular blood with diffuse or no SAH

To improve the objective assessment of the severity of SAH, the WFNS Scale was developed in 1988. Stratification is achieved by grading the level of consciousness of the patient based on the GCS, as well as any possible motor deficit.

Table 5. Modified Fisher Rating Scale

Modified Fisher					
Group	*No SAH*	*Focal or diffuse, thin SAH*	*Focal or diffuse, thick SAH*	*Intraventricular SAH*	
0	+	-	-	-	No subarachnoid or intraventricular blood
1	-	+	-	-	Thin, diffuse or focal SAH, no intraventricular blood
2	-	+	-	+	Thin, diffuse or focal SAH with intraventricular blood
3	-	-	+	-	Thick, diffuse or focal SAH, no intraventricular blood
4	-	-	+	+	Thick, diffuse or focal SAH with intraventricular blood

In addition to rating SAH severity clinically, there are also imaging-based classification systems. Grading in this case is mostly undertaken using the Fisher Rating Scale (Table 4) and Modified Fisher Rating Scale (Table 5) [7, 8]. The volume and distribution of the blood in the initial CCT can certainly act as predictors for the occurrence of clinically relevant vasospasm, and thus correlate with a poor neurological outcome. Assignment to Fisher 4 with intraparenchymal or intraventricular blood thus implies the highest risk of vasospasm.

Table 6. Glasgow Outcome Scale

Glasgow Outcome Score		
Grade		*Clinical description*
1	Death	Severe injury or death without recovering consciousness
2	Persistent vegetative status	Severe damage with prolonged state of unresponsiveness and a lack of higher mental functions
3	Severe disability	Severe injury with permanent need for help with activities of daily living
4	Moderate disability	No need for assistance in everyday life, employment is possible but may require special equipment
5	(Almost) complete recovery	Slight damage with minor neurological and psychological deficits

To describe the outcome objectively, the Glasgow Outcome Score (GOS, see Table 6) is often used in patients with SAH as well as in other patients with brain injuries [9]. The degree of disability in the patient that results from the effects of SAH are thus described, but the neurological deficits are not precisely differentiated. Moreover, the GOS only inadequately determines psychological disorders and cognitive impairment.

In addition to the SAH classification systems described above, there are others which in everyday practice are used only seldom or only on a regional level. Those of particular interest are the Claassen CT Rating Scale, which describes the distribution of the blood on CCT in greater detail than the Fisher Grade and likewise permits estimation of the risk of vasospasm, and the SAH grading system developed by Ogilvy and Carter in 1998. Patient age, HH grade, Fisher grade and aneurysm size are thereby included in these assessments. Both scales permit a slightly more exact risk estimation but are far more complicated to use and to analyse [10, 11].

References

[1] Rosen DS, Macdonald RL. Subarachnoid hemorrhage grading scales: a systematic review. *Neurocritical care.* 2005;2(2):110-8. PubMed PMID: 16159052.

[2] Teasdale G, Jennett B. Assessment of coma and impaired consciousness. A practical scale. *Lancet.* 1974 Jul 13;2(7872):81-4. PubMed PMID: 4136544.

[3] Hunt WE, Hess RM. Surgical risk as related to time of intervention in the repair of intracranial aneurysms. *J Neurosurg*. 1968 Jan;28(1):14-20. PubMed PMID: 5635959.

[4] Report of World Federation of Neurological Surgeons Committee on a Universal Subarachnoid Hemorrhage Grading Scale. *Journal of neurosurgery.* 1988 Jun;68(6): 985-6. PubMed PMID: 3131498.

[5] Wostrack M, Sandow N, Vajkoczy P, Schatlo B, Bijlenga P, Schaller K, et al. Subarachnoid haemorrhage WFNS grade V: is maximal treatment worthwhile? *Acta neurochirurgica*. 2013 Apr;155(4):579-86. PubMed PMID: 23397308.

[6] Hunt WE, Kosnik EJ. Timing and perioperative care in intracranial aneurysm surgery. *Clinical neurosurgery*. 1974;21:79-89. PubMed PMID: 4608645.

[7] Fisher CM, Kistler JP, Davis JM. Relation of cerebral vasospasm to subarachnoid hemorrhage visualized by computerized tomographic scanning. *Neurosurgery*. 1980 Jan;6(1):1-9. PubMed PMID: 7354892.

[8] Frontera JA, Claassen J, Schmidt JM, Wartenberg KE, Temes R, Connolly ES, Jr., et al. Prediction of symptomatic vasospasm after subarachnoid hemorrhage: the modified fisher scale. *Neurosurgery*. 2006 Jul;59(1):21-7; discussion -7. PubMed PMID: 16823296.

[9] Jennett B, Bond M. Assessment of outcome after severe brain damage. *Lancet*. 1975 Mar 1;1(7905):480-4. PubMed PMID: 46957.

[10] Claassen J, Vu A, Kreiter KT, Kowalski RG, Du EY, Ostapkovich N, et al. Effect of acute physiologic derangements on outcome after subarachnoid hemorrhage. *Critical care medicine*. 2004 Mar;32(3):832-8. PubMed PMID: 15090970.

[11] Ogilvy CS, Carter BS. A proposed comprehensive grading system to predict outcome for surgical management of intracranial aneurysms. *Neurosurgery*. 1998 May;42(5):959 -68; discussion 68-70. PubMed PMID: 9588539.

In: Spontaneous Subarachnoid Haemorrhage
Editors: Thomas Kapapa and Ralph König
ISBN: 978-1-63485-270-8

Chapter 7

SYMPTOMS, EXTRACRANIAL MANIFESTATIONS

Petra Schödel and Karl-Michael Schebesch
Department of Neurosurgery,
University of Regensburg, Regensburg, Germany

ABSTRACT

The sudden development of intense headache (thunderclap headache) is usually the first symptom of aneurysmal subarachnoid haemorrhage: "worst headache of my life." The headaches are often accompanied by clouding of consciousness and even coma. Loss of consciousness can be just temporary following Subarachnoid Haemorrahge, but can also result in persistent coma and even death. Nuchal rigidity is one of the key symptoms. Localised pressure resulting from a ruptured aneurysm as well as an innocent aneurysm can lead to cranial nerve deficits. Depending on its location and extent of an intracerebral haemorrhage it can lead to focal neurological deficits such as hemiparesis or aphasia, as well as epileptic seizures. However, there are a certain number of more rare extracranial symptoms.

The sudden development of intense headache (thunderclap headache) is usually the first symptom of aneurysmal subarachnoid haemorrhage [1]. This type of headache will even be described by migraine patients as the "worst headache of my life" or the "feeling that my skull is being split in two by an axe." Retrospectively, approximately 30%-40% of patients report headaches of increased intensity in the preceding weeks which are interpreted as being related to mild SAH ("warning bleed") or a growing aneurysm [2, 3]. In addition to a thunderclap headache, severe nuchalgia and occasionally back pain along the entire length of the spine can also develop.

The headaches are often accompanied by clouding of consciousness and even coma. They can be caused by increased intracranial pressure, acute hydrocephalus, direct parenchymal brain damage from intracerebral bleeding or ischaemia associated with SAH, or even seizures. This loss of consciousness can be just temporary following SAH, but can also result in persistent coma and even death. Secondary clouding of consciousness over the course of the disease can be an expression of secondary haemorrhage, or also increased intracranial pressure with CSF stasis.

Clinical examination of the patient will usually reveal marked nuchal rigidity not long after SAH. Meningeal irritation is indicated by the patient's avoidance of light and sensitivity to noise. Nausea and vomiting can also occur. The Lasègue, Kernig and Brudzinski signs may be positive.

Given the close proximity of the cranial nerves and arteries of the circle of Willis, localised pressure resulting from a ruptured aneurysm as well as an innocent aneurysm can lead to cranial nerve deficits. There have been reports in particular of oculomotor nerve palsy from aneurysms in the left and right posterior communicating artery, abducens nerve palsy from aneurysms in the cavernous sinus, or scotomas from large aneurysms in the internal carotid artery or anterior communicating artery.

A ruptured aneurysm causes intracerebral bleeding, which depending on its location and extent can lead to focal neurological deficits such as hemiparesis or aphasia, as well as epileptic seizures.

Ocular bleeding, especially into the vitreous body, is likely to occur as a result of stasis in the intraocular veins which arises due to an increase in intracranial pressure during and after the aneurysm has ruptured. This condition, known as Terson syndrome, is found in approx. 10%-20% of all SAH patients and is associated with a higher rate of mortality. If visual disorders develop due to Terson syndrome, vitrectomy may be necessary over the course [4, 5].

In addition to all these symptoms, which result from changes in the brain and dura precipitated by the aneurysm and SAH, there are a certain number of more rare extracranial symptoms.

Cardiac problems of any nature are a secondary symptom of SAH and occur in approx. 14% of patients. From basic ECG changes to tachyarrhythmias and bradyarrhythmias, and even elevated troponin and heart attacks - anything is possible [6]. A rare cardiac complication is Takotsubo-like cardiomyopathy, which probably develops due to increased catecholamine release during the acute phase of SAH [7]. This left-ventricular dyskinesia abates as a rule after a few weeks. Neurogenic pulmonary oedema can develop from SAH-induced cardiac dysfunction, but also from treatment-related hypervolaemia. Furthermore, hyperglycaemia and marked electrolyte disorders, such as hyponatraemia and hypokalaemia, can result from SAH [8].

References

[1] van Gijn J, Rinkel GJ. Subarachnoid haemorrhage: diagnosis, causes and management. *Brain : a journal of neurology*. 2001 Feb;124(Pt 2):249-78. PubMed PMID: 11157554.

[2] Verweij RD, Wijdicks EF, van Gijn J. Warning headache in aneurysmal subarachnoid hemorrhage. A case-control study. *Archives of neurology*. 1988 Sep;45(9):1019-20. PubMed PMID: 3274041.

[3] Juvela S. Minor leak before rupture of an intracranial aneurysm and subarachnoid hemorrhage of unknown etiology. *Neurosurgery*. 1992 Jan;30(1):7-11. PubMed PMID: 1738458.

[4] Stiebel-Kalish H, Turtel LS, Kupersmith MJ. The natural history of nontraumatic subarachnoid hemorrhage-related intraocular hemorrhages. *Retina*. 2004 Feb;24(1):36-40. PubMed PMID: 15076942.

[5] Wietholter S, Steube D, Stotz HP. [Terson syndrome: a frequently missed ophthalmologic complication in subarachnoid hemorrhage]. *Zentralblatt fur Neurochirurgie*. 1998;59(3):166-70. PubMed PMID: 9816667. Terson-Syndrom: Haufig ubersehene ophthalmologische Komplikation bei Subarachnoidalblutung.

[6] Ahmadian A, Mizzi A, Banasiak M, Downes K, Camporesi EM, Thompson Sullebarger J, et al. Cardiac manifestations of subarachnoid hemorrhage. Heart, lung and vessels. 2013;5(3):168-78. PubMed PMID: 24364008. *Pubmed Central* PMCID: 3848675.

[7] Inamasu J, Nakatsukasa M, Mayanagi K, Miyatake S, Sugimoto K, Hayashi T, et al. Subarachnoid hemorrhage complicated with neurogenic pulmonary edema and takotsubo-like cardiomyopathy. *Neurologia medico-chirurgica*. 2012;52(2):49-55. PubMed PMID: 22362283.

[8] Chen S, Li Q, Wu H, Krafft PR, Wang Z, Zhang JH. The harmful effects of subarachnoid hemorrhage on extracerebral organs. *BioMed research international*. 2014;2014:858496. PubMed PMID: 25110700. Pubmed Central PMCID: 4109109.

In: Spontaneous Subarachnoid Haemorrhage
Editors: Thomas Kapapa and Ralph König
ISBN: 978-1-63485-270-8

Chapter 8

Admission, Diagnostic Imaging, Acute Hydrocephalus

Thomas Schmidt
Department of Neurosurgery, Evangelic Hospital Oldenburg,
Medical Campus University of Oldenburg, Germany

Abstract

A patient with subarachnoid haemorrhage can be at extremely high risk on the clinical spectrum or appear to be almost asymptomatic on admission. Medical management must be able to quickly adapt to this clinical scenario and the rapid progression of the condition that under certain circumstances can occur. Therefore, the neurological and radiological scales for evaluating patients with subarachnoid haemorrhage should be used routinely. The life-threatening complications that accompany subarachnoid haemorrhage must be immediately identified, corrected, and avoided with a view to rebleeding from the ruptured haemorrhage. Modern methods of computed tomography permit diagnosis of subarachnoid haemorrhage in the first few hours after onset of the symptoms in particular. A non-aneurysmal cause for spontaneous subarachnoid haemorrhage is found in only 15% of cases.

Keywords: grading scales, diagnostic imaging, aneurysm rerupture, acute hydrocephalus, epileptic seizures

Initial Neurocritical Care – Medical Evaluation

Patients with suspected or proven subarachnoid haemorrhage admitted to a neurovascular unit should immediately undergo targeted neurological evaluation to determine the scope and urgency of further diagnostic and therapeutic efforts. Initial management involves primary clinical stabilisation of the patient, ascertainment of the correct diagnosis, definitive treatment of the aneurysm and avoidance of complications. If patients have survived the first few hours of subarachnoid haemorrhage, they are subsequently at risk of three major neurological complications: rebleeding of the ruptured aneurysm, acute hydrocephalus, and delayed cerebral ischaemia.

Once the patient has been admitted, attention should first be given to his/her level of consciousness and any neurological deficits. At this point about half of the patients are already comatose. [1, 2] The loss of consciousness at onset of the symptoms is also a strong indication of a ruptured aneurysm and does not typically occur in perimesencephalic subarachnoid haemorrhage. [3] These patients are at risk of respiratory failure. Intubation and mechanical ventilation should ensure adequate oxygenation, maintain the pH in the normal range and prevent hypercapnia.

Alert patients usually describe the headaches as the worst they have ever had in their lives, focussing in particular on their extremely sudden onset. A preceding "sentinel" headache is reported by 10% to 43% of patients. [4] The headaches are mostly associated with one or more concomitant symptoms including nausea and vomiting, meningism, temporary loss of consciousness, cranial nerve disorders and neurological deficits.

Grading Scales

The initial clinical severity of subarachnoid haemorrhage is in itself a significant predictor for the outcome of the condition. [5] The severity should therefore be clinically determined as soon as possible using the Glasgow Coma Scale [6], the Hunt and Hess Scale [7], and the WFNS Scale [8]. Whereas the GCS is used to judge the clinical level of consciousness regardless of the underlying cause, the HH and WFNS scales were developed specifically for clinically stratifying SAH (Following Chapter). Use of these scales provides a clear clinical determination of the patients condition, whilst the parameters of the HH Scale are influenced heavily by the examiner's subjective opinion.

The Fischer Scale [9] was developed as a means of assessing the risk of vasopasm and cerebral ischaemia from baseline CCT. The subsequently adapted and less subjective Modified Fisher Scale [10] evaluates the volume of cisternal and intraventricular blood more specifically as part of its risk assessment (following Chapter).

Epileptic Seizures and SAH

Epileptic seizures occur in approx. 8% of patients after subarachnoid haemorrhage, 90% of which are observed within the first 24 hours. [11-13] Epileptic seizures occur at a later stagme in 3% to 7% of patients. [14, 15] In retrospective studies, intracerebral haematoma, rebleeding, a ruptured aneurysm of the middle cerebral artery, the thickness of the subarachnoid blood clot, an unfavourable neurological status and cerebral infarction have been identified as risk factors for the occurrence of epileptic seizures in the early phase of subarachnoid haemorrhage. [14-18] The significance in terms of the impact on the prognosis of a patient with epileptic seizures in the early phase of subarachnoid haemorrhage is not clear. In some studies, epileptic seizures were not found to influence the outcome. [13, 15, 19] A correlation to a poor clinical outcome was established in a retrospective study, however. [20] Although prophylactic anticonvulsant medication after subarachnoid haemorrhage has not as yet been found to produce a favourable therapeutic outcome, prophylactic antiepileptic treatment is used widely for preventing the risk of rebleeding from an untreated ruptured aneurysm during an epileptic seizure. This concept is furiously debated, meaning that a general recommendation for prophylactic anticonvulsant treatment cannot be pronounced [21].

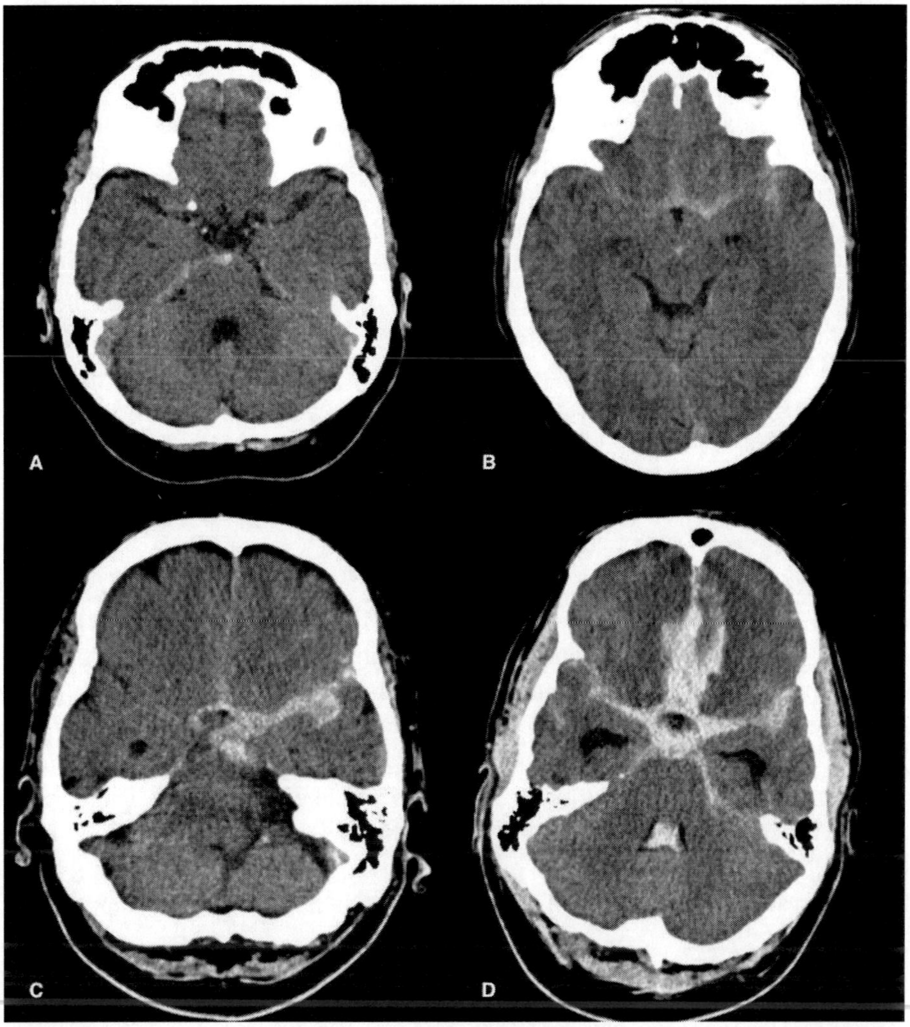

Figure 1. According to the modified Fisher scale the CT-Scans of four different patients with subarachnoid hemorrhage (A-D) demonstrate an increasing clot burden at the basal cisterns. A: Grade I hemorrhage with minimal blood at the interpeduncular cistern. B: Also grade I haemorrhage, but significant more CSF-spaces are filled with blood. C: Subarachnoid haemorrhage grade IV with substantial blood in the sylvian fissure on the left. D: CT also reveals intraventricular blood and intraparenchymal hematoma corresponding grade V.

DIAGNOSTIC IMAGING

Once the patient with subarachnoid haemorrhage has received primary clinical care, appropriate diagnostic imaging should be arranged without further delay to detect the actual cause of the given symptoms. In doing so, it is important not only to establish the diagnosis of subarachnoid haemorrhage in itself, but also to detect a life-threatening situation that could potentially exist due to space-occupying subdural or intracerebral haematoma, decompensated hydrocephalus or severe cerebral swelling.

Computed Tomography

Non-contrast computed tomography is the first examination when SAH is clinically suspected and is at the same time the diagnostic imaging method of choice. Hyperdense blood in the basal cisterns and fissures is a characteristic feature of SAH on cranial CT (CCT). However, the haemorrhage is not necessarily confined to the subarachnoid space, but can also involve the ventricles, subdural space and brain parenchyma, consistent with intracerebral haemorrhage (Figure 1). The sensitivity is affected by the volume of blood, the time since symptom onset, the scanner properties and the experience of the examining radiologist. CT produces false negative results in approx. 2.5% – 7% of aneurysmal SAHs. On the day the haemorrhage occurs, extravasal blood can be detected in more than 95% of patients. [22, 23] As blood can be flushed out of the cerebrospinal cavities relatively quickly, the sensitivity of cranial CT drops to 50% on the seventh day following the haemorrhage [24].

Lumbar Puncture

In a small group of patients with negative cranial CT and transient sudden headache, metabolites of haemoglobin can be identified within the first 12 hours by lumbar puncture and intracranial aneurysm, in fact, in a subsequent angiography. Therefore, a lumbar puncture is certainly indicated in patients with a clinical event and negative cranial CT, even when the cerebrospinal fluid findings are normal in a majority of the examinations. The puncture itself should be performed with great care and ensue within a suitable time frame, no earlier than six hours after the onset of symptoms. This seems to be easier than it is in reality in order to obtain reliable results. The traditional three-glass test is not considered appropriate in this regard [25].

Computed Tomographic Angiography (CTA)

CT angiography has now become more valuable in the first-line work-up of spontaneous SAH than catheter angiography. On the one hand, the sensitivity of CTA in detecting an intracranial aneurysm is the same as that of catheter angiography. [26, 27] In addition, CTA has other apparent advantages that have contributed to this development. These include its less invasive nature compared to DSA, lower costs, reduced time and effort, as well as the simultaneous ability to depict the bony structures at the base of the skull. However, despite the modern scanner technology, the negative predictive value is only 82% to 96% [28, 29], meaning that CTA cannot completely replace DSA even today. It is with aneurysms of less than 3 mm in size that the diagnostic confidence is reduced [30-32].

DSA and Three-Dimensional Rotational Angiography

Angiography of the cerebral arteries is not only intended to detect one or more aneurysms as the underlying cause of spontaneous SAH, but also provides further essential information about the exact configuration of the aneurysm and its adjacent angioarchitecture, which is needed in order to decide on the appropriate treatment option of surgical clipping and endovascular coiling. Even when a cerebral aneurysm was not detected in non-invasive diagnostic testing, DSA led to a change in treatment strategy in 19% to 30% of patients [33].

Angiography is invasive, however. The risk of transient or permanent neurological complications during an angiogram of the cerebral vessels after subarachnoid haemorrhage is 1.8%, [34] and that of intraprocedural rebleeding from the ruptured aneurysm 1%-2% [35, 36].

In approx. 15% of spontaneous subarachnoid haemorrhage cases, primary diagnostic testing including conventional angiography does not detect an aneurysm of the cerebral arteries. Repetition of conventional angiography after 10 to 14 days is mandatory in such a case, since in a substantial number of patients a missed aneurysm can be subsequently detected [37].

MRI

Because of the high diagnostic significance of computed tomography in the acute phase of subarachnoid haemorrhage, the shorter examination times and the simple workflow required for the intensive care patient, the number of MRI studies in the initial diagnostic testing of subarachnoid haemorrhage is very low. Fresh subarachnoid bleeding within the first 12 hours after symptom onset can be detected in FLAIR sequences. [38-40] MRI reaches a sensitivity comparable to that of CT [38, 40].

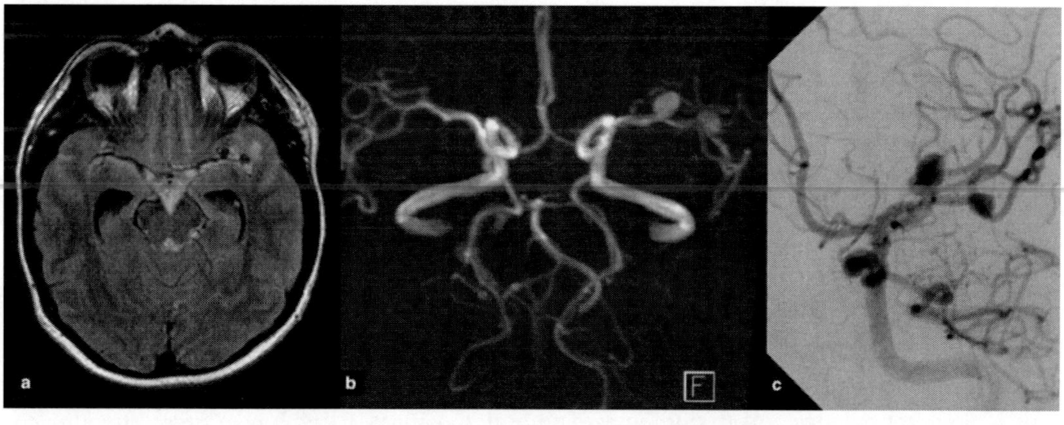

Figure 2. MRI of a 36-year-old women in the 22th week of pregnancy suffering by acute onset of severe headache and vomiting. In a fresh T2-hyperintensive subarachnoid haemorrhage in the basal cistern can be detected in FLAIR sequences. 3D-MIP reconstructed TOF-MRA (b) shows two saccular aneurysms at the M1- and M2-segment of middle cerebral artery on the left. Diagnosis was confirmed on DSA and aneurysm were successfully occluded by endovascular coiling subsequently.

Table 1. Non-aneurysmatic causes of spontaneous SAH

Cerebrovascular lesions
- Arterial dissection - Arteriovenous malformation (BAVM) - Dural arteriovenous fistula - Intracerebral cavernoma - Sinus vein thrombosis - Cerebral amyloid angiopathy - Moyamoya
Inflammatory vascular lesions
- Wegener's granulomatosis - Polyarteritis nodosa - Churg-Strauss syndrome - Behçet's disease - Other types of vasculitis - Mycotic aneurysms
Spinal vascular lesions
- Saccular aneurysm of the anterior spinal artery - Arteriovenous malformation (SAVM) - Dural arteriovenous fistula - Spinal cavernoma
Medicines
- Cocaine consumption - Overdose of anticoagulants
Other causes
- Sickle cell disease - Coagulopathies - Pituitary apoplexy - Meningeal carcinomatosis - Intracranial tumours

Due to the loss of hyperdensity of blood and signal intensity in CT in the days following SAH, the diagnostic significance of MRI in the detection of subarachnoid blood with FLAIR and T2* sequences increases and becomes better than with CT [41].

In avoiding exposure to radiation, MRI is thus a suitable alternative to CT in patients who during pregnancy experience subarachnoid haemorrhage. (Figure 2) In addition, a supplementary cranial and cervical MRI scan is necessary if in the initial diagnostic testing of spontaneous subarachnoid haemorrhage, including catheter angiography, no source of haemorrhage was detectable and other causes have to be ruled out. (Table 1) In approx. 14% of this patient population, other findings are compiled using MRI which substantially alter the further treatment plan in approx. 6% of patients [42].

PREVENTION OF REBLEEDING

Rebleeding from a ruptured aneurysm after subarachnoid haemorrhage is linked with a mortality of up to 74% [43, 44] and with a significantly poorer functional outcome in surviving patients. A significant factor in the acute phase of the illness is that the risk of rebleeding is at its highest in the first 12 hours and occurs within the first 24 hours 13.6% to 48.6% of cases. [1, 45-48] In fact, about one third of recurrent haemorrhages occur within the first three hours and about one half within the first six hours. Rebleeding during this early time window also appears to have a more negative impact on the clinical outcome than rebleeding at a later stage. [48] After the first day, the further risk of rebleeding is evenly distributed and is about 2% per day, 40% after one month, [1] and 50% after six months [49].

Numerous factors have an influence on the risk of rebleeding. Poor neurological status on admission, [45, 50] initial loss of consciousness, the size of the aneurysm, [50-52] and hypertension above 160 mm Hg [45, 52] as well as a lengthy period until definitive aneurysm treatment increase the risk of rebleeding. Early treatment of the aneurysm can reduce the risk of rebleeding [53, 54].

Antifibrinolytic treatment with tranexamic acid or epsilon-aminocaproic acid has proven effective in protecting against rebleeding after an aneurysm has ruptured. [55-57] However, because of the increased risk of secondary vasospasm and cerebral ischaemia, the overall clinical outcome is not positively affected, [58, 59] meaning that this treatment has not found a place in clinical practice. Nevertheless, it may be feasible under certain circumstances [60].

ACUTE HYDROCEPHALUS

The occurrence of acute hydrocephalus as a result of subarachnoid haemorrhage is a frequent complication and in an initially awake patient typically causes subsequent gradual deterioration in the level of consciousness. Figures related to frequency vary between 15% and 87%. [60-62] An initial enlargement of the ventricles, especially the temporal horns, is frequently attempted but regresses within the first two days. In fact, in about 50% of patients with acute hydrocephalus the clinical symptoms regressed spontaneously in the first 24 hours without any specific intervention. [63] (Figure 3) Acute hydrocephalus is to be seen as an independent risk factor for a poor clinical outcome [64, 65].

Pathophysiologically, there are two mechanisms behind the development of acute hydrocephalus. Firstly, the circulation of cerebrospinal fluid is displaced into the ventricles and basal cisterns by intraventricular or subarachnoid blood, [66] and secondly, reabsorption of the cerebrospinal fluid at the level of the arachnoid granulations is decreased. In contrast, the later chronic hydrocephalus is the result of secondary, reactive fibrosis and adhesion of the leptomeninges, which restrict the CSF circulation. [67-70] The hypothesis that subarachnoid haemorrhage increases the production of cerebrospinal fluid is furiously debated in the literature and to date has not been proven with any certainty [71-74].

Risk factors for acute hydrocephalus from subarachnoid haemorrhage are intraventricular bleeding, a substantial volume of blood in the subarachnoid space, increasing loss of consciousness, increased patient age, and an aneurysm located in the posterior circulation [75, 76].

Proven and symptomatic hydrocephalus is treated with an external ventricular drain and more rarely in clinical practice with lumbar drainage or a series of lumbar punctures. After an external ventricular drain has been inserted, an improvement in the patient's neurological condition is generally seen due to the reduction in intracranial pressure. [77-79] A recently published prospective cohort study came to the conclusion that use of an external drain must be regarded as an independent risk factor for rebleeding. [80] In this context, preliminary retrospective studies also identified an increased risk of rebleeding. [79, 81] However, there are also studies that did not report an increased risk of rebleeding after placement of an external drain for treatment of hydrocephalus following subarachnoid haemorrhage [82, 83].

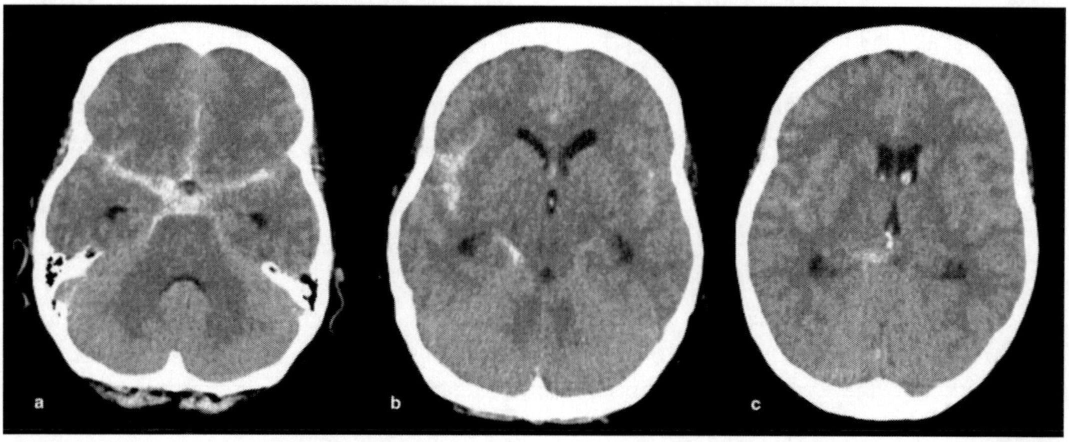

Figure 3. CT (a-c) demonstrates acute hydrocephalus of a 42-year-old individual following subarchnoid hemorrhage. However the were no significant clinical symptoms related to hydrocephalus and initial enlargement of the ventricles regresses within the first two days without any specific intervention.

References

[1] Brilstra EH, Rinkel GJ, Algra A, van Gijn J. Rebleeding, secondary ischemia, and timing of operation in patients with subarachnoid hemorrhage. *Neurology*. 2000 Dec 12;55 (11):1656–60.

[2] Fontanarosa PB. Recognition of subarachnoid hemorrhage. *Ann Emerg Med.* 1989 Nov;18 (11):1199–205.

[3] Dupont SA, Lanzino G, Wijdicks EFM, Rabinstein AA. The use of clinical and routine imaging data to differentiate between aneurysmal and nonaneurysmal subarachnoid hemorrhage prior to angiography. Clinical article. *J Neurosurg. American Association of Neurological Surgeons*; 2010 Oct;113 (4):790–4.

[4] Polmear A. Sentinel headaches in aneurysmal subarachnoid haemorrhage: what is the true incidence? A systematic review. *Cephalalgia.* 2003 Dec;23 (10):935–41.

[5] Rosen DS, Macdonald RL. Subarachnoid hemorrhage grading scales: a systematic review. *Neurocrit Care*. 2005;2 (2):110–8.

[6] Teasdale G, Jennett B. Assessment of coma and impaired consciousness. A practical scale. *Lancet.* 1974 Jul 13;2 (7872):81–4.

[7] Hunt WE, Hess RM. Surgical risk as related to time of intervention in the repair of intracranial aneurysms. *J Neurosurg. Journal of Neurosurgery Publishing Group;* 1968 Jan;28 (1):14–20.

[8] Report of World Federation of Neurological Surgeons Committee on a Universal Subarachnoid Hemorrhage Grading Scale. *J Neurosurg*. 1988 Jun;68 (6):985–6.

[9] Fisher CM, Kistler JP, Davis JM. Relation of cerebral vasospasm to subarachnoid hemorrhage visualized by computerized tomographic scanning. *Neurosurgery.* 1980 Jan;6 (1):1–9.

[10] Frontera JA, Claassen J, Schmidt JM, Wartenberg KE, Temes R, Connolly ES, et al. Prediction of symptomatic vasospasm after subarachnoid hemorrhage: the modified fisher scale. *Neurosurgery*. 2006 Jul;59 (1):21–7–discussion21–7.

[11] Hasan D, Schonck RS, Avezaat CJ, Tanghe HL, van Gijn J, van der Lugt PJ. Epileptic seizures after subarachnoid hemorrhage. Ann Neurol. Wiley Subscription Services, Inc., A Wiley Company; 1993 Mar;33 (3):286–91.

[12] Baker CJ, Prestigiacomo CJ, Solomon RA. Short-term perioperative anticonvulsant prophylaxis for the surgical treatment of low-risk patients with intracranial aneurysms. *Neurosurgery*. 1995 Nov;37 (5):863–70–discussion870–1.

[13] Rhoney DH, Tipps LB, Murry KR, Basham MC, Michael DB, Coplin WM. Anticonvulsant prophylaxis and timing of seizures after aneurysmal subarachnoid hemorrhage. *Neurology*. 2000 Jul 25;55 (2):258–65.

[14] Lin C-L, Dumont AS, Lieu A-S, Yen C-P, Hwang S-L, Kwan A-L, et al. Characterization of perioperative seizures and epilepsy following aneurysmal subarachnoid hemorrhage. *J Neurosurg. Journal of Neurosurgery Publishing Group*; 2003 Dec;99 (6):978–85.

[15] Choi K-S, Chun H-J, Yi H-J, Ko Y, Kim Y-S, Kim J-M. Seizures and Epilepsy following Aneurysmal Subarachnoid Hemorrhage : Incidence and Risk Factors. *J Korean Neurosurg Soc*. 2009 Aug;46 (2):93–8.

[16] Kvam DA, Loftus CM, Copeland B, Quest DO. Seizures during the immediate postoperative period. *Neurosurgery*. 1983 Jan;12 (1):14–7.

[17] Ukkola V, Heikkinen ER. Epilepsy after operative treatment of ruptured cerebral aneurysms. *Acta neurochirurgica*. 1990;106 (3-4):115–8.

[18] Huttunen J, Kurki MI, Und Zu Fraunberg von M, Koivisto T, Ronkainen A, Rinne J, et al. Epilepsy after aneurysmal subarachnoid hemorrhage: A population-based, long-term follow-up study. *Neurology*. Lippincott Williams and Wilkins; 2015 Jun 2;84 (22):2229–37.

[19] Fung C, Balmer M, Murek M, Z'Graggen WJ, Abu-Isa J, Ozdoba C, et al. Impact of early-onset seizures on grading and outcome in patients with subarachnoid hemorrhage. *J Neurosurg. American Association of Neurological Surgeons*; 2015 Feb;122 (2):408–13.

[20] Butzkueven H, Evans AH, Pitman A, Leopold C, Jolley DJ, Kaye AH, et al. Onset seizures independently predict poor outcome after subarachnoid hemorrhage. *Neurology*. 2000 Nov 14;55 (9):1315–20.

[21] Lanzino G, D'Urso PI, Suarez J, Participants in the International Multi-Disciplinary Consensus Conference on the Critical Care Management of Subarachnoid Hemorrhage. Seizures and anticonvulsants after aneurysmal subarachnoid hemorrhage. *Neurocrit Care*. 2011 Sep;15 (2):247–56.

[22] Boesiger BM, Shiber JR. Subarachnoid hemorrhage diagnosis by computed tomography and lumbar puncture: are fifth generation CT scanners better at identifying subarachnoid hemorrhage? *J Emerg Med.* Elsevier; 2005 Jul;29 (1):23–7.

[23] van der Wee N, Rinkel GJ, Hasan D, van Gijn J. Detection of subarachnoid haemorrhage on early CT: is lumbar puncture still needed after a negative scan? *J Neurol Neurosurg Psychiatr.* BMJ Group; 1995 Mar;58 (3):357–9.

[24] Edlow JA, Caplan LR. Avoiding pitfalls in the diagnosis of subarachnoid hemorrhage. *N Engl J Med.* 2000 Jan 6;342 (1):29–36.

[25] Buruma OJ, Janson HL, Bergh Den FA, Bots GT. Blood-stained cerebrospinal fluid: traumatic puncture or haemorrhage? J Neurol Neurosurg Psychiatr. *BMJ Group*; 1981 Feb;44 (2):144–7.

[26] Jayaraman MV, Mayo-Smith WW, Tung GA, Haas RA, Rogg JM, Mehta NR, et al. Detection of intracranial aneurysms: multi-detector row CT angiography compared with DSA. Radiology. *Radiological Society of North America*; 2004 Feb;230 (2):510–8.

[27] Villablanca JP, Jahan R, Hooshi P, Lim S, Duckwiler G, Patel A, et al. Detection and characterization of very small cerebral aneurysms by using 2D and 3D helical CT angiography. *AJNR Am J Neuroradiol.* 2002 Aug;23 (7):1187–98.

[28] Papke K, Kuhl CK, Fruth M, Haupt C, Schlunz-Hendann M, Sauner D, et al. Intracranial aneurysms: role of multidetector CT angiography in diagnosis and endovascular therapy planning. *Radiology. Radiological Society of North America;* 2007 Aug;244 (2):532–40.

[29] Li Q, Lv F, Li Y, Luo T, Li K, Xie P. Evaluation of 64-section CT angiography for detection and treatment planning of intracranial aneurysms by using DSA and surgical findings. *Radiology. Radiological Society of North America*, Inc; 2009 Sep;252 (3):808–15.

[30] McKinney AM, Palmer CS, Truwit CL, Karagulle A, Teksam M. Detection of aneurysms by 64-section multidetector CT angiography in patients acutely suspected of having an intracranial aneurysm and comparison with digital subtraction and 3D rotational angiography. *American Journal of Neuroradiology. American Society of Neuroradiology*; 2008 Mar;29 (3):594–602.

[31] Donmez H, Serifov E, Kahriman G, Mavili E, Durak AC, Menkü A. Comparison of 16-row multislice CT angiography with conventional angiography for detection and evaluation of intracranial aneurysms. Eur *J Radiol.* Elsevier; 2011 Nov;80 (2):455–61.

[32] Bechan RS, van Rooij SB, Sprengers ME, Peluso JP, Sluzewski M, Majoie CB, et al. CT angiography versus 3D rotational angiography in patients with subarachnoid hemorrhage. Neuroradiology. Springer Berlin Heidelberg; 2015 Sep 4;:1–8.

[33] Tomycz L, Bansal NK, Hawley CR, Goddard TL, Ayad MJ, Mericle RA. "Real-world" comparison of non-invasive imaging to conventional catheter angiography in the diagnosis of cerebral aneurysms. *Surg Neurol Int.* 2011;2 (1):134.

[34] Cloft HJ, Joseph GJ, Dion JE. Risk of cerebral angiography in patients with subarachnoid hemorrhage, cerebral aneurysm, and arteriovenous malformation: a meta-analysis. *Stroke.* 1999 Feb 1;30 (2):317–20.

[35] Saitoh H, Hayakawa K, Nishimura K, Okuno Y, Teraura T, Yumitori K, et al. Rerupture of cerebral aneurysms during angiography. *AJNR Am J Neuroradiol.* 1995 Mar;16 (3):539–42.

[36] Koenig GH, Marshall WH, Poole GJ, Kramer RA. Rupture of intracranial aneurysms during cerebral angiography: report of ten cases and review of the literautre. *Neurosurgery.* 1979 Sep;5 (3):314–24.

[37] Suarez JI, Tarr RW, Selman WR. Aneurysmal subarachnoid hemorrhage. *N Engl J Med.* 2006 Jan 26;354 (4):387–96.

[38] Noguchi K, Ogawa T, Seto H, Inugami A, Hadeishi H, Fujita H, et al. Subacute and chronic subarachnoid hemorrhage: diagnosis with fluid-attenuated inversion-recovery MR imaging. *Radiology.* 1997 Apr;203 (1):257–62.

[39] Küker W, Thiex R, Block F. Hyperacute perimesencephalic subarachnoid hemorrhage: demonstration of blood extravasation with MRI. *J Comput Assist Tomogr.* 1999 Jul;23 (4):521–3.

[40] Wiesmann M, Mayer TE, Yousry I, Medele R, Hamann GF, Brückmann H. Detection of hyperacute subarachnoid hemorrhage of the brain by using magnetic resonance imaging. *J Neurosurg. Journal of Neurosurgery Publishing Group*; 2002 Apr;96 (4):684–9.

[41] Mitchell P, Wilkinson ID, Hoggard N, Paley MN, Jellinek DA, Powell T, et al. Detection of subarachnoid haemorrhage with magnetic resonance imaging. *J Neurol Neurosurg Psychiatr.* BMJ Group; 2001 Feb;70 (2):205–11.

[42] Rogg JM, Smeaton S, Doberstein C, Goldstein JH, Tung GA, Haas RA. Assessment of the value of MR imaging for examining patients with angiographically negative subarachnoid hemorrhage. AJR American journal of roentgenology. *American Public Health Association*; 1999 Jan;172 (1):201–6.

[43] Juvela S. Rebleeding from ruptured intracranial aneurysms. *Surgical Neurology.* 1989 Nov;32 (5):323–6.

[44] Hijdra A, Vermeulen M, van Gijn J, van Crevel H. Rerupture of intracranial aneurysms: a clinicoanatomic study. *J Neurosurg.* 1987 Jul;67 (1):29–33.

[45] Ohkuma H, Tsurutani H, Suzuki S. Incidence and significance of early aneurysmal rebleeding before neurosurgical or neurological management. *Stroke.* 2001 May;32 (5):1176–80.

[46] Fujii Y, Takeuchi S, Sasaki O, Minakawa T, Koike T, Tanaka R. Ultra-early rebleeding in spontaneous subarachnoid hemorrhage. *J Neurosurg. Journal of Neurosurgery Publishing Group*; 1996 Jan;84 (1):35–42.

[47] Inagawa T, Kamiya K, Ogasawara H, Yano T. Rebleeding of ruptured intracranial aneurysms in the acute stage. *Surgical Neurology.* 1987 Aug;28 (2):93–9.

[48] Tanno Y, Homma M, Oinuma M, Kodama N, Ymamoto T. Rebleeding from ruptured intracranial aneurysms in North Eastern Province of Japan. A cooperative study. *J Neurol Sci.* Elsevier; 2007 Jul 15;258 (1-2):11–6.

[49] Jane JA, Kassell NF, Torner JC, Winn HR. The natural history of aneurysms and arteriovenous malformations. *J Neurosurg. Journal of Neurosurgery Publishing Group*; 1985 Mar;62 (3):321–3.

[50] Naidech AM, Janjua N, Kreiter KT, Ostapkovich ND, Fitzsimmons B-F, Parra A, et al. Predictors and impact of aneurysm rebleeding after subarachnoid hemorrhage. *Arch Neurol. American Medical Association;* 2005 Mar;62 (3):410–6.

[51] Boogaarts HD, van Lieshout JH, van Amerongen MJ, de Vries J, Verbeek ALM, Grotenhuis JA, et al. Aneurysm diameter as a risk factor for pretreatment rebleeding: a meta-analysis. *J Neurosurg.* 2015 Apr;122 (4):921–8.

[52] Guo L-M, Zhou H-Y, Xu J-W, Wang Y, Qiu Y-M, Jiang J-Y. Risk Factors Related to Aneurysmal Rebleeding. *World Neurosurgery*. 2011 Sep;76 (3-4):292–8.

[53] Kassell NF, Torner JC, Haley EC, Jane JA, Adams HP, Kongable GL. The International Cooperative Study on the Timing of Aneurysm Surgery. Part 1: Overall management results. *J Neurosurg. Journal of Neurosurgery Publishing Group;* 1990 Jul;73 (1):18–36.

[54] Diringer MN, Bleck TP, Claude Hemphill J, Menon D, Shutter L, Vespa P, et al. Critical Care Management of Patients Following Aneurysmal Subarachnoid Hemorrhage: Recommendations from the Neurocritical Care Society's Multidisciplinary Consensus Conference. *Neurocrit Care*. 2011 Jul 20;15 (2):211–40.

[55] Roos Y. Antifibrinolytic treatment in subarachnoid hemorrhage: a randomized placebo-controlled trial. STAR Study Group. *Neurology*. 2000 Jan 11;54 (1):77–82.

[56] Kassell NF, Torner JC, Adams HP. Antifibrinolytic therapy in the acute period following aneurysmal subarachnoid hemorrhage. Preliminary observations from the Cooperative Aneurysm Study. *J Neurosurg. Journal of Neurosurgery Publishing Group*; 1984 Aug;61 (2):225–30.

[57] Vermeulen M, Lindsay KW, Murray GD, Cheah F, Hijdra A, Muizelaar JP, et al. Antifibrinolytic treatment in subarachnoid hemorrhage. *N Engl J Med*. 1984 Aug 16;311 (7):432–7.

[58] Roos Y, Rinkel G, Vermeulen M, Algra A, van Gijn J. Antifibrinolytic therapy for aneurysmal subarachnoid hemorrhage: a major update of a cochrane review. Stroke. Lippincott Williams and Wilkins; 2003 Sep;34 (9):2308–9.

[59] Hillman J, Fridriksson S, Nilsson O, Yu Z, Saveland H, Jakobsson K-E. Immediate administration of tranexamic acid and reduced incidence of early rebleeding after aneurysmal subarachnoid hemorrhage: a prospective randomized study. *J Neurosurg. Journal of Neurosurgery Publishing Group;* 2002 Oct;97 (4):771–8.

[60] Connolly ES, Rabinstein AA, Carhuapoma JR, Derdeyn CP, Dion J, Higashida RT, et al. Guidelines for the Management of Aneurysmal Subarachnoid Hemorrhage: A Guideline for Healthcare Professionals From the American Heart Association/American Stroke Association. *Stroke*. 2012 May 25;43 (6):1711–37.

[61] Zaidi HA, Montoure A, Elhadi A, Nakaji P, McDougall CG, Albuquerque FC, et al. Long-term Functional Outcomes and Predictors of Shunt-Dependent Hydrocephalus After Treatment of Ruptured Intracranial Aneurysms in the BRAT Trial. *Neurosurgery*. 2015 May;76 (5):608–15.

[62] Shah AH, Komotar RJ. Pathophysiology of Acute Hydrocephalus After Subarachnoid Hemorrhage. WNEU. Elsevier Inc; 2015 Aug 22;80 (3-4):304–6.

[63] Suarez-Rivera O. Acute hydrocephalus after subarachnoid hemorrhage. *Surgical Neurology*. 1998 May;49 (5):563–5.

[64] Giraldo EA, Mandrekar JN, Rubin MN, Dupont SA, Zhang Y, Lanzino G, et al. Timing of clinical grade assessment and poor outcome in patients with aneurysmal subarachnoid hemorrhage. *J Neurosurg. American Association of Neurological Surgeons*; 2012 Jul;117 (1):15–9.

[65] Karamanakos PN, Und Zu Fraunberg von M, Bendel S, Huttunen T, Kurki M, Hernesniemi J, et al. Risk factors for three phases of 12-month mortality in 1657 patients from a defined population after acute aneurysmal subarachnoid hemorrhage. WNEU. Elsevier; 2012 Dec;78 (6):631–9.

[66] Hasan D, Tanghe HL. Distribution of cisternal blood in patients with acute hydrocephalus after subarachnoid hemorrhage. Ann Neurol. Wiley Subscription Services, Inc., A Wiley Company; 1992 Apr;31 (4):374–8.

[67] KIBLER RF, COUCH RS, CROMPTON MR. Hydrocephalus in the adult following spontaneous subarachnoid haemorrhage. *Brain*. 1961 Mar;84:45–61.

[68] Brydon HL, Bayston R, Hayward R, Harkness W. The effect of protein and blood cells on the flow-pressure characteristics of shunts. *Neurosurgery*. 1996 Mar;38 (3):498–504–discussion505.

[69] Blasberg R, Johnson D, Fenstermacher J. Absorption resistance of cerebrospinal fluid after subarachnoid hemorrhage in the monkey; effects of heparin. *Neurosurgery*. 1981 Dec;9 (6):686–91.

[70] Vermeij FH, Hasan D, Vermeulen M, Tanghe HL, van Gijn J. Predictive factors for deterioration from hydrocephalus after subarachnoid hemorrhage. *Neurology*. 1994 Oct;44 (10):1851–5.

[71] Kosteljanetz M. Cerebrospinal fluid production in subarachnoid haemorrhage. *Br J Neurosurg*. 1988;2 (2):161–7.

[72] Black PM, Tzouras A, Foley L. Cerebrospinal fluid dynamics and hydrocephalus after experimental subarachnoid hemorrhage. *Neurosurgery*. 1985 Jul;17 (1):57–62.

[73] Kanat A, Turkmenoglu O, Aydin MD, Yolas C, Aydin N, Gursan N, et al. Toward Changing of the Pathophysiologic Basis of Acute Hydrocephalus After Subarachnoid Hemorrhage: A Preliminary Experimental Study. WNEU. Elsevier Inc; 2015 Aug 22;80 (3-4):390–5.

[74] Niemela M, Marbacher S. Acute Hydrocephalus After Subarachnoid Hemorrhage—Can It Be Caused by Water Vesicles of Choroid Plexuses? WNEU. Elsevier Inc; 2015 Aug 22;80 (3-4):307–8.

[75] Graff-Radford NR, Torner J, Adams HP, Kassell NF. Factors associated with hydrocephalus after subarachnoid hemorrhage. A report of the Cooperative Aneurysm Study. *Arch Neurol*. 1989 Jul;46 (7):744–52.

[76] Mohr G, Ferguson G, Khan M, Malloy D, Watts R, Benoit B, et al. Intraventricular hemorrhage from ruptured aneurysm. Retrospective analysis of 91 cases. *J Neurosurg. Journal of Neurosurgery Publishing Group*; 1983 Apr;58 (4):482–7.

[77] Ransom ER, Mocco J, Komotar RJ, Sahni D, Chang J, Hahn DK, et al. External ventricular drainage response in poor grade aneurysmal subarachnoid hemorrhage: effect on preoperative grading and prognosis. *Neurocrit Care*. 2007;6 (3):174–80.

[78] Rajshekhar V, Harbaugh RE. Results of routine ventriculostomy with external ventricular drainage for acute hydrocephalus following subarachnoid haemorrhage. Acta neurochirurgica. 1992;115 (1-2):8–14.

[79] Hasan D, Vermeulen M, Wijdicks EF, Hijdra A, van Gijn J. Management problems in acute hydrocephalus after subarachnoid hemorrhage. *Stroke*. 1989 Jun;20 (6):747–53.

[80] van Donkelaar CE, Bakker NA, Veeger NJGM, Uyttenboogaart M, Metzemaekers JDM, Luijckx G-J, et al. Predictive Factors for Rebleeding After Aneurysmal Subarachnoid Hemorrhage: Rebleeding Aneurysmal Subarachnoid Hemorrhage Study. *Stroke*. Lippincott Williams and Wilkins; 2015 Aug;46 (8):2100–6.

[81] Paré L, Delfino R, Leblanc R. The relationship of ventricular drainage to aneurysmal rebleeding. *J Neurosurg. Journal of Neurosurgery Publishing Group;* 1992 Mar;76 (3):422–7.

[82] McIver JI, Friedman JA, Wijdicks EFM, Piepgras DG, Pichelmann MA, Toussaint LG, et al. Preoperative ventriculostomy and rebleeding after aneurysmal subarachnoid hemorrhage. *J Neurosurg. Journal of Neurosurgery Publishing Group;* 2002 Nov;97 (5):1042–4.

[83] Hellingman CA, van den Bergh WM, Beijer IS, van Dijk GW, Algra A, van Gijn J, et al. Risk of rebleeding after treatment of acute hydrocephalus in patients with aneurysmal subarachnoid hemorrhage. Stroke. Lippincott Williams and Wilkins; 2007 Jan;38 (1):96–9.

In: Spontaneous Subarachnoid Haemorrhage
Editors: Thomas Kapapa and Ralph König
ISBN: 978-1-63485-270-8

Chapter 9

Endovascular Treatment of Aneurysms. Pre-, Peri- and Post-Interventional Management

G. Friedrich Götz
Medical School Hanover, Hanvover, Germany

Abstract

Endovascular treatment is a minimally invasive procedure for occluding cerebral aneurysms. The number of aneurysms undergoing endovascular treatment in different hospitals and countries is astonishingly varied. The ISAT study has demonstrated that interventional treatment offers an advantage over surgical treatment in the management of ruptured intracranial cerebral aneurysms. In the treatment of unruptured intracranial aneurysms, surgical and endovascular procedures are equally effective, but in incidental middle cerebral artery bifurcation aneurysms clipping is superior. Continuing advances in interventional tools has resulted not only in a reduction of the complication rate, but also an expansion of the therapeutic spectrum to include complex aneurysms.

Keywords: subarachnoid haemorrhage (SAH), coils, balloon remodelling, intracranial stent, stent-assisted coiling, flow diverter, antiplatelet treatment, MR angiography, follow-up, ISAT, barrow institute study

Endovascular treatment is a minimally invasive procedure for occluding cerebral aneurysms, which can be space-occupying, symptomatic or incidental. This interventional procedure is the treatment of choice for aneurysms which in neurosurgical terms are difficult to reach – especially those at the basilar tip. The prospective, randomised ISAT study [1] has demonstrated that interventional treatment offers an advantage over surgical treatment in the management of ruptured intracranial aneurysms. Endovascular treatment leads more rarely to a slight drop in the post-therapeutic GCS and to post-therapeutic epilepsy [2]. In the treatment of unruptured intracranial aneurysms, surgical and endovascular procedures are equally effective, but in incidental MCA (middle cerebral artery) bifurcation aneurysms clipping is superior [3, 4]. The number of aneurysms undergoing endovascular treatment in different hospitals and countries is astonishingly varied, however. Continuing advances in interventional tools has resulted not only in a reduction of the complication rate, but also an expansion of the therapeutic spectrum to include complex aneurysms. Endovascular treatment comprises a variety of different therapeutic approaches such as coil embolisation of the aneurysmal sac or other method of embolisation, flow modulation in the parent artery, as well as implantation of devices for bridging the aneurysm neck. Therapy can be customised by using varied combinations of these technical aids. Thanks to special interventional tools, continuing miniaturisation and optimised biocompatibility, and increasing experience worldwide, the number of aneurysms that cannot be treated interventionally has been minimised.

Proximal vessel occlusion and diversion of the blood flow in aneurysms of the intracranial vertebral artery and the cavernous internal carotid artery today represent an established, yet seldom employed therapeutic concept. The procedure can induce thrombosis of the aneurysm, and prevent both an increase in size and rupture. Interventional vascular occlusion with balloons, coils or, more effectively, so-called vascular plaques, is superior to surgical vessel ligation, since during angiography collateral cerebral perfusion can be evaluated.

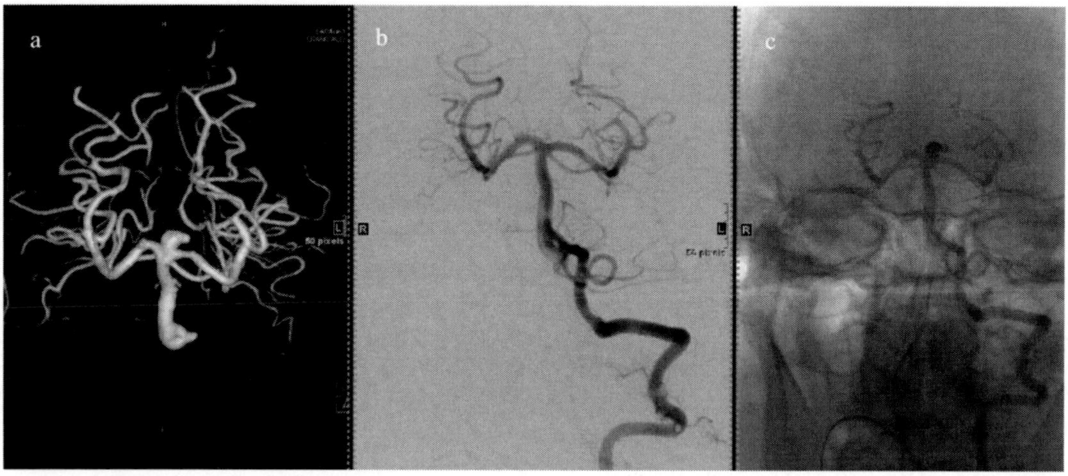

Figure 1. Endovascular treatment with coils: . 58 male with Subarachnoid Haemorrhage Hunt and Hess grade 2. a) 3D digital subtraction angiography, b + c) subtracted and unsubtracted frontal projection after embolisation with two coils.

Conventional endovascular treatment entails filling the lumen with coils to occlude the aneurysm. Berry-shaped aneurysms with a narrow neck (smaller than 4 mm) and favourable dome-to-neck ratio (larger than 1.4 mm), respectively, can be treated with coils only and without having to permanently modulate the coagulation. After carefully probing the aneurysm with a microcatheter the three-dimensional expanding coils are inserted in decreasing order of diameter. Small and short coils can be used to ensure that they fit snugly against the parent vessel. The aim is to pack the aneurysm as densely as possible with coils, reduce perfusion of the aneurysm to zero and thus induce thrombosis and subsequent fibrosis. The rate of complications from coil embolisation is less than 10%; this includes thromboembolic and haemorrhagic complications at less than 5% and 2%, respectively. The permanent occlusion of an aneurysm depends not only on the density with which the implanted coils are packed (up to 40% of the aneurysm lumen are filled with coils), but also on the flow properties in the parent vessel and stability of the wall. The occlusion rate is stratified in accordance with the Raymond classification into complete (class 1), residual perfusion of the aneurysm neck (class 2, equivalent to 90%-95%) and incomplete (class 3, marked remnant/reperfusion >90%) [5] (Figure 1).

The technique in use the longest for improving the treatment options for wide-necked intracranial aneurysms is remodelling [6]. It involves brief inflation of a balloon in the parent artery so as to stabilise the coils in the aneurysm. To use a balloon catheter and microcatheter simultaneously, a wide-bore or second distal access and/or guide catheter is required. Prior to balloon insufflation, a bolus dose of heparin is usually injected intravenously. This method, which requires considerable technical dexterity, permits dense packing of the coils and, as a result, safe and stable occlusion of broad-based aneurysms. Another advantage of this technique is that it provides protection for the efferent blood vessels in close proximity to the base of the aneurysm, especially at the MCA bifurcation, the A1/A2 junction, the posterior communicating artery and the basilar tip, and permits action to be taken immediately in response to a ruptured vessel (Figure 2).

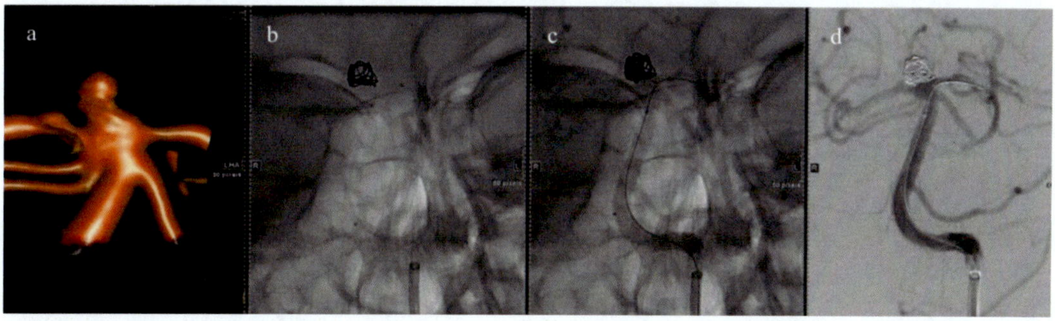

Figure 2. Balloon remodelling: 44 female with an aneurysm of the basilary tip and a history of Subarachnoid Haemorrhage Hunt and Hess Score 4 and of coil embolisation. Modified Rankin Scale 0. a) 3D DSA b) Working projection with balloon catheter (Eclipse 6 x 9, Balt®) at the aneurysm fundus (the markers indicate the length of the balloon) and microcatheter tip at the base of the aneurysm. c + d) unsubtracted and subtracted DSA. Embolisation of the basal reperfusion with a coil using balloon inflation for scaffolding.

Permanent implants in the parent artery generally necessitate modulation of coagulation over a prolonged period. This also applies to the latest generation of intracranial stents, the thrombogenicity of which is much lower than with older models. Hence, stent-protected coil embolisation as a treatment for ruptured aneurysms can only be recommended to a limited extent. Wherever possible, coils are used exclusively in the treatment of an acute aneurysm rupture.

The premedication used most commonly prior to permanent implantation of a device in the cerebral vasculature entails a daily dose of 100-300 mg aspirin and 75 mg clopidogrel for a minimum of five days, or a loading dose of 450 mg clopidogrel and 100 mg aspirin the evening beforehand. To monitor the regular intake and the efficacy of the medication, specific coagulation analysis is recommended immediately before the intervention. If the standard medication does not satisfactorily modulate the coagulation, either an increased dose or alternative drug (e.g., ticagrelor) can be used.

The development of flexible intracranial stents, which are available in an open-cell or closed-cell design, and are interwoven or laser-cut, has expanded the endovascular possibilities for treating wide-necked, complex aneurysms. The stent mesh not only prevents the coils placed into the aneurysm from herniation into the parent artery, but also positively alters the flow properties at the neck of the aneurysm. This should help to reduce the number of aneurysms incompletely embolised at the base and, in turn, the frequency of recurrence. This theoretic advantage is certainly consistent with the results reported in numerous case studies, but has not yet been confirmed by a randomised prospective trial.

Elective stent-assisted coil embolisation necessitates modulation of the coagulation as described above. If emergency stent implantation is required to correct prolapsed coil loops or to treat peri-interventional vascular dissection, 500 mg of intravenous aspirin and an intravenously effective platelet aggregation inhibitor as a bolus and subsequent infusion should be administered during the procedure. Long-term medication should be initiated with a loading dose of clopidogrel (e.g., 450 mg via gastric tube) at the periprocedural stage.

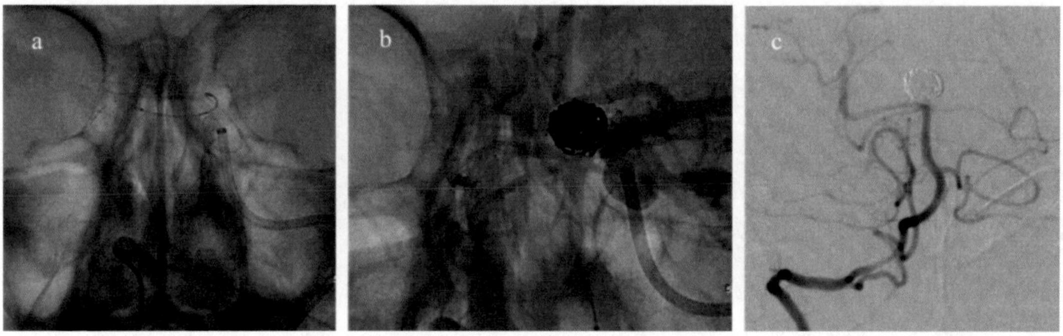

Figure 3. Stent assisted coiling: 66 male who presented with an incidental basilar tip aneurysm and vertebrobasilar arteriosclerotic stenosis. a) Stent implantation (LVIS junior 3.5 x 18 Microvention®) via the left posterior communicating artery into the right posterior cerebral artery b) Post coil embolization c) Treatment outcome after 6 months (subtracted DSA after right vertebral artery injection).

Coiling with stent assistance can be performed in one or two stages. To accurately deploy the stent, a stable access route is required – ideally consisting of a guide, distal coaxial and microcatheter. Using the jailing technique, the microcatheter placed in the aneurysm is fixed with the subsequently deployed stent and then carefully removed after coiling is complete. As with remodelling, this approach requires two microcatheters to be inserted simultaneously in the parent vessel. Alternatively, the stent can be implanted first and coiling performed six weeks later at the earliest. With this method, it is necessary to probe the aneurysm through the tines of the stent. This can be done even with small and flat aneurysms once the stent has stabilised. Sequential stent implantation and coiling during an intervention is less advisable, since probing the aneurysm can cause the stent to become misaligned if it has not yet stabilised (Figure 3).

Wide-necked aneurysms located in the carotid T, the MCA bifurcation or basilar tip have an unfavorable haemodynamic, the so called water hammer effect [7]. The recanalisation rate after coil embolisation, generally known to be high in these aneurysms, is induced by coil compaction and progressive aneurysmal growth. Reconstruction of the base of the aneurysm and preservation of the efferent arteries pose a particular challenge. Special techniques and materials are required to treat such aneurysms.

The base of the aneurysm can be reconstructed by inserting two microstents to form an X or Y shape. The resulting haemodynamic effects vary depending on the design of the stent and implant geometry [7]. The stents can be implanted in two stages by probing the mesh once the first stent has stabilised, or in one procedure. Different technical variations for vascular reconstruction have been described [8]. The microcatheter for coil embolisation must either be navigated through the struts of the stent into the aneurysm, or be placed in the aneurysm using the jailing technique prior to deployment of the stent. Protection of the efferent arteries allowsdense coil packing, which is necessary for preventing recanalization (Figure 4).

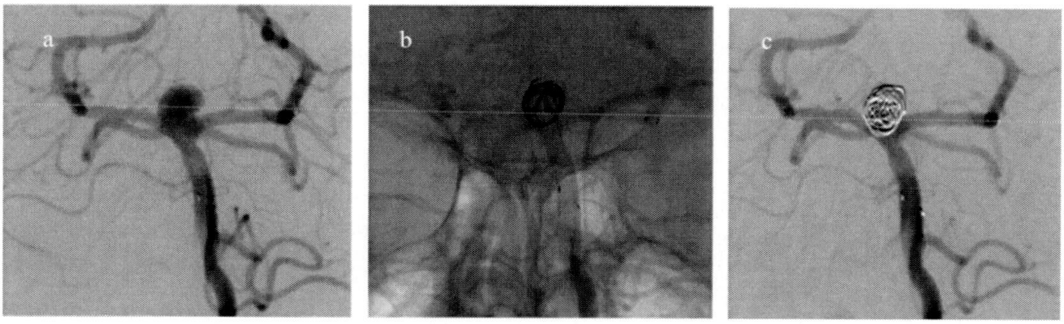

Figure 4. Y stenting: 46 female presenting with a wide-necked, incidental basilar tip aneurysm and a history of familial subarachnoid haemorrhage. a) frontal projection of an angiogram. Stent implantation firstly from the right, secondly on the left posterior cerebral artery to the basilar artery (Solitaire® 4 x 20), b) Unsubtracted DSA with Y- stenting in situ and the first coil inside the aneurysm. c) Subtracted DSA after embolisation with two coils.

Intra- and extra-aneurysmal placement of a stent and subsequent coil embolisation is referred to as the waffle-cone technique [9, 10]. The expandable end of the self-expanding microstent is designed for reconstructing and modelling the aneurysm fundus and stabilising the coil.

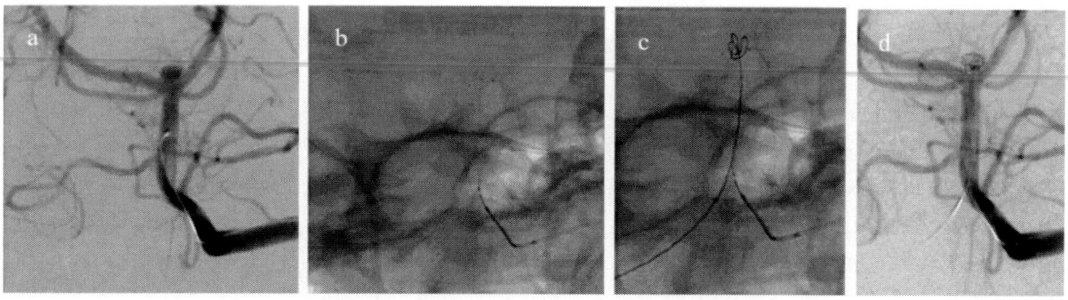

Figure 5. Waffle cone technique: 28 male with a wide-necked basilar tip aneurysm. Implantation of a pCONus (®) device and embolisation of the aneurysm with four coils. a) subtracted angiogram, working position. b) unsubtracted projection after expansion of the pCONus® 4-25-5 from the neck of the aneurysm to the basilar artery. c) unsubtracted projection with a second microcatheter placed inside the aneurysm d) subtracted angiogram after implantation of four coils, prior to detachment of pCONus.

A stent-like device with a distal portion that unfolds like a flower is suitable in particular for treating wide-necked bifurcation aneurysms [11, 12]. The distal end, which opens out into a disc shape, is used to secure the aneurysm fundus, whilst the proximal end ensures stabilisation in the parent artery. Stable anchorage facilitates probing of the aneurysm and coiling. Compared to X and Y stenting, the waffle-cone technique using the described device is easier to perform and is regularly done within one treatment procedure (Figure 5).

Flow diverters are flexible, self-expanding stent-like devices with a more dense wire mesh. They modulate the blood flow in the parent vessel, reduce inflow of blood into the aneurysm. Consequently they, or when Combined with loosely packed coils flow diverters promote occlusion of the aneurysm. The high mesh density of flow diverters results in low porosity of these implants. Porosity is a measure of permeability to liquid, and describes the ratio of the free surface not covered by struts to the total surface. A flow diverter is most effective if it is densely woven with as little material as possible. The goal is achieved technologically if the product offers low permeability combined with high flexibility and good wall apposition.

Compared to intracranial microstents, the denser wire mesh of flow diverters inevitably results in relatively high thrombogenicity. It is essential to adequately modulate the coagulation at the time of implantation. Following the intervention, treatment with aspirin and Plavix should continue for a minimum of 3-6 months. Since late thromboembolic complications have been reported [13, 14], consideration should be given to modulating the coagulation for an even longer period in individual cases.

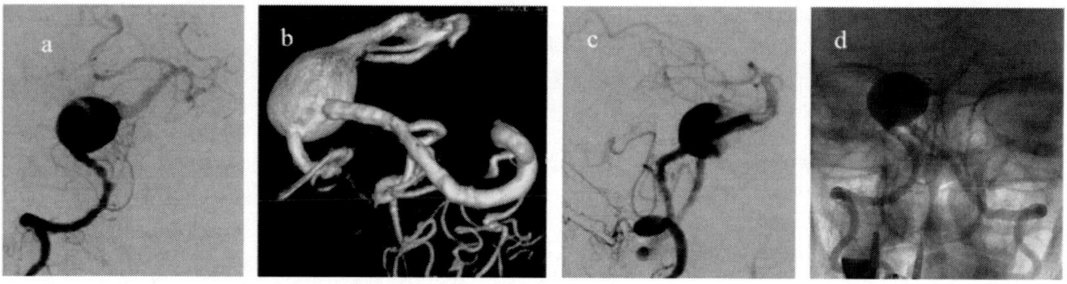

Figure 6. Arteriosclerotic fusiform vertebrobasilar aneurysm: 60 female with progressive brain stem symptoms. a) Angiogramm after injection of the right vertebral artery. b) 3D digital subtraction angiography. The terminal segments of both vertebral arteries and the basilar artery are incorporated in the aneurysm sac. c + d) Subtracted and unsubtracted DSA after implantation of a stent (Leo® 4.5 x 75) and a flow diverter (Silk® 5.5 x 50).

Flow diverters are suitible for the management of wide-necked and dysplastic aneurysms. They offer promise in the treatment of dissecting aneurysms and blood blister-like aneurysms that are extremely difficult to manage [15, 16]. Despite the initial euphoria, clinically viable therapeutic outcomes with fusiform aneurysms can only be expected if such treatment is strictly indicated. Large vertebrobasilar, fusiform aneurysms are a particular therapeutic challenge given the numerous efferent perforators, as well as the lack of mural stability and parietal thrombi. Vascular reconstruction with a stable, self-expanding stent and additional implantation of a flow diverter may be necessary in the treatment of extremely wide, fusiform aneurysms. Although causal therapy would appear to be possible with such a device, peri-interventional mortality is significant and good long-term outcome has been achieved rarely (Figure 6).

A hazardous scenario arises if an aneurysm ruptures after implantation of a flow diverter [17]. This can possibly be caused by a small amount of blood continuing to flow into the aneurysm but the outflow being blocked, thus increasing the intra-aneurysmal pressure. This potential complication can probably be ameliorated by partially coiling the aneurysm. The rational use of flow diverters is hindered by the fact that the pathophysiological effects are not fully understood, combined with a lack of randomised studies [14, 18] as opposed to numerous case studies and small retrospective series.

A cork-like implant made of interwoven nitinol fibres that unfolds inside the aneurysm is also suitable for treating wide-necked aneurysms. The wire, ball-like device is selected in a suitable size based on the maximum transverse diameter of the aneurysm. It can be modelled to fit the wall to the parent artery perfectly prior to electrolytic detachment. Perfusion of the aneurysm often ceases immediately after the implant has unfolded. An advantage with this technique is the possibility to use it in the event of acute rupture of an aneurysm, since modulation of the coagulation is not essential [19, 20] (Figure 7).

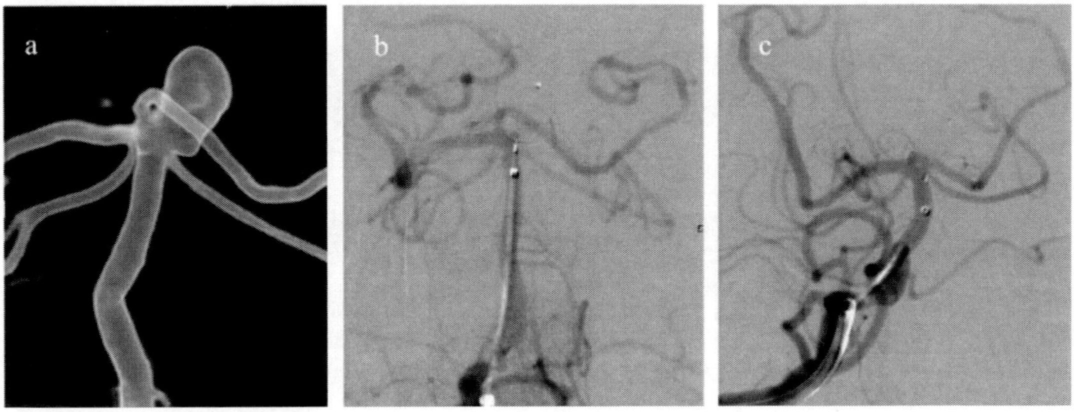

Figure 7. WEB® (woven endobridge): in superior cerebellar aneurysms. 59 female, history of sentinel bleeding and a wide-necked basilar artery aneurysm between the origin of the superior cerebellar and posterior cerebral arteries on the left.. a) 3D digital subtraction angiography. b) DSA after implantation of a WEB® SL 2-8-S device. Immediate cessation of aneurysm perfusion. c) Angiogram after electrolytic detachment of the device and complete occlusion of the aneurysm.

Post-Interventional Measures

If coiling has been completed successfully without complications, post-interventional pharmacological modulation of the coagulation is not necessary. If individual tines prolapse into the carrier vessel, intravenous or subcutaneous heparin can be prescribed for five days; aspirin is likely to be equally effective.

Aspirin (100-300 mg) and clopidogrel (75 mg) are essential for modulating the coagulation when implanting stents and flow diverters. When prescribing dual antiplatelet therapy, additional gastric protection is usually recommended. After implanting intracranial stents, drug therapy is switched no sooner than eight weeks later to long-term aspirin and is continued for a minimum of one year.

Dual antiplatelet therapy should last longer if a flow diverter has been implanted. Reports of late thromboembolic complications [12, 13] call the six-month limitation of intensive anticoagulation into doubt. It is therefore advisable to consider the benefits and risks in each individual case. Most authors recommend lifelong continuation of aspirin after dual antiplatelet therapy once a flow diverter has been implanted. The thrombogenicity of the implants can be expected to decrease in future thanks to improved surface technology.

MRI is used preferentially in the follow-up of aneurysms after coil embolisation [19-23]. High-resolution, thin-section 3D TOF sequences are used by most practitioners. Analysis must not be restricted to MIP reformations, but must account for the individual axial images.

The coil-filled aneurysm is displayed on 3D TOF MRA as a compact, attenuated signal. The contrast to the flow signal in the adjacent artery is high. Segments of the aneurysm that are still perfused and not excluded from the circulation exhibit a bright signal and can be identified precisely from the 3D TOF images. Visual assessment of the treatment outcome is most reliable if it is done by two examiners using a three-part scale [24] (Figure 8).

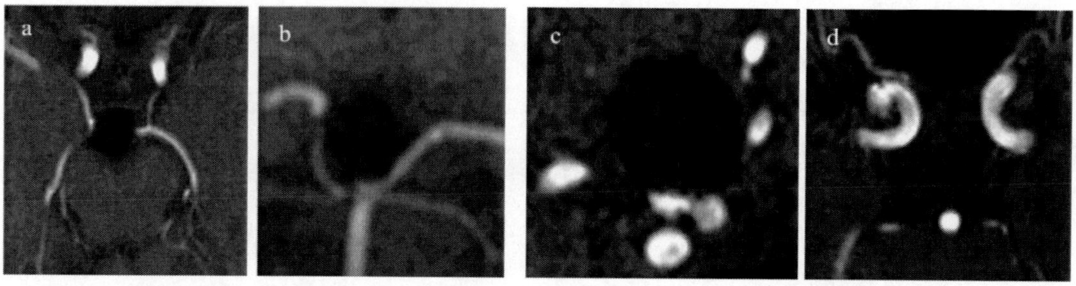

Figure 8. MRA after endovascular treatment: (a+b) 3D TOF MRA (3 Tesla) thick-slice MIP reformations complete exclusion with a homogenous signal void inside a basilar tip aneurysm post coiling. c + d) 3D TOF MRA (3 Tesla). Axial source images of a 72 male show an area of recurrence at the neck of an opthalmic ACI aneurysm on the right.

Contrast-enhanced head and neck angiography is less often used for post-interventional assessment of aneurysms. In the current literature, 3D TOF MR angiography is reported to offer greater sensitivity with rather than without contrast enhancement [21, 23]. The use of a contrast agent does not ensure that a distinction can be made between flow and a contrast-enhanced thrombus, however. In the authors`s opinion the minimal gain in sensitivity is therefore accompanied by a decrease in specificity. Infectious complications or an inflammation of the aneurysm wall are absolute indications for the application of contrast agents.

Although all intracranial stents and flow diverters are MR-compatible, image distortion of varying degrees does occur with the individual implants. The implants of a number of manufacturers cause a large void in the signal [21] and hamper the assessment of the carrier vessel and aneurysm region. Others permit identification of the parent vessel, but might mistake the artefact of the device for stenosis. Artifacts also depend on the field strength of the used MRI system and can be so misleading that conventional DSA will be required in order to elucidate the situation. Despite the high material density, unexpectedly small artifacts occur with intrasaccular flow disrupters on MRI, meaning that in principle non-invasive follow-up is possible. For the woven endobridge intra-arterial catheter angiography is recommended three months after implantation, since early reperfusion of aneurysms was not detected by MRI in all cases [20].

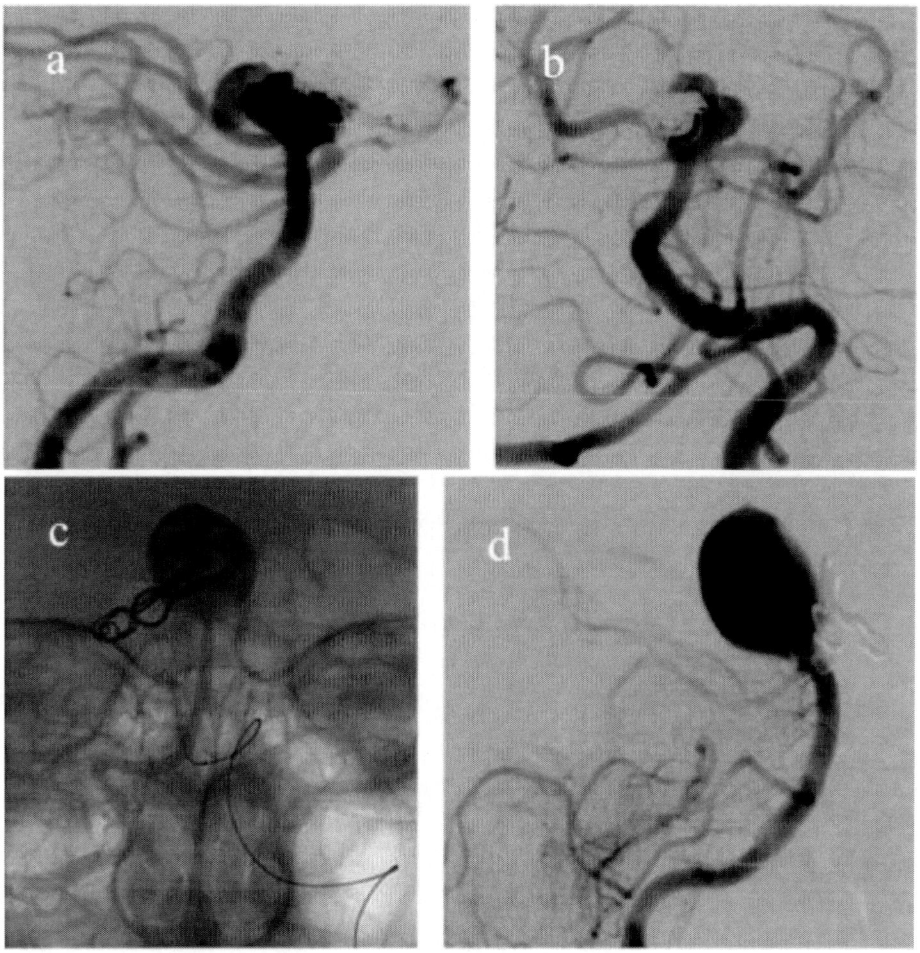

Figure 9. Recurrence after therapy: a+ b) 49 female with a history of SAH I and embolisation of a basilar tip aneurysm with coils. Recurrent SAH and regrowth of the aneurysm 9 years later. Digital subtraction angiography with frontal and lateral projection c + d) 52 male presents with headaches and aneurysm recurrence. History ofSAH and clipping in 1992 for basilar tip aneurysm, no follow-up since.; Unsubtracted and subtracted DSA, frontal and lateral views, prior to stent assisted coiling.

The modified Raymond classification is often also applied in the evaluation of the treatment outcome after using other devices than coils. It can take up to six months to completely occlude a wide-necked aneurysm with a flow diverter. Therefore, the last angiogram taken on the day of the procedure to assess the therapeutic outcome will not be conclusive, since a further reduction as well as an increase in the perfusion of the aneurysm can result [15]. MRA usually is scheduled at 6-12 months after endovascular aneurysm treatment. The timing should be scheduled individually, however, depending on the course of the intervention and the implants used. If MRA follow-up reveals a change over the final angiogram taken at intervention, it is advisable to perform intraarterial DSA for confirmation and to weigh up therapeutic consequences. In all cases in which stable occlusion of the aneurysm is achieved, cerebral catheter angiography is not necessary. Depending on the type of materials implanted, MRA may not be sufficient to reliably evaluate the therapeutic outcome.

The recanalisation rate after endovascular coiling is reported at up to 40% and is much higher than after clipping [2-4, 25, 26]. Remarkably, this treatment outcome evidently correlates only vaguely with the number of recurrent bleeds [26, 27]. Complete occlusion of an aneurysm with coils might be not necessary for cure and continuing protection against rebleeding. The decision whether reintervention for incompletely occluded aneurysms is indicated should be made on a personalized basis. As long as valid data on the long-term outcome of endovascular aneurysm treatment remain sparse [26, 27], follow-up examinations are still mandatory. Recommendations for follow-up also account for the occurrence of de novo aneurysms, which are reported at a rate of up to 1% per year.

Recurrence can occur after both endovascular and surgical treatment due to aneurysmal growth associated with arteriopathy (Figure 9). Recanalisation and recurrent SAH following endovascular treatment are observed more often in smokers than in non-smokers.

REFERENCES

[1] Molyneux A, Kerr R, International Subarachnoid Aneurysm Trial Collaborative G, Stratton I, Sandercock P, Clarke M, et al. International Subarachnoid Aneurysm Trial (ISAT) of neurosurgical clipping versus endovascular coiling in 2143 patients with ruptured intracranial aneurysms: a randomized trial. *Journal of stroke and cerebrovascular diseases: the official journal of National Stroke Association.* 2002 Nov-Dec;11 (6):304-14. PubMed PMID: 17903891.

[2] Ayling OG, Ibrahim GM, Drake B, Torner JC, Macdonald RL. Operative complications and differences in outcome after clipping and coiling of ruptured intracranial aneurysms. *Journal of neurosurgery.* 2015 Sep;123 (3):621-8. PubMed PMID: 26047409.

[3] Ruan C, Long H, Sun H, He M, Yang K, Zhang H, et al. Endovascular coiling vs. surgical clipping for unruptured intracranial aneurysm: A meta-analysis. *British journal of neurosurgery.* 2015 Aug;29 (4):485-92. PubMed PMID: 26037936.

[4] Smith TR, Cote DJ, Dasenbrock HH, Hamade YJ, Zammar SG, El Tecle NE, et al. Comparison of the Efficacy and Safety of Endovascular Coiling Versus Microsurgical Clipping for Unruptured Middle Cerebral Artery Aneurysms: A Systematic Review and Meta-Analysis. *World neurosurgery.* 2015 Oct;84 (4):942-53. PubMed PMID: 26093360.

[5] Raymond J, Guilbert F, Weill A, Georganos SA, Juravsky L, Lambert A, et al. Long-term angiographic recurrences after selective endovascular treatment of aneurysms with detachable coils. *Stroke; a journal of cerebral circulation.* 2003 Jun;34 (6):1398-403. PubMed PMID: 12775880.

[6] Pierot L, Cognard C, Spelle L, Moret J. Safety and efficacy of balloon remodeling technique during endovascular treatment of intracranial aneurysms: critical review of

the literature. *AJNR American journal of neuroradiology.* 2012 Jan;33 (1):12-5. PubMed PMID: 21349960.

[7] Kono K, Terada T. Hemodynamics of 8 different configurations of stenting for bifurcation aneurysms. *AJNR American journal of neuroradiology.* 2013 Oct;34 (10):1980-6. PubMed PMID: 23578668.

[8] Brassel F, Melber K, Schlunz-Hendann M, Meila D. Kissing-Y stenting for endovascular treatment of complex wide necked bifurcation aneurysms using Acandis Acclino stents: results and literature review. *Journal of neurointerventional surgery.* 2015 May 18. PubMed PMID: 25987589.

[9] Horowitz M, Levy E, Sauvageau E, Genevro J, Guterman LR, Hanel R, et al. Intra/extra-aneurysmal stent placement for management of complex and wide-necked-bifurcation aneurysms: eight cases using the waffle cone technique. *Neurosurgery.* 2006 Apr;58 (4 Suppl 2):ONS-258-62; discussion ONS-62. PubMed PMID: 16582648.

[10] Lee SM, Kim YJ, Ho Ko J. The effectiveness of the waffle-cone technique in treating complex intracranial aneurysms. *Interventional neuroradiology: journal of peritherapeutic neuroradiology, surgical procedures and related neurosciences.* 2015 Aug;21 (4):470-8. PubMed PMID: 26092438.

[11] Gory B, Aguilar-Perez M, Pomero E, Turjman F, Weber W, Fischer S, et al. pCONus Device for the Endovascular Treatment of Wide-Neck Middle Cerebral Artery Aneurysms. *AJNR American journal of neuroradiology.* 2015 Sep;36 (9):1735-40. PubMed PMID: 26206810.

[12] Henkes H, Weber W. The Past, Present and Future of Endovascular Aneurysm Treatment. *Clinical neuroradiology.* 2015 Oct;25 Suppl 2:317-24. PubMed PMID: 26031430.

[13] Rossen JD, Chalouhi N, Wassef SN, Thomas J, Abel TJ, Jabbour PM, et al. Incidence of cerebral ischemic events after discontinuation of clopidogrel in patients with intracranial aneurysms treated with stent-assisted techniques. *Journal of neurosurgery.* 2012 Nov;117 (5):929-33. PubMed PMID: 22957528.

[14] Shankar JJ, Tampieri D, Iancu D, Cortes M, Agid R, Krings T, et al. SILK flow diverter for complex intracranial aneurysms: a Canadian registry. *Journal of neurointerventional surgery.* 2015 May 18. PubMed PMID: 25987591.

[15] Mpotsaris A, Skalej M, Beuing O, Eckert B, Behme D, Weber W. Long-term occlusion results with SILK flow diversion in 28 aneurysms: Do recanalizations occur during follow-up? *Interventional neuroradiology: journal of peritherapeutic neuroradiology, surgical procedures and related neurosciences.* 2015 Jun;21 (3):300-10. PubMed PMID: 26015522.

[16] Nossek E, Chalif DJ, Chakraborty S, Lombardo K, Black KS, Setton A. Concurrent use of the Pipeline Embolization Device and coils for intracranial aneurysms: technique, safety, and efficacy. *Journal of neurosurgery.* 2015 Apr;122 (4):904-11. PubMed PMID: 25658781.

[17] Turowski B, Macht S, Kulcsar Z, Hanggi D, Stummer W. Early fatal hemorrhage after endovascular cerebral aneurysm treatment with a flow diverter (SILK-Stent): do we need to rethink our concepts? *Neuroradiology.* 2011 Jan;53 (1):37-41. PubMed PMID: 20339842.

[18] Wakhloo AK, Lylyk P, de Vries J, Taschner C, Lundquist J, Biondi A, et al. Surpass flow diverter in the treatment of intracranial aneurysms: a prospective multicenter

study. *AJNR American journal of neuroradiology*. 2015 Jan;36 (1):98-107. PubMed PMID: 25125666.

[19] Behme D, Berlis A, Weber W. Woven EndoBridge Intrasaccular Flow Disrupter for the Treatment of Ruptured and Unruptured Wide-Neck Cerebral Aneurysms: Report of 55 Cases. *AJNR American journal of neuroradiology*. 2015 Aug;36 (8):1501-6. PubMed PMID: 25953761.

[20] Mine B, Tancredi I, Aljishi A, Alghamdi F, Beltran M, Herchuelz M, et al. Follow-up of intracranial aneurysms treated by a WEB flow disrupter: a comparative study of DSA and contrast-enhanced MR angiography. *Journal of neurointerventional surgery*. 2015 May 21. PubMed PMID: 25999378.

[21] Attali J, Benaissa A, Soize S, Kadziolka K, Portefaix C, Pierot L. Follow-up of intracranial aneurysms treated by flow diverter: comparison of three-dimensional time-of-flight MR angiography (3D-TOF-MRA) and contrast-enhanced MR angiography (CE-MRA) sequences with digital subtraction angiography as the gold standard. *Journal of neurointerventional surgery*. 2014 Oct 28. PubMed PMID: 25352582.

[22] Lane A, Vivian P, Coulthard A. Magnetic resonance angiography or digital subtraction catheter angiography for follow-up of coiled aneurysms: do we need both? *Journal of medical imaging and radiation oncology*. 2015 Apr;59 (2):163-9. PubMed PMID: 25857748.

[23] Levent A, Yuce I, Eren S, Ozyigit O, Kantarci M. Contrast-Enhanced and Time-of-Flight MR Angiographic Assessment of Endovascular Coiled Intracranial Aneurysms at 1.5 T. *Interventional neuroradiology: journal of peritherapeutic neuroradiology, surgical procedures and related neurosciences*. 2014 Dec;20 (6):686-92. PubMed PMID: 25496678. Pubmed Central PMCID: 4295240.

[24] Ernst M, Yoo AJ, Kriston L, Schonfeld MH, Vettorazzi E, Fiehler J. Is visual evaluation of aneurysm coiling a reliable study end point? Systematic review and meta-analysis. *Stroke; a journal of cerebral circulation*. 2015 Jun;46 (6):1574-81. PubMed PMID: 25944331.

[25] Mascitelli JR, Oermann EK, Mocco J, Fifi JT, Paramasivam S, Stapleton CJ, et al. Predictors of success following endovascular retreatment of intracranial aneurysms. *Interventional neuroradiology: journal of peritherapeutic neuroradiology, surgical procedures and related neurosciences*. 2015 Aug;21 (4):426-32. PubMed PMID: 26092439.

[26] Spetzler RF, McDougall CG, Zabramski JM, Albuquerque FC, Hills NK, Russin JJ, et al. The Barrow Ruptured Aneurysm Trial: 6-year results. *Journal of neurosurgery*. 2015 Sep;123 (3):609-17. PubMed PMID: 26115467.

[27] Molyneux AJ, Birks J, Clarke A, Sneade M, Kerr RS. The durability of endovascular coiling versus neurosurgical clipping of ruptured cerebral aneurysms: 18 year follow-up of the UK cohort of the International Subarachnoid Aneurysm Trial (ISAT). *Lancet*. 2015 Feb 21;385 (9969):691-7. PubMed PMID: 25465111. Pubmed Central PMCID: 4356153.

In: Spontaneous Subarachnoid Haemorrhage
Editors: Thomas Kapapa and Ralph König
ISBN: 978-1-63485-270-8

Chapter 10

SURGICAL THERAPY OF ANEURYSMS

Ralph König
Department of Neurosurgery,
University of Ulm, 89312 Günzburg, Germany

ABSTRACT

The following chapter addresses several peculiarities with regard to surgery for ruptured intracranial aneurysms. Furthermore the chapter tries to give an insight in newer developments of neurovascular, especially aneurysm surgery: tailored approaches, retractorless neurosurgery, endoscopic and endoscope assisted aneurysm surgery. Furthermore it provides an overview of intraoperative imaging and electrophysiology in aneurysm surgery.

Keywords: aneurysm surgery, retractorless neurosurgery, tailored approaches, intraoperative angiography, intraoperative electrophysiology

INTRODUCTION

"Endovascular therapy has changed the practice of vascular neurosurgery forever" [1]. Albeit the subject of best treatment for ruptured aneurysms of the anterior circulation remains controversial [2-6] there is accumulating evidence that patients undergoing surgical clipping after acute subarachnoid hemorrhage (aSAH) demonstrate substantial postoperative decline of their clinical condition [7]. More precisely, Ayling [8], in a post hoc analysis of perioperative complications from the CONCIOUS-1 Study demonstrated a greater perioperative decline in GCS after clipping compared to coiling. Additionally patients clipped for ruptured aneurysms seem to have higher rates of delayed ischemic deficits (DCI) compared to those treated endovascularly [9, 10].

As a consequence of those data, particularly since the International Subarachnoid Hemorrhage Trial (ISAT) [11] the number of ruptured aneurysms treated endovascularly increased steadily. A paradigm shift in acute management of patients with ruptured aneurysms occurred in many neurovascular centers around the world [12]. In spite of this general development one should not lose sight of the fact that the most appropriate treatment for an individual patient might be different in various treatment centers, as the level of endovascular or surgical experience varies. Furthermore in the presence of SAH endovascular procedures that require dual antiplatelet therapy (stent remodeling, flow diversion) should be avoided, as this has important ramifications for necessary subsequent surgical procedures (CSF-diversion, central venous lines, ICP measurement, tracheotomy).

Regardless of any further developments in endovascular therapy there will be ruptured aneurysms that require surgical treatment. Therefore aneurysm clipping will retain importance in the future. Also, more or less in obscurity and silent aneurysm surgery refined in the recent years:

- Application and adaption of tailored minimally invasive skull base approaches
- Retractorless surgery [13, 14]
- Endoscopic and endoscope-assisted techniques [15, 16]
- Intraoperative neuromonitoring [17, 18]
- Intraoperative imaging and visualization techniques [19] [20-22]

CLIPPING OF RUPTURED ANEURYSMS

Clipping of ruptured aneurysms is the other side of the same coin. Albeit the objective is the same, complete clipping of the aneurysm without a remnant and compromise of parent vessels, surgery for ruptured aneurysms has various specific characteristics compared to unruptured ones.

- First timing of treatment: Based on the results of the cooperative study the optimum time for definitive aneurysm treatment shifted from late (>7 days after aSAH) to early (<3 days after aSAH) (Kassell: 1990di; 23). Today, to further reduce the risk of recurrent haemorrhage from ruptured aneurysms a policy of urgent treatment within the first 24 hours after bleeding is pursued. But this might not be the end of the story as there seems to be some evidence for emergency treatment of ruptured aneurysms [24].
- Second, the "angry, red, swollen brain": In the presence of SAH the brain is vulnerable and swollen, due to brain edema, acute hydrocephalus and potential intracerebral haemorrhage. The subarachnoid cisterns are filled up with clotted blood and anatomy might be distorted from space-occupying intracerebral hematoma. Therefore to gain space and to get access to the relevant pathology is hampered, particularly as premature intraoperative rupture threatens to complicate the procedure. Generous indication for CSF diversion, either by ventricular or lumbar drainage helps to relax the brain, as suction of CSF from the basal cisterns is made difficult by clotted blood. Further osmotic therapy administered by the anaesthetist may help to create a slack brain. Temporary mild hyperventilation may additionally help if the aforementioned measures fail [25].

- Third, temporary clipping: temporary clipping is used frequently especially during surgery for ruptured aneurysms. On the one hand it is used to deal with intraoperative rupture, which occurs between 7 and 35%, depending on various aneurysm and surgeon specific factors (Batjer: 1986wq; Fridriksson: 2002if; 26). On the other it is a helpful adjunct in the final dissection of the aneurysm dome and clip application, especially in larger aneurysms. Griessenauer, in the so far largest study about the effect of temporary clipping in ruptured aneurysms concluded, that limited temporary clipping did not affect clinical outcome in patients with aSAH [27]. Perfect interaction and communication between the between the anaesthesiological and surgical team helps to reduce potential harmful effects of temporary artery occlusion.
- Fourth, posthaemorrhagic hydrocephalus: surgery with or without opening of the lamina terminalis during the procedure does not have any positive effect on shunt dependency after aSAH, but on the contrary seem to result in an elevated risk for shunt dependency compared to endovascular therapy [28]. Apart from that aneurysm location, especially ruptured anterior cerebral artery ACA aneurysms, and the amount of blood are predictors for persistent posthaemorrhagic hydrocephalus.

Minimally Invasive or Tailored Approaches to Aneurysms

In public the term "minimal invasive surgery" unfortunately is connoted in particular with small skin incisions. This does not necessarily imply, that a minimal invasive procedure is minimal invasive in handling with crucial structures e.g., the brain. In this respect minimal invasive surgery may turn out to be rather invasive and harmful. Therefore the term keyhole approach (or tailored approach), as coined by Axel Perneczky [29] seems to be a more appropriate designation for the concept of moving away from standard approaches ("one size fits all"), but instead come down to small approaches, which take into account the individual anatomy and pathology of each case. e.g., a tailored approach for a ruptured ACM aneurysm with associated space occupying temporal intracerebral haemorrhage might not be a osteoplastic supraorbital craniotomy, but a decompressive craniectomy.

A crucial prerequisite for tailored approaches is excellent preoperative planning based on multimodal (e.g., MRI, CT, DSA) neuroradiological cross-sectional and 3D imaging. In order to realise multimodality planning for complex neurovascular procedures computerized planning is helpful. Meanwhile even coregistration of projectional DSA data with 3D datasets allows for 4-D planning, taking into account the fourth dimension: time (Smartbrush Angio, Brainlab AG, Feldkirchen). Based on 3-D imaging development of surgical simulation tools using virtual or physical models proceed [30]. Concerning to this especially 3D printing techniques appear as a promising tool in the future [31-33].

Retractorless Surgery

By now the potentially harmful effects of static brain retraction have been well described and the underlying cellular and molecular mechanisms of injury were unveiled [34-37]. In their publication entitled "The quiet revolution: retractorless surgery for complex vascular and skull base lesions", Spetzler and Sanai [13] described a technique to overcome fixed retraction by dynamic retraction with surgical instruments. Especially the sucker and suction hand play a critical role as a mobile, "roving retractor" [1]. The sucker complements the dissecting instrument providing e.g., countertraction while cutting arachnoid bands with microscissors. Along with an extensive arachnoidal dissection, careful patient positioning allowing for gravity retraction of the brain this technique allows for a limited retractor-induced tissue injury even in complex vascular and skull base lesions.

To put it in the right light: limited use of retractors, e.g., in the final stage of aneurysm clipping after careful dissection is not a problem. But use of fixed retraction should be reduced to the minimum.

Intraoperative Imaging and Visualization

The idea of intraoperative angiography (IOA) goes back to almost 50 years now [38, 39]. The rationale is based on the studies of Drake [40], dealing with the "…late consequences of incomplete surgical treatment of cerebral aneurysms". The potential benefit is obvious: prompt and correctable detection of inadvertent aneurysm residuals and parent vessel or branch occlusion respectively.

In the so far largest contemporary study of IOA dealing with IOA performed during surgical treatment of 976 aneurysms Chalouhi et al. [19] described a clip revision rate of 8.2%. Reasons for clip readjustment were residual aneurysm in 54, 7%, parent vessel occlusion in 42.9% and a combination of both in 2.4% of cases.

Albeit the benefits of IOA seem to be clear the critique never silenced: besides safety concerns, accuracy, duration and costs appeared as main arguments against routine use of IOA in aneurysm surgery. Further the development of intraoperative microscope-based Indocyanine Green Angiography (ICG) seemed to make IOA superfluous.

- Safety concerns: Complications, especially permanent stroke rate due to IOA reported in the literature exceed by far that of routine cerebral angiography [41]. The prevailing mechanism thereby is vessel injury (dissection) on catheter access caused by distorted vessel anatomy due to patient positioning and thromboembolic events [42-44]. However, most of those publications date back 20 years. Further development and distribution of imaging technology e.g., enable intelligent catheter navigation from groin to neck, therefore reducing the risk of vessel injury. In their review of 1093 consecutive cases, Chalouhi et al. [19] for instance report about 0,99% of transient or minor complications, none resulting in permanent morbidity.
- Diagnostic accuracy: Diagnostic accuracy of IOA has always been one important criticism as the rate of false negative findings range up to 8.7%. Similar to complications ongoing technical development and integration of modern flat panel diagnostic imaging devices into the operation theatre with the possibility of 3D-rotational angiography helped to overcome that issue. Apart from very few exceptions image quality of IOA come about standard diagnostic angiography [45, 46].

- Duration and costs: in health care systems always under pressure to control costs IOA is not economically advantageous, as it extends operation time by at least 15 to 20 minutes. But, in a more comprehensive view calculating the incremental cost-utility ration for routine IOA Kallmes et al. [47] proved IOA to be cost-effective in a manner consistent with low morbidity as it helps prevent clinically relevant cerebral infarctions.
- IOA in the era of ICG: development of microscope-based ICG was an important landmark in neurovascular surgery [20]. ICG enables for simple, easy intraoperative control of vessel patency and aneurysm obliteration. However, thorough evaluation of ICG in aneurysm surgery yielded some disconcordance between ICG and intra- or postoperative control angiograms. Reasons include the "field of view" problem of ICG and its weakness for low-flow detection (e.g., residual inflow to an aneurysm) [48-50].

Devoid of intraoperative imaging modalities yielding comparable diagnostic accuracy, nowadays associated with a low complication rate IOA still remains a valuable tool in neurovascular surgery, especially in aneurysm surgery. Klopfenstein [51], in a comparison of routine and selective use of IOA during aneurysm surgery concluded, that "given the frequency of significant disease that remains undetected if IOA is used on a selective basis and the low complication rate associated with the procedure, the use of IOA should be considered in the majority of aneurysm cases". To put it into the right light: we are far away of considering IOA as a standard in aneurysm surgery. But it proves to be very helpful, especially in large aneurysms, tailored approaches and aneurysms previously treated endovascularly.

Intraoperative Electrophysiology

In a series of 50 unruptured large and giant aneurysms Takebayashi [52] evaluated the utility of MEP monitoring (direct cortical stimulation) with a focus on the correlation of MEP changes during surgery and postoperative motor function. The study demonstrated a good correlation of MEP recordings and postoperative motor outcome: Preserved MEPs during surgery were always correlated with good motor outcome regardless of duration of temporary vessel occlusion. On the other hand permanent loss of MEPs during the surgical course was always followed by severe and permanent motor deficits.

Unfortunately the validity of intraoperative monitoring during vascular neurosurgical procedures is considered rather low compared to brain tumor surgery. Wicks et al. [53] for example, in a recent consecutive series of 691 patients determining accuracy of SSEP changes in predicting postoperative stroke rate reported positive and negative predictive values of 30% and 94% respectively. In Szelenyi's series using MEP recordings [54, 55] a relatively high rate of false negative results with motor evoked potentials (MEP) (postoperative motor deficits without intraoperative MEP changes) occurred. These findings were especially ascribed to delayed neurological deficits caused by lacunar infarction from perforating arteries. Hence development of lacunar infarcts may take longer than 12 hours [56] these could not be detected with intraoperative recordings.

Though intraoperative neuromonitoring during cerebral aneurysm surgery is not standard today, especially MEP recordings seem to be a rather robust prognostic factor for postoperative motor outcome. SEP´s and MEP´s may give real-time feedback regarding the individual ischemic tolerance e.g., during temporary clipping. Although not always possible, alterations in monitoring may initiate an alternative surgical strategy (e.g., clip alteration, additional bypass) and therefore have the potential to improve operative safety [54].

References

[1] Lawton MT. Seven Aneurysms. Tenets and Techniques for Clipping, Thieme, New York, Stuttgart, 2011: 1-240.

[2] McDougall, CG; Spetzler, RF; Zabramski, JM; Partovi, S; Hills, NK; Nakaji, P; et al. The Barrow Ruptured Aneurysm Trial. *J Neurosurg*., 2012 Jan, 116(1), 135–44.

[3] Spetzler, RF; McDougall, CG; Albuquerque, FC; Zabramski, JM; Hills, NK; Partovi, S; et al. The Barrow Ruptured Aneurysm Trial: 3-year results. *J Neurosurg*., 2013 Jul, 119(1), 146–57.

[4] Spetzler, RF; McDougall, CG; Zabramski, JM; Albuquerque, FC; Hills, NK; Russin, JJ; et al. The Barrow Ruptured Aneurysm Trial: 6-year results. *J Neurosurg*., 2015 Sep, 123(3), 609–17.

[5] Ayling, OGS; Ibrahim, GM; Drake, B; Torner, JC; Macdonald, RL. Operative complications and differences in outcome after clipping and coiling of ruptured intracranial aneurysms. *J Neurosurg*., 2015 Sep, 123(3), 621–8.

[6] Moon, K; Levitt, MR; Almefty, RO; Nakaji, P; Albuquerque, FC; Zabramski, JM; et al. Treatment of Ruptured Anterior Communicating Artery Aneurysms: Equipoise in the Endovascular Era? *Neurosurgery*., 2015 Oct, 77(4), 566–71.

[7] Mahaney, KB; Todd, MM; Bayman, EO; Torner, JC. IHAST Investigators. Acute postoperative neurological deterioration associated with surgery for ruptured intracranial aneurysm: incidence, predictors, and outcomes. *J Neurosurg*., 2012 Jun, 116(6), 1267–78.

[8] Ayling, OGS; Ibrahim, GM; Drake, B; Torner, JC; Macdonald, RL. Operative complications and differences in outcome after clipping and coiling of ruptured intracranial aneurysms. *J Neurosurg*., 2015 Sep, 123(3), 621–8.

[9] Dehdashti, AR; Mermillod, B; Rufenacht, DA; Reverdin, A; de Tribolet, N. Does treatment modality of intracranial ruptured aneurysms influence the incidence of cerebral vasospasm and clinical outcome? Cerebrovasc Dis. Karger Publishers, 2004, 17(1), 53–60.

[10] Dorhout Mees, SM; Kerr, RS; Rinkel, GJE; Algra, A; Molyneux, AJ. Occurrence and impact of delayed cerebral ischemia after coiling and after clipping in the International Subarachnoid Aneurysm Trial (ISAT). *J Neurol.* Springer-Verlag, 2012 Apr, 259(4), 679–83.

[11] Molyneux, A; Kerr, R; Stratton, I; Sandercock, P; Clarke, M; Shrimpton, J; et al. International Subarachnoid Aneurysm Trial (ISAT) of neurosurgical clipping versus endovascular coiling in 2143 patients with ruptured intracranial aneurysms: a randomised trial. *Lancet*., 2002 Oct 26, 360(9342), 1267–74.

[12] Lin, N; Cahill, KS; Frerichs, KU; Friedlander, RM; Claus, EB. Treatment of ruptured and unruptured cerebral aneurysms in the USA: a paradigm shift. *J Neurointerv Surg*. BMJ Publishing Group Ltd, 2012 May, 4(3), 182–9.

[13] Spetzler, RF; Sanai, N. The quiet revolution: retractorless surgery for complex vascular and skull base lesions. *J Neurosurg*., 2012 Feb, 116(2), 291–300.

[14] Lanzino, G. Retractorless brain surgery. *J Neurosurg*., 2012 Feb, 116(2), 290–0.

[15] Fischer, G; Oertel, J; Perneczky, A. Endoscopy in aneurysm surgery. *Neurosurgery*., 2012 Jun, 70(2 Suppl Operative), 184–90–discussion190–1.

[16] Yoshioka, H; Kinouchi, H. The Roles of Endoscope in Aneurysmal Surgery. *Neurol Med Chir (Tokyo)*., 2015, 55(6), 469–78.

[17] Yue, Q; Zhu, W; Gu, Y; Xu, B; Lang, L; Song, J; et al. Motor evoked potential monitoring during surgery of middle cerebral artery aneurysms: a cohort study. *WNEU*. Elsevier, 2014 Dec, 82(6), 1091–9.

[18] Nakaji, P. Motor-evoked potentials in cerebral aneurysm surgery. *WNEU*. Elsevier, 2015 Feb, 83(2), 162–3.

[19] Chalouhi, N; Theofanis, T; Jabbour, P; Dumont, AS; Fernando Gonzalez, L; Starke, RM; et al. Safety and efficacy of intraoperative angiography in craniotomies for cerebral aneurysms and arteriovenous malformations: a review of 1093 consecutive cases. *Neurosurgery*., 2012 Dec, 71(6), 1162–9.

[20] Raabe, A; Beck, J; Gerlach, R; Zimmermann, M; Seifert, V. Near-infrared indocyanine green video angiography: a new method for intraoperative assessment of vascular flow. *Neurosurgery*., 2003 Jan, 52(1), 132–9–discussion139.

[21] Raabe, A; Nakaji, P; Beck, J; Kim, LJ; Hsu, FPK; Kamerman, JD; et al. Prospective evaluation of surgical microscope-integrated intraoperative near-infrared indocyanine green videoangiography during aneurysm surgery. *J Neurosurg. Journal of Neurosurgery Publishing Group*, 2005 Dec, 103(6), 982–9.

[22] Raabe, A; Beck, J; Seifert, V. Technique and image quality of intraoperative indocyanine green angiography during aneurysm surgery using surgical microscope integrated near-infrared video technology. Zentralbl Neurochir. © Georg Thieme Verlag Stuttgart · New York, 2005 Feb, 66(1), 1–6–discussion7–8.

[23] de Gans, K; Nieuwkamp, DJ; Rinkel, GJE; Algra, A. Timing of aneurysm surgery in subarachnoid hemorrhage: a systematic review of the literature. *Neurosurgery*., 2002 Feb, 50(2), 336–40–discussion340–2.

[24] Zipfel, GJ. Editorial: Ultra-early surgery for aneurysmal subarachnoid hemorrhage. *J Neurosurg*., 2015 Feb, 122(2), 381–2.

[25] Velly, LJ; Bilotta, F; Fàbregas, N; Soehle, M; Bruder, NJ; Nathanson, MH; et al. Anaesthetic and ICU management of aneurysmal subarachnoid haemorrhage: A survey of European practice. *Eur J Anaesthesiol*., 2015 Mar, 32(3), 168–76.

[26] Leipzig, TJ; Morgan, J; Horner, TG; Payner, T; Redelman, K; Johnson, CS. Analysis of intraoperative rupture in the surgical treatment of 1694 saccular aneurysms. *Neurosurgery*., 2005 Mar, 56(3), 455–68–discussion 455–68.

[27] Griessenauer, CJ; Poston, TL; Shoja, MM; Mortazavi, MM; Falola, M; Tubbs, RS; et al. Peer-Review Reports. *WNEU*. Elsevier Inc, 2013 Jun 17, 1–9.

[28] Yamada, S; Ishikawa, M; Yamamoto, K; Ino, T; Kimura, T; Kobayashi, S; et al. Aneurysm location and clipping versus coiling for development of secondary normal-

pressure hydrocephalus after aneurysmal subarachnoid hemorrhage: Japanese Stroke DataBank. *J Neurosurg*., 2015 Jul 31, 1–7.

[29] Perneczky, A; Kindel, S; Kanno, T; Tschabitscher, M; Reisch, R. Keyhole Approaches in Neurosurgery. *S*pringer Science and Business Media, 2009. 1 p.

[30] Marinho, P; Thines, L; Verscheure, L; Mordon, S; Lejeune, JP; Vermandel, M. Recent advances in cerebrovascular simulation and neuronavigation for the optimization of intracranial aneurysm clipping. *Computer Aided Surgery*., 2015 Apr 12, 17(2), 47–55.

[31] Abla, AA; Lawton, MT. Three-dimensional hollow intracranial aneurysm models and their potential role for teaching, simulation, and training. *WNEU.* Elsevier, 2015 Jan, 83(1), 35–6.

[32] Weinstock, P; Prabhu, SP; Flynn, K; Orbach, DB; Smith, E. Optimizing cerebrovascular surgical and endovascular procedures in children via personalized 3D printing. *J Neurosurg Pediatr. American Association of Neurological Surgeons*, 2015 Jul 31, 1–6.

[33] Aoun, RJN; Hamade, YJ; Zammar, SG; Patel, NP; Bendok, BR. Futuristic 3D Printing and Personalized Neurosurgery. *WNEU.* Elsevier, 2015 Aug 20, 0(0).

[34] Rosenørn, J; Diemer, NH. Reduction of regional cerebral blood flow during brain retraction pressure in the rat. *J Neurosurg. Journal of Neurosurgery Publishing Group*, 1982 Jun, 56(6), 826–9.

[35] Rosenørn, J; Diemer, NH. The influence of intermittent versus continuous brain retractor pressure on regional cerebral blood flow and neuropathology in the rat. *Acta Neurochir*., 1988, 93(1-2), 13–7.

[36] Rosenørn, J; Diemer, NH. The influence of the profile of brain retractors on regional cerebral blood flow in the rat. *Acta Neurochir*., 1987, 87(3-4), 140–3.

[37] Xu, W; Mellergård, P; Ungerstedt, U; Nordström, C-H. Local changes in cerebral energy metabolism due to brain retraction during routine neurosurgical procedures. *Acta Neurochir.* Springer-Verlag, 2002 Jul, 144(7), 679–83.

[38] Bartal, AD; Tirosh, MS; Weinstein, M. Angiographic control during total excision of a cerebral arteriovenous malformation. Technical note. *J Neurosurg*., 1968 Aug, 29(2), 211–3.

[39] Lazar, ML; Watts, CC; Kilgore, B; Clark, K. Cerebral angiography during operation for intracranial aneurysms and arteriovenous malformations. Technical note. *J Neurosurg*., 1971 May, 34(5), 706–8.

[40] Drake, CG; Vanderlinden, RG. The late consequences of incomplete surgical treatment of cerebral aneurysms. *J Neurosurg*., 1967 Sep, 27(3), 226–38.

[41] Chiang, VL; Gailloud, P; Murphy, KJ; Rigamonti, D; Tamargo, RJ. Routine intraoperative angiography during aneurysm surgery. *J Neurosurg*., 2002 Jun, 96(6), 988–92.

[42] Vitaz, TW; Gaskill-Shipley, M; Tomsick, T; Tew, JM. Utility, safety, and accuracy of intraoperative angiography in the surgical treatment of aneurysms and arteriovenous malformations. *AJNR Am J Neuroradiol*., 1999 Sep, 20(8), 1457–61.

[43] Martin, NA; Bentson, J; Viñuela, F; Hieshima, G; Reicher, M; Black, K; et al. Intraoperative digital subtraction angiography and the surgical treatment of intracranial aneurysms and vascular malformations. *J Neurosurg*., 1990 Oct, 73(4), 526–33.

[44] Martin, N; Doberstein, C; Bentson, J; Viñuela, F; Dion, J; Becker, D. Intraoperative angiography in cerebrovascular surgery. *Clin Neurosurg*., 1991, 37, 312–31.

[45] Schaller, K; Cabrilo, I; Pereira, VM; Bijlenga, P. [Hybrid operation theatre from the perspective of neurosurgery]. *Chirurg.*, 2013 Dec, 84(12), 1041–7.

[46] Kotowski, M; Sarrafzadeh, A; Schatlo, B; Boex, C; Narata, AP; Pereira, VM; et al. Intraoperative angiography reloaded: a new hybrid operating theater for combined endovascular and surgical treatment of cerebral arteriovenous malformations: a pilot study on 25 patients. *Acta Neurochir.*, 2013 Nov, 155(11), 2071–8.

[47] Kallmes, DF; Kallmes, MH. Cost-effectiveness of angiography performed during surgery for ruptured intracranial aneurysms. *AJNR Am J Neuroradiol.*, 1997 Sep, 18(8), 1453–62.

[48] Caplan, JM; Sankey, E; Yang, W; Radvany, MG; Colby, GP; Coon, AL; et al. Impact of indocyanine green videoangiography on rate of clip adjustments following intraoperative angiography. *Neurosurgery.*, 2014 Oct, 75(4), 437–43–disucssion444.

[49] Kulwin, C; Cohen-Gadol, AA. False-negative indocyanine green videoangiography among complex unruptured middle cerebral artery aneurysms: the importance of further aneurysm inspection. *Br J Neurosurg.*, 2014 Oct, 28(5), 658–62.

[50] Sharma, M; Ambekar, S; Ahmed, O; Nixon, M; Sharma, A; Nanda, A; et al. The utility and limitations of intraoperative near-infrared indocyanine green videoangiography in aneurysm surgery. *WNEU.* Elsevier, 2014 Nov, 82(5), e607–13.

[51] Klopfenstein, JD; Spetzler, RF; Kim, LJ; Feiz-Erfan, I; Han, PP; Zabramski, JM; et al. Comparison of routine and selective use of intraoperative angiography during aneurysm surgery: a prospective assessment. *J Neurosurg.*, 2004 Feb, 100(2), 230–5.

[52] Takebayashi, S; Kamiyama, H; Takizawa, K; Kobayashi, T; Saitoh, N. The Significance of Intraoperative Monitoring of Muscle Motor Evoked Potentials during Unruptured Large and Giant Cerebral Aneurysm Surgery. *Neurol Med Chir (Tokyo).*, 2014, 54(3), 180–8.

[53] Wicks, RT; Pradilla, G; Raza, SM; Hadelsberg, U; Coon, AL; Huang, J; et al. Impact of changes in intraoperative somatosensory evoked potentials on stroke rates after clipping of intracranial aneurysms. *Neurosurgery.*, 2012 May, 70(5), 1114–24–discussion1124.

[54] Szelényi, A; Langer, D; Kothbauer, K; De Camargo, AB; Flamm, ES; Deletis, V. Monitoring of muscle motor evoked potentials during cerebral aneurysm surgery: intraoperative changes and postoperative outcome. *J Neurosurg. American Association of Neurological Surgeons*, 2006 Nov, 105(5), 675–81.

[55] Szelényi, A; Langer, D; Beck, J; Raabe, A; Flamm, ES; Seifert, V; et al. Transcranial and direct cortical stimulation for motor evoked potential monitoring in intracerebral aneurysm surgery. *Neurophysiol Clin.*, 2007 Dec, 37(6), 391–8.

[56] Steinke, W; Ley, SC. Lacunar stroke is the major cause of progressive motor deficits. Stroke. Lippincott Williams and Wilkins, 2002 Jun, 33(6), 1510–6.

In: Spontaneous Subarachnoid Haemorrhage
Editors: Thomas Kapapa and Ralph König
ISBN: 978-1-63485-270-8

Chapter 11

DECOMPRESSIVE CRANIECTOMY AND ANEURYSMAL SUBARACHNOID HAEMORRHAGE

Stefan Röhrer
Department of Neurosurgery, University of Ulm, Ulm, Germeny

ABSTRACT

Cerebral vasospasm is a redoubtable complication of subarachnoid hemorrhage. Due to this cerebral infarction may be the consequence. At worst, a space-occupying infarct can develop and threaten patients life additionally which will necessitate decompressive craniectomy.

It is known that decompressive craniectomy can reduce the increased intracranial pressure, but this is often fraught with severe complications.

Keywords: cerebral vasospasm, subarachnoid hemorrhage, decompressive hemicraniectomy, cerebral oedema

PATHOPHYSIOLOGY OF CEREBRAL OEDEMA

Cerebral oedemas are categorised as being either cytotoxic or vasogenic. Pathophysiologically, cytotoxic cerebral oedema develops as a result of swollen glial cells, as well as disruption to the membranous ion pump (sodium-potassium pump) and intracellular autoregulation. The result is an enlargement of the intracellular space of the brain owing to an influx of sodium into the cells, with water and chloride ions being drawn into the intracellular environment. This type of cerebral oedema mostly occurs with intracerebral bleeding, and cerebral infarctions respectively. The worst possible consequence of the cerebral vasospasms that develop due to a ruptured cerebral aneurysm is cerebral hypoperfusion with consecutive cerebral infarctions. Such infarctions can lead to cytotoxic cerebral oedema, which in turn can result in life-threatening swelling of the brain. Conversely, vasogenic cerebral oedema develops from an impairment of the blood-brain barrier, as well as from increased permeability of the capillary vessels, which can cause the increased influx of fluid into the interstitium and, in turn, to an enlargement of the extracellular space. This can be caused by traumatic brain injury, abscesses, or brain tumours.

Indication for Decompressive Hemicraniectomy

In case of traumatic brain injury, decompressive hemicraniectomy is indicated in the event of space-occupying haemorrhage, and space-occupying cerebral oedema with a midline shift on CCT imaging of >5 mm respectively. It is indicated moreover for treating intracranial pressure that is increased to more than 25 mm Hg for 30 minutes and resistant to therapy, as well as cerebral perfusion pressure that is decreased to <50-60 mm Hg at the same time as rising intracranial pressure values.

In case of cerebral infarctions, decompressive craniectomy is indicated due to the development of a mass from secondary swelling of the infarcted cerebral tissue consistent with cytotoxic cerebral oedema. The positive clinical aspects were demonstrated by the DESTINY study.

Cerebral vasospasms with cerebral perfusion deficit can be a secondary consequence of aneurysmal subarachnoid haemorrhage. Cerebral infarctions are a tertiary complication here; at worst, a space-occupying infarct can develop which, depending on the size and the space consumed, will necessitate decompressive craniectomy.

It is known that decompressive craniectomy can reduce the increased intracranial pressure following traumatic brain injury [1] as well as after malignant middle cerebral artery infarctions [2, 3]. Cerebral oedema can accompany the initial bleed in the event of aneurysmal subarachnoid haemorrhage, but can also develop later as a result of cerebral vasospasms and consecutive infarctions. Irrespective of the point at which cerebral oedema occurs, it is known to worsen the outcome of the patient after subarachnoid haemorrhage [4, 5]. Treatment of this life-threatening form of oedema is essential, though this is often also fraught with severe complications such as infections, axonal injury or hygromas. Given that the functional outcome is unclear, especially with severe subarachnoid haemorrhage (WFNS IV-V) accompanied by extremely high intracranial pressure, aggressive therapy in the form of decompressive craniectomy is a topic of hot debate. Between 1999 and 2008, Güresir et al. studied a total of 939 patients with aneurysmal subarachnoid haemorrhage. Decompressive craniectomy was performed in 79 of these patients. The study concluded that decompressive craniectomy is an effective method of treatment for patients with increased intracranial pressure. It was also demonstrated that surgery to treat the pressure is indicated irrespective of the time at which it occurs. Such treatment can be undertaken regardless of the pathophysiology of the elevated intracranial pressure (haemorrhage, infarction or swelling) [6].

References

[1] Bullock M. R., Chesnut R., Ghajar J., Gordon D., Hartl R., Newell D. W. et al. 2006. Surgical management of acute subdural hematomas. *Neurosurgery*, 58: 16-24.

[2] Schwab S., Steiner T., Aschoff A., Schwarz S., Steiner H. H., Jansen O. et al. 1998. Early hemicraniectomy in patients with complete middle cerebral artery infarction. *Stroke*, 29: 1888-1893.

[3] Vahedi K., Hofmeijer J., Juettler E., Vicaut E., George B., Algra A. et al. 2007. Early decompressive surgery in malignant infarction of the middle cerebral artery: a pooled analysis of three randomised controlled trials. *Lancet Neurol*, 6: 215-222.

[4] Broderick J. P., Brott T. G., Duldner J. E., Tomsick T., Leach A. et al. 1994. Initial and recurrent bleeding are the major causes of death following subarachnoid hemorrhage. *Stroke*, 25: 1342-1347.

[5] Ferguson S., Macdonald R. L. 2007. Predictors of cerebral infarction in patients with aneurysmal subarachnoid hemorrhage. *Neurosurgery*, 60: 658-667.

[6] Güresir E., Schuss P., Vatter H., Raabe A., Seifert V., Beck J. 2009. Decompressive craniectomy in subarachnoid hemorrhage; *Neurosurg Focus*, 26 E4.

In: Spontaneous Subarachnoid Haemorrhage
Editors: Thomas Kapapa and Ralph König

ISBN: 978-1-63485-270-8

Chapter 12

Intensive Care: General Considerations

Thomas Kerz
Department of Neurosurgery,
Johannes Gutenberg University of Mainz,
Mainz, Germany

Abstract

There are special features of the intensive medical care of patients with SAH that are essential to outcome. American as well as European recommendations do exist, and the American Neurocritical Care Society has also published its own recommendations [1-3]. Nevertheless, a recently published survey revealed that treatments offered to such patients vary considerably. This chapter tries to summarize evidence-based recommendations relevant to therapy, sedation, blood pressure, fluids and electrolytes.

Keywords: Subarachnoid haemorrhage, intensive care therapy, cerebral vasospasm, hyponatremia, cerebral blood flow

1. Sedation

By minimising sedation in ventilated patients, the length of stay in intensive care and ventilation time can be reduced [4]. If sedation is too deep, clinical examination of neurological patients is difficult and important findings may be obscured. On the other hand, insufficient sedation can result in increased cerebral oxygen consumption and elevated intracranial pressure. Most studies and recommendations focus on patients in mixed intensive care units, whereas only few studies have been published in regard to sedated patients with neurological damage. Therefore and until further studies are available, the recommendations for patients in general ICUs should be followed. In patients in neurological intensive care, analgesia-based sedation (fentanyl or remifentanil) has achieved greater pain relief than sedatives (propofol or midazolam), albeit with an equal rate of unscheduled extubations [5].

Significant interindividual pharmacokinetic effects have been reported for midazolam in neurological patients. In one study, midazolam or its active metabolite, 1-hydroxymidazolam glucuronide, was still detectable 67 h on average after ending the midazolam infusion. By measuring the concentrations, a higher percentage of patients with neurological damage could be distinguished from those with delayed recovery, since approx. three quarters of the patients with no measurable drug concentration died due to neurological damage or were severely affected, whereas approx. three quarters of the patients with measurable concentrations recovered completely [5].

In neurological patients without an increase in intracranial pressure requiring sedation for less than five days, daily neurological evaluation could be performed sooner after sedation with remifentanil, if necessary together with propofol or midazolam, than after analgesia with fentanyl or morphine [6]. In patients with increased intracranial pressure or those requiring deep sedation due to unstable intracerebral pathologies, conventional sedatives can be administered. In a meta-analysis, no single regimen was found to offer any particular benefit over another [7]. Ketamine is no longer contraindicated – in fact, the substance is beneficial due to its sedative and analgesic properties [8]. After termination of sedation, O_2 consumption and energy turnover each increase by about 50% [5]. Withdrawal delirium is observed in approx. 15%-50% of all patients on general intensive care units [9]. No information is available on its frequency in neurointensive care patients. If vigilance deteriorates, a cranial CT scan should generally be taken to investigate the cause (hydrocephalus, secondary haemorrhage, ischaemia, etc.).

A comparison of dexmedetomidine and propofol in patients with SAH revealed that the incidence of bradycardia and hypotension is identical [10]. Whereas dexmedetomidine is often used in awake operations and has been found to convey cerebroprotective effects in animal studies, its potentially negative effect on cerebral blood flow (CBF) in humans has not yet been fully explained. Hence, no firm recommendation can be made as to its use in sedating patients with neurological conditions [11].

Inhalational anaesthetics lead to decoupling of $CMRO_2$ (cerebral metabolic rate of oxygen) and CBF, by decreasing the former and increasing the latter. In doing so, they could play a protective role against vasospasm-induced ischaemia. Isoflurane has resulted in an insignificant increase in ICP, but significant decreases in mean arterial pressure (MAP) and cerebral perfusion pressure (CPP, 6.5 and 6.3 mm Hg, respectively), despite raising the vasopressor dose [12]. The mean blood flow rates in the middle cerebral artery remained unchanged. In another study that compared isoflurane with propofol, regional CBF measured by thermodiffusion was markedly increased [13]. In approximately one third of patients, sevoflurane resulted in severe adverse reactions, including an elevation in ICP and a drop in MAP and CPP, necessitating discontinuation of drug administration [14].

Conclusion: All sedatives conventionally used in intensive care patients can also be applied in SAH patients.

2. Blood Pressure and Fluids

Blood pressure and cardiac output play a pivotal role in terms of cerebral perfusion. Acute SAH is regularly associated with reduced cerebral autoregulation. Hence, CBF is directly related to MAP and cannot be maintained at a constant level by the cerebral vessels.

Triple H therapy, consisting of hypervolaemia, hypertension and haemodilution, has long been used as a means of increasing CBF in the presence of vasospasm. In the only available randomised study on this subject, however, hypervolaemia did not lead to an improvement either in CBF or the neurological outcome [5]. Prophylactic volume expansion and hyperdynamic therapy, even when introduced before development of vasospasm and after securing the aneurysm, also had no positive effect on CBF and no clinical benefit as compared to normovolaemia [15]. Only isolated case reports have demonstrated that such therapy is beneficial. The target values in such a case were a systolic pressure of 160 mm Hg before clipping the aneurysm and 240 mm Hg after, respectively [16]. However, significant adverse effects have also been reported: pulmonary oedema, hyponatraemia, secondary haemorrhage and coagulopathies. With respect to blood pressure management, randomised studies are lacking. Whereas dopamine was used in most of the earlier studies, phenylephrine, dobutamine or noradrenaline have been the focus of more recent studies, and vasopressin was also studied in another. Case series and cohort studies suggest that CBF is increased by approx. 10 ml · 100g-1 · ml-1 as a result of adjusting hypertensive blood pressure levels (systolic 160-200 mm Hg). Miller et al. reported an 88% improvement in the neurological deficits of their patients if hypertensive treatment was not commenced until after onset of the symptoms [17]. Neurological improvement was noted in 71% of patients in another study in which normovolaemic hypertension was modified to 25%-50% above the normal arterial systolic blood pressure by dopamine and dobutamine [18]. In line with these findings, CBF and cerebral oxygen tension ($PtiO_2$) increased as a result of hypertensive therapy [19], whilst hypervolaemia was associated with an increased rate of adverse reactions (pulmonary oedema, heart failure) [20]. Two studies have demonstrated that the CBF can be increased in patients with severe SAH by administering hypertonic saline [21, 22]. With respect to blood pressure and the treatment of concomitant Takotsubo cardiomyopathy [23, 24], levosimendan [25] or intra-aortic counterpulsation [26, 27] have been used in isolated cases. Therapeutic anticoagulation is necessary in case of the latter, however. In patients with further aneurysms in addition to a haemorrhaged and occluded aneurysm, induced hypertension with CPP values between 80 and 120 mm Hg (MAP 90-130 mm Hg) was not associated with an increased rate of bleeding [28]. Noradrenaline was mainly used in this study, if needed in combination with dopamine or dobutamine.

The study group of the Neurocritical Care Society recommends maintaining euvolaemia and avoiding prophylactic hypervolaemia. Isotonic solutions should be used for fluid replacement. If a negative fluid balance persists, hydrocortisone or fludrocortisone can be considered [2]. In general, higher blood pressure is accompanied by increased CBF; most studies noted an improvement in the neurological deficit in approx. two thirds of patients.

Conclusion: Isotonic solutions should be used for replacing fluids. Euvolaemia should be the goal.

3. Electrolytes

Hyponatraemia is the most common form of electrolyte imbalance in SAH. It can occur with euvolaemia, hypervolaemia or hypovolaemia. The most common cause for euvolaemic or hypervolaemic hyponatraemia is the inadequate secretion of antidiuretic hormone (ADH). Since it is not always possible to detect an excessive ADH concentration, the term "syndrome of inadequate antidiuresis" (SIAD) has been coined lately. Other signs are a urine osmolality of > 100 mOsm/kg and a urinary sodium concentration of > 30 mmol/L. The levels generally return to normal if water is restricted. To measure the increased reabsorption rate of sodium, fractional sodium excretion (> 0.5%) is appropriate but can be falsified by the administration of diuretics. Fractional uric acid excretion has a positive predictor rate for SIAD of 100% at a cut-off of > 12% and is not distorted by diuretics [5].

Hypovolaemic hyponatraemia thus is usually accompanied by a urinary sodium concentration of < 30 mmol/L, fractional sodium excretion of < 0.5%, and fractional uric acid excretion of < 12%. Differentiation is complicated, however, as excessive diuresis and excessive reabsorption of free water sometimes occur simultaneously [29].

Determination of volume status is crucial to therapy, since hypervolaemic patients require diuresis whereas in euvolaemia it would lead to unwanted fluid deficiency. Drug-wise, fludrocortisone and hydrocortisone can be administered. Hypertonic saline solutions or enteral administration of saline are likewise possible. Vasopressin receptor antagonists, such as tolvaptan, lead to ofree water clearance but can also cause excessive diuresis and therefore should only be used whilst closely monitoring the volume status [5].

Studies and meta-analyses have not found prophylactic treatment with magnesium to be beneficial in preventing a delayed ischaemic neurological deficit (DIND, [30]). The benefit in terms of avoiding hypomagnesaemia also has not been adequately demonstrated [31].

Conclusion: A thorough investigation of the causes and appropriate therapy are required if hyponatraemia is to be avoided. Magnesium replacement cannot be recommended.

References

[1] Bederson JB, Connolly ES, Jr., Batjer HH, Dacey RG, Dion JE, Diringer MN, et al. Guidelines for the management of aneurysmal subarachnoid hemorrhage: a statement for healthcare professionals from a special writing group of the Stroke Council, American Heart Association. Stroke. 2009;40(3):994-1025.

[2] Diringer MN, Bleck TP, Claude Hemphill J, 3rd, Menon D, Shutter L, Vespa P, et al. Critical care management of patients following aneurysmal subarachnoid hemorrhage: recommendations from the Neurocritical Care Society's Multidisciplinary Consensus Conference. Neurocrit Care. 2011;15(2):211-40.

[3] Steiner T, Juvela S, Unterberg A, Jung C, Forsting M, Rinkel G, et al. European Stroke Organization guidelines for the management of intracranial aneurysms and subarachnoid haemorrhage. Cerebrovasc Dis. 2013;35(2):93-112.

[4] Velly LJ, Bilotta F, Fabregas N, Soehle M, Bruder NJ, Nathanson MH, et al. Anaesthetic and ICU management of aneurysmal subarachnoid haemorrhage: a survey of European practice. Eur J Anaesthesiol. 2015;32(3):168-76.

[5] Barr J, Fraser GL, Puntillo K, Ely EW, Gelinas C, Dasta JF, et al. Clinical practice guidelines for the management of pain, agitation, and delirium in adult patients in the intensive care unit. Crit Care Med. 2013;41(1):263-306.

[6] Egerod I, Jensen MB, Herling SF, Welling KL. Effect of an analgo-sedation protocol for neurointensive patients: a two-phase interventional non-randomized pilot study. Crit Care. 2010;14(2):R71.

[7] McKenzie CA, McKinnon W, Naughton DP, Treacher D, Davies G, Phillips GJ, et al. Differentiating midazolam over-sedation from neurological damage in the intensive care unit. Crit Care. 2005;9(1):R32-6.

[8] Karabinis A, Mandragos K, Stergiopoulos S, Komnos A, Soukup J, Speelberg B, et al. Safety and efficacy of analgesia-based sedation with remifentanil versus standard hypnotic-based regimens in intensive care unit patients with brain injuries: a randomised, controlled trial [ISRCTN50308308]. Crit Care. 2004;8(4):R268-80.

[9] Roberts DJ, Hall RI, Kramer AH, Robertson HL, Gallagher CN, Zygun DA. Sedation for critically ill adults with severe traumatic brain injury: a systematic review of randomized controlled trials. Crit Care Med. 2011;39(12):2743-51.

[10] Himmelseher S, Durieux ME. Revising a dogma: ketamine for patients with neurological injury? Anesth Analg. 2005;101(2):524-34, table of contents.

[11] Bruder N, Lassegue D, Pelissier D, Graziani N, Francois G. Energy expenditure and withdrawal of sedation in severe head-injured patients. Crit Care Med. 1994;22(7):1114-9.

[12] Jaber S, Chanques G, Altairac C, Sebbane M, Vergne C, Perrigault PF, et al. A prospective study of agitation in a medical-surgical ICU: incidence, risk factors, and outcomes. Chest. 2005;128(4):2749-57.

[13] Erdman MJ, Doepker BA, Gerlach AT, Phillips GS, Elijovich L, Jones GM. A comparison of severe hemodynamic disturbances between dexmedetomidine and propofol for sedation in neurocritical care patients. Crit Care Med. 2014;42(7):1696-702.

[14] Farag E. Dexmedetomidine in the neurointensive care unit. Discov Med. 2010;9(44):42-5.

[15] Bosel J, Purrucker JC, Nowak F, Renzland J, Schiller P, Perez EB, et al. Volatile isoflurane sedation in cerebrovascular intensive care patients using AnaConDa((R)): effects on cerebral oxygenation, circulation, and pressure. Intensive Care Med. 2012;38(12):1955-64.

[16] Villa F, Iacca C, Molinari AF, Giussani C, Aletti G, Pesenti A, et al. Inhalation versus endovenous sedation in subarachnoid hemorrhage patients: effects on regional cerebral blood flow. Crit Care Med. 2012;40(10):2797-804.

[17] Purrucker JC, Renzland J, Uhlmann L, Bruckner T, Hacke W, Steiner T, et al. Volatile sedation with sevoflurane in intensive care patients with acute stroke or subarachnoid haemorrhage using AnaConDa(R): an observational studydagger. Br J Anaesth. 2015;114(6):934-43.

[18] Lennihan L, Mayer SA, Fink ME, Beckford A, Paik MC, Zhang H, et al. Effect of hypervolemic therapy on cerebral blood flow after subarachnoid hemorrhage : a randomized controlled trial. Stroke. 2000;31(2):383-91.

[19] Egge A, Waterloo K, Sjoholm H, Solberg T, Ingebrigtsen T, Romner B. Prophylactic hyperdynamic postoperative fluid therapy after aneurysmal subarachnoid hemorrhage: a

clinical, prospective, randomized, controlled study. Neurosurgery. 2001;49(3):593-605; discussion -6.

[20] Kassell NF, Peerless SJ, Durward QJ, Beck DW, Drake CG, Adams HP. Treatment of ischemic deficits from vasospasm with intravascular volume expansion and induced arterial hypertension. Neurosurgery. 1982;11(3):337-43.

[21] Miller JA, Dacey RG, Jr., Diringer MN. Safety of hypertensive hypervolemic therapy with phenylephrine in the treatment of delayed ischemic deficits after subarachnoid hemorrhage. Stroke. 1995;26(12):2260-6.

[22] Otsubo H, Takemae T, Inoue T, Kobayashi S, Sugita K. Normovolaemic induced hypertension therapy for cerebral vasospasm after subarachnoid haemorrhage. Acta Neurochir (Wien). 1990;103(1-2):18-26.

[23] Muench E, Horn P, Bauhuf C, Roth H, Philipps M, Hermann P, et al. Effects of hypervolemia and hypertension on regional cerebral blood flow, intracranial pressure, and brain tissue oxygenation after subarachnoid hemorrhage. Crit Care Med. 2007;35(8):1844-51; quiz 52.

[24] Raabe A, Beck J, Keller M, Vatter H, Zimmermann M, Seifert V. Relative importance of hypertension compared with hypervolemia for increasing cerebral oxygenation in patients with cerebral vasospasm after subarachnoid hemorrhage. J Neurosurg. 2005;103(6):974-81.

[25] Tseng MY, Al-Rawi PG, Czosnyka M, Hutchinson PJ, Richards H, Pickard JD, et al. Enhancement of cerebral blood flow using systemic hypertonic saline therapy improves outcome in patients with poor-grade spontaneous subarachnoid hemorrhage. J Neurosurg. 2007;107(2):274-82.

[26] Tseng MY, Al-Rawi PG, Pickard JD, Rasulo FA, Kirkpatrick PJ. Effect of hypertonic saline on cerebral blood flow in poor-grade patients with subarachnoid hemorrhage. Stroke. 2003;34(6):1389-96.

[27] Lee VH, Connolly HM, Fulgham JR, Manno EM, Brown RD, Jr., Wijdicks EF. Takotsubo cardiomyopathy in aneurysmal subarachnoid hemorrhage: an underappreciated ventricular dysfunction. J Neurosurg. 2006;105(2):264-70.

[28] Wybraniec MT, Mizia-Stec K, Krzych L. Neurocardiogenic injury in subarachnoid hemorrhage: A wide spectrum of catecholamin-mediated brain-heart interactions. Cardiol J. 2014;21(3):220-8.

[29] Busani S, Rinaldi L, Severino C, Cobelli M, Pasetto A, Girardis M. Levosimendan in cardiac failure after subarachnoid hemorrhage. J Trauma. 2010;68(5):E108-10.

[30] Apostolides PJ, Greene KA, Zabramski JM, Fitzgerald JW, Spetzler RF. Intra-aortic balloon pump counterpulsation in the management of concomitant cerebral vasospasm and cardiac failure after subarachnoid hemorrhage: technical case report. Neurosurgery. 1996;38(5):1056-9; discussion 9-60.

[31] Lazaridis C, Pradilla G, Nyquist PA, Tamargo RJ. Intra-aortic balloon pump counterpulsation in the setting of subarachnoid hemorrhage, cerebral vasospasm, and neurogenic stress cardiomyopathy. Case report and review of the literature. Neurocrit Care. 2010;13(1):101-8.

[32] Platz J, Guresir E, Vatter H, Berkefeld J, Seifert V, Raabe A, et al. Unsecured intracranial aneurysms and induced hypertension in cerebral vasospasm: is induced hypertension safe? Neurocrit Care. 2011;14(2):168-75.

[33] Fenske W, Stork S, Koschker AC, Blechschmidt A, Lorenz D, Wortmann S, et al. Value of fractional uric acid excretion in differential diagnosis of hyponatremic patients on diuretics. J Clin Endocrinol Metab. 2008;93(8):2991-7.

[34] Audibert G, Steinmann G, de Talance N, Laurens MH, Dao P, Baumann A, et al. Endocrine response after severe subarachnoid hemorrhage related to sodium and blood volume regulation. Anesth Analg. 2009;108(6):1922-8.

[35] Murphy T, Dhar R, Diringer M. Conivaptan bolus dosing for the correction of hyponatremia in the neurointensive care unit. Neurocrit Care. 2009;11(1):14-9.

[36] Reddy D, Fallah A, Petropoulos JA, Farrokhyar F, Macdonald RL, Jichici D. Prophylactic magnesium sulfate for aneurysmal subarachnoid hemorrhage: a systematic review and meta-analysis. Neurocrit Care. 2014;21(2):356-64.

[37] de Rooij NK, Rinkel GJ, Dankbaar JW, Frijns CJ. Delayed cerebral ischemia after subarachnoid hemorrhage: a systematic review of clinical, laboratory, and radiological predictors. Stroke. 2013;44(1):43-54.

In: Spontaneous Subarachnoid Haemorrhage
Editors: Thomas Kapapa and Ralph König
ISBN: 978-1-63485-270-8

Chapter 13

INTENSIVE CARE: MONITORING

Werner Klingler[1,2] and Dirk Repkewitz[2]
[1]Division of Neurophysiology, Ulm University, Ulm, Germany
[2]Department of Neuroanaesthesiology, Neurosurgical Ulm University hospital, Guenzburg, Germany

ABSTRACT

Besides direct and indirect cerebral lesions, subarachnoid haemorrhage (SAH) may cause severe alterations of metabolism as well as cardiac, pulmonary and other medical complications. Specialized intensive care is required to improve neurological outcome and overall survival. This chapter covers monitoring of patients suffering from SAH in the intensive care unit (ICU). Prudent observation and evaluation of these parameters helps to manage the course of disease.

INTRODUCTION

Intensive care in specialized neurocritical care centers is associated with a lower mortality and better outcome in SAH compared to general ICU's (Kurtz et al. 2011). Multimodal cerebral monitoring including clinical examination, assessment of cerebral perfusion, intracranial pressure and other specific parameters is essential for an individualized treatment plan and for prevention of secondary brain injury (Figure 1). This chapter focuses on ICU monitoring after the initial SAH. In this critical time interval there is a high risk for re-bleeding, epileptic seizures and/or delayed cerebral ischemia (DCI) due to vasospasm. Indeed, vasospasm can occur up to roughly 20 days after the initial event and is assoiated to mortality, functional and cognitive disability (Le Roux et al. 2014, Lantigua et al. 2015).

Despite the brain weighs only roughly 2% of lean body mass, it is allocated 20% of cardiac output at rest. Perfusion and oxygenation are crucial for cerebral energy metabolism, which is primarily based on glucose degradation and the respiratory chain. Early detection of an imbalance between cerebral oxygen supply and demand is relevant to outcome in these patients (Diringer et al. 2009).

Clinical Examination

Whereas the initial presentation of SAH is characterized by severe headache, meningism and neurological impairment, the later course of symptoms varies significantly, most notably during ICU treatment. Here, detection of re-bleeding and vasospasm is of vital importance. Clinical examination of SAH patients is fast and focuses on vital signs, level of consciousness and motor responses. Asymmetric motor responses or partial epileptic seizures may be an indication of focal brain lesion hinting towards vasospasm. In awake patients one of the first signs of a developing vasospasm usually are cognitive deficits such as an attention deficit or change in conscious state. Quantification of the level of consciousness is best achieved by structured assessment of sedation and agitation. Several clinical grading scales have been developed. The Glasgow Coma Scale is widely known, however it is only validated for traumatic brain injury. Instead, the Richmond Agitation Sedation Scale (RASS) is designed for ICU use and has the advantage of a high validity and interrater reliability (Ely et al. 2003).

In unconscious patients, a key element is the examination of the pupillary light reflex, which integrates the optic and oculomotor nerves and brainstem nuclei. Instrument-based documentation of pupillary function is commercially available. The oculomotor nerve partially controls eye movements and activates the ciliary muscle, via parasympathetic fibers, i.e., miosis. The oculomotor nerve trails along the base of the brain and is especially vulnerable to direct pressure lesions or secondary damage. Up to one third of SAH patients show intraocular hemorrhage, known as Terson´s syndrome. This phenomenon likely occurs due to elevated ICP. Other symptoms of elevated ICP include cephalgia, nausea and vomiting including cranial nerve palsies. Indeed, persistent ocular divergence, ocular bobbing, lack of pupillary light reflex, unequal or irregular pupils are signs of severe brain damage and associated with poor neurological prognosis. Damage of the autonomous nuclei in the brainstem leads to pathological breathing patterns, cardiac arrhythmia and finally death (Miyata et al. 2014).

Monitoring of the Intracranial Pressure (ICP)

ICP monitoring allows an estimation of cerebral perfusion by calculating the perfusion pressure as the difference between mean arterial pressure and ICP (see chapter 13).

In over 90% of SAH patients some degree of elevated ICP is found, mainly within the first 8 days after the bleeding. The Hunt and Hess grade correlates with the degree of ICP elevation. Mortality is increased in those patients, which have significantly elevated post-SAH ICP levels (Lv et al. 2015). Hence, ICP monitoring is advisable in those patients showing clinical or radiographic signs and symptoms of elevated ICP, especially in sedated patients (chapter 9). Invasive ICP monitoring is used significantly more frequently in neurocritical care units compared to general ICU´s. Whether ICP-directed therapy is causative for better outcome in these specialized units has not been shown yet (Kurtz et al. 2011). There are several methods for assessment of ICP. Most centers use ventricular catheters, which have the advantage of potential use for CSF drain in order to reduce intracranial volume and also to obtain material for microbiological analysis. Other possibilities include the insertion of a small pressure sensor via a small drill trepanation. The sensor can be placed in the epidural, subdural, subarachnoid or parenchymatous space (Diringer et al. 2011)

TRANSCRANIAL DOPPLER ULTRASONOGRAPHY (TCD)

Roughly 30 – 70% of SAH patients show radiographic evidence of vasospasm, but only half of those experience neurological symptoms. Clinical signs of vasospasm fluctuate and often are unspecific. The frequent use of sedatives in SAH patients further limits clinical evaluation (Kistka et al. 2013, Le Roux et al. 2014). Vasospasm is detected by cerebral angiography with high sensitivity and specificity. TCD bridges the gap between physiological and radiological examination. The main advantage of TCD is its non-invasive nature and bedside evaluation. However, analysis is limited to the blood supply originating from trunk of the middle cerebral artery. Technical problems such as inadequate insonation window or interrater variability account for moderate sensitivity, especially in the assessment of the outflow into the anterior cerebral artery. In other words, TCD is an easy applicable method with a high predictive value for vasospasm detection predominantly of the middle cerebral artery. Increased flow velocities (> 120cm/s), most notably in combination with clinical suspicion of vasospasm, should prompt additional investigations such as diagnostic imaging (see chapter 9).

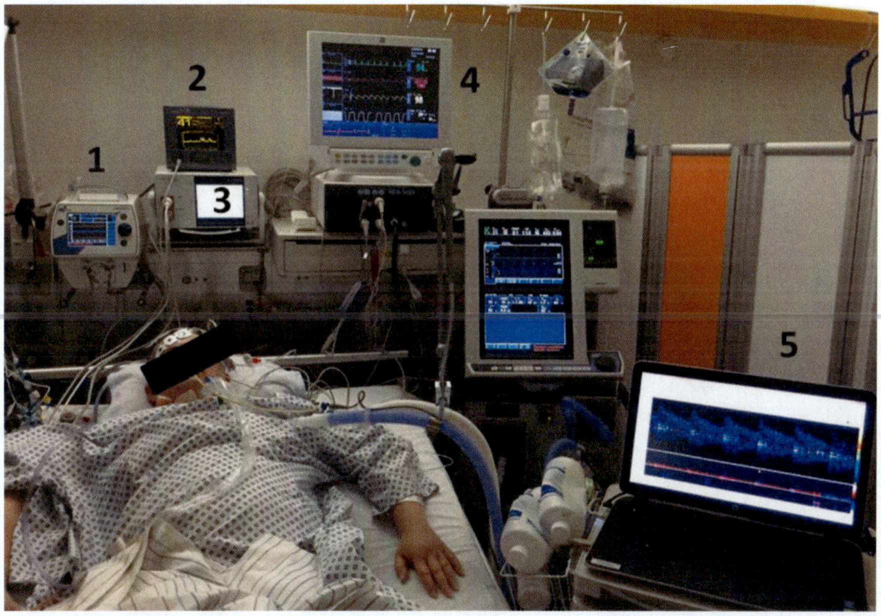

Figure 1. Neurocritical care including intracranial pressure monitoring and brain oxygenation monitoring [1], processed EEG [2], continous cardiac output monitoring [3], ECG, invasive blood pressure, SpO_2, pCO_2, temperature monitoring [4] and TCD [5].

Near-Infrared Spectroscopy (NIRS)

NIRS is another non-invasive method for estimation of cerebral perfusion. Absorption of specific near-infrared wavelengths (700-1000nm) depends on tissue oxygenation and mitochondrial oxygen metabolism. Thereby cerebral hypoperfusion, e.g., in carotid surgery or temporary clipping, can be detected intraoperatively. In the ICU, NIRS may detect vasospasm but also impairment of cerebral autoregulation. However, NIRS electrodes mainly cover the frontal lobe and are vulnerable to sweat and other obstacles impairing electrical impedance (Zweifel et al. 2010).

Brain Oxygenation Measurements and Cerebral Microdialysis

Even if cerebral perfusion pressure and other parameters are normal, neuronal metabolism may be impaired in SAH. In these conditions, an accumulation of acidic metabolites as well as a drop of brain tissue oxygenation ($ptiO_2$) and pH can be observed by tissue microdialysis. Several studies suggest a link between regional ptiO2 and vasospasm respectively impaired autoregulation. However, sample sizes are small and results not fully consistent (Kistka et al. 2012). Several metabolic markers can be measured using microdialysis. Glycolytic metabolites include glucose, lactate and pyruvate. Neuronal degradation goes along with an increase in glutamate, nitrite and taurine concentrations. These parameters as well as the lactate/pyruvate ratio may even be prognostic markers for neurological outcome (Sarrafzadeh et al. 2004). A pre-requisite and limitation is the necessity of an invasive implantation of a microcathether into the relevant brain region and the sensors are only monitoring a localized region of the brain. A modification of the above described microcatheters is a thermal diffusion flowmetry probe. This intracerebral microcathether contains a temperature sensitive electrode, which detects heat signals emitted by a gold electrode of the same device. The time delay is a measure for local cerebral blood flow (Kistka et al. 2013).

Biomarkers

The occurrence of neuronal degradation products, enzymes and specific proteins in the cerebro-spinal fluid (CSF) of SAH patients supports the concept of monitoring these biomarkers for prognostication and vasospasm detection. A well recognized feature of SAH is a centrally mediated sympathetic response. Indeed, increased CSF and blood levels of epinephrine are independent prognostic predictors of poor prognosis. One of the best studied biomarkers in SAH is the calcium-binding glial protein S100β. Brain lesions of various aetiology lead to release of S100β, which is not only found in elevated concentrations in the CSF but to a lesser extent also in peripheral blood. S100β may be a prognostic biomarker of SAH, but it does not seem to be a specific indicator for vasospasm or DCI. Neuroinflammatory response is a key element in the pathophysiology of SAH. Indeed, acute phase proteins such as C-reactive protein or cytokines, e.g., TNF-α and IL-1β are variably and asynchronously upregulated in SAH. IL-1β and other cytokines are endogenous pyrogens that impair thermoregulation. Other proteins, which are released in brain damage, are for example neuron-specific enolase, apolipoprotein E, amyloid β protein and creatine kinase BB. High CSF concentrations of those proteins may indicate poor outcome. A promising approach is the investigation of vasogenic biomarkers because there are indications, that vascular endothelial growth factor and the vasoconstrictive substance endothelin-1 is elevated in SAH (Hong et al. 2014). In conclusion, analysis of biomarkers may help for the differentiation between re-bleeding and vasospasm. Currently, its use in SAH is still limited due to the need for sophisticated laboratory technology and lack of point of care specificity.

Electrophysiological Monitoring

Vasospasm and non-convulsive epileptic seizures are frequent complications of SAH but difficult to detect in the unconscious patient. Electroencephalography (EEG) is a tool to assess electrical brain activity. The electrical signal of the EEG recording is based on summation of depolarization events in neighbouring brain cells, most notably of postsynaptic potentials of apical cortical neurons. In contrast to the ECG waveform, the registration is characterized by scattered potentials. Amplitude and and frequency of the EEG signal are indirect markers for synchronicity of neuronal excitation (Table 1). A decrease in the Alpha/Delta frequency band ratio is associated with delayed cerebral ischemia due to vasospasm (Claassen et al. 2004). EEG can also detect epileptic seizures, which in SAH patients are often a hint for aneurysmal re-bleeding. Non-convulsive seizures occur in 10-20% of comatose SAH patients and in some patients may explain unconsciousness (Kistka et al. 2013, Lantigua et al. 2015).

The question arises, whether the main goal for the prevention of DCI may be achieved by using modified EEG recordings, which are already in use for the analysis of the depth of sedation and have the advantage of easy interpretation. Processed EEG parameters, such as the bispectral index and the suppression ratio have been shown to have prognostic value concerning neurological outcome following hypoxic brain damage (Selig et al. 2014). Potential use of such devices in stroke/vasospasm detection is currently under investigation. Similarly the use of evoked potentials is still controversial for outcome prognosis or early detection of vasospasm in the ICU, although evoked potentials are frequently used during aneurysm surgery to indicate a loss of neuronal function respectively diminished local blood perfusion (Wachter et al. 2011). All discussed electrophysiological methods are difficult to integrate in the ICU due to technical pitfalls such as electrical noise fields, nursing care as well as requiring specific expertise for the application and interpretation of the complex signals (Le Roux et al. 2014).

Table 1. EEG-frequency bands and level of consciousness

Frequency range	*Label*	*Symbol*	*Level of consciousness*
0,5-4 Hz	Delta	δ	deep sedation, trance
4-8 Hz	Theta	θ	hypnosis
8-13 Hz	Alpha	α	awake, closed eyes
13-30 Hz	Beta	ß	awake, concentrated, REM sleeping cycle
30-42 Hz	Gamma	γ	high information flow

Reduced metabolic activity due to e.g., hypoxia or sedative drugs results in synchronisation of potentials and reduction of EEG frequency.

Cardio-Respiratory Monitoring

Arterial blood pressure is a hemodynamic index, most relevant for goal-directed therapy in SAH patients (chapter 13). Correct evaluation of blood pressure is not simple, there are pitfalls in the technical assessment but also since the pressure pulse waveform depends on the point of measurement. Invasive blood pressure monitoring is superior to non-invasive methods both in terms of accuracy and time restraints (Kim et al. 2014). The insertion of an arterial line is rarely associated with complications such as infection, bleeding or thrombosis. Non-invasive blood pressure readings disguise hypotensive intervals by overestimating systolic arterial blood pressure resulting in elevated ICU mortality compared to invasive blood pressure monitoring (Lehman et al. 2013).

Physiologically, systolic arterial blood pressure is roughly 20mmHg to 40mmHg higher in the legs than in the arms even in supine position. Systolic blood pressure rises and blood flow velocity decreases with increasing distance from the heart, which results in different pulse waveforms. Hence, the mean arterial pressure (MAP) as the geometric mean of the pulse wave is the best parameter for therapeutic decisions. Continuous cardiac output monitoring and evaluation of stroke volume variability may be helpful in some patients, most notably for evaluation of the dilemma volume versus adrenergic drugs (Lehman et al. 2013).

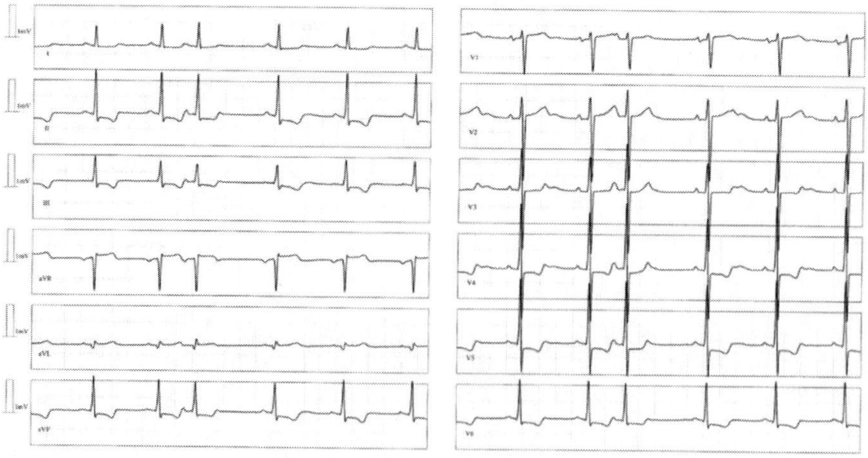

Figure 2. ECG alterations in SAH. Dysrhythmia and ST-segment abnormalities.

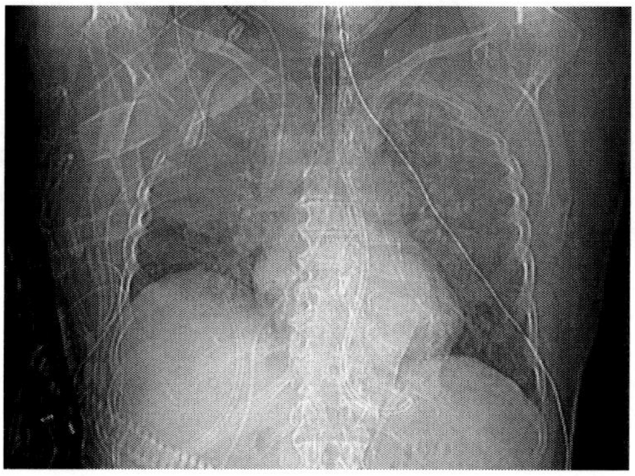

Figure 3. Neurogenic pulmonary edema.

ICU monitoring further requires continuous electrocardiographic (ECG) monitoring, because 50-100% of patients present cardiac arrhythmia and/or signs of myocardial ischemia as a consequence of the SAH induced adrenergic surge (Cushing´s reflex). ST-segment abnormalities (Figure 2) may be the primary reason for hospital admission. Myocardial stress markers, such as Troponin, N-terminal end of the prohormone brain natriuretic peptide (NTproBNP) and CK-MB may be elevated in SAH patients. Similarily, lung insufficiency of variable degree is a well recognized complication of SAH and causes up to 30% of deaths after SAH. Mascia (2009) introduced a double hit model of lung injury after severe brain lesion. The initial adrenergic reaction hits the lung by constriction of pulmonary veins resulting in pulmonary hypertension, increasing hydrostatic pressure, cardiac burden and ventilation/perfusion deficit. The second hit is mediated by a systemic inflammatory response syndrome, which not only causes an increase of the permeability in the blood-brain barrier, but also causes leaky lung capillaries. Inflammatory neuropeptides activate neutrophil infiltration into the lungs, which cause further deterioration of pulmonary function. The lungs are then even more vulnerable to mechanical stress of invasive ventilation. Apart from neurogenic pulmonary edema (Figure 3) there are other reasons impairing pulmonary function such as respiratory tract infections, aspiration, pulmonary embolisation and drugs influencing pulmonary shunt (Mascia 2009, Diringer et al. 2011, Lantigua et al. 2015). Vasodilating drugs, most notably nimodipine, hamper the physiological vasoconstriction of non- or low-ventilated alveoli, thus increasing pulmonary shunt. The above mentioned mechanisms might be one reason, why lungs are rarely viable for organ donation after severe brain injury Furthermore, pCO2 has to be monitored closely in SAH because of its key role in controlling cerebral blood flow (chapter 15).

General Considerations

General considerations in SAH include monitoring of hemoglobin and of the coagulation system for obvious reasons. A key factor in SAH monitoring are glucose levels, because there is strong evidence that hypo- as well as hyperglycemia is associated to poor neurological outcome. Further parameters include hormones and electrolyte levels (chapter 13). Tight monitoring of temperature in indispensable in SAH patients as thermoregulation is impaired in this group of patients. Neurogenic, non-infectious fever usually occurs within the first 3 days of admission and has a higher incidence poor grade SAH and in those patients with intraventricular bleeding. Common causes of infectious fever include cathether infections, respiratory tract infections or ventriculitis. Aggressive temperature control is indispensable and achieved by pharmacological and physical cooling including intravascular cooling cathethers. Surprisingly, therapeutic hypothermia has failed to show a benefit in SAH (Karnatovskaia et al. 2014). Other medical complications include thrombocytopenia, hepatic and renal dysfunction. The gastrointestinal function is often impaired due to adrenergic reflexes and neurogenic inflammatory response. Osmotic stimulation of peristalsis and early enteral nutrition is beneficial to prevent secondary complications as gastrointestinal bleeding or ileus (Diringer et al. 2011, Le Roux et al. 2014, Lantigua et al. 2015).

Summary Statement

Survival and neurological outcome after SAH depends on specific complications such as vasospasm and re-bleeding but also on a variety of general medical parameters. Specific monitoring is essential for management of SAH patients. Detection of vasospasm is essential but not trivial, because all discussed methods have limitations. Recognition and treatment of the typical medical complications of SAH is another key element in the management of SAH-patients. Hence, multimodal monitoring and specific neurocritical care is a decisive factor for overall outcome.

References

Claassen, J; Hirsch, LJ; Kreiter, KT; Du, EY; Connolly, ES; Emerson, RG; Mayer, SA. Quantitative continuous EEG for detecting delayed cerebral ischemia in patients with poor-grade subarachnoid hemorrhage. *Clin Neurophysiol.*, 2004 Dec, 115(12), 2699-710.

Diringer, MN; Bleck, TP; Claude Hemphill, J; 3rd, Menon, D; Shutter, L; Vespa, P; Bruder, N; Connolly, ES; Jr, Citerio, G; Gress, D; Hänggi, D; Hoh, BL; Lanzino, G; Le Roux, P; Rabinstein, A; Schmutzhard, E; Stocchetti, N; Suarez, JI; Treggiari, M; Tseng, MY; Vergouwen, MD; Wolf, S; Zipfel, G. Neurocritical Care Society. Critical care management of patients following aneurysmal subarachnoid hemorrhage: recommendations from the Neurocritical Care Society's Multidisciplinary Consensus Conference. *Neurocrit Care.*, 2011 Sep, 15(2), 211-40

Ely, E; Truman, B; Shintani, A; Thomason, J; Wheeler, A; Gordon, S; Francis, J; Speroff, T; Gautam, S; Margolin, R; Sessler, C; Dittus, R; Bernard, G. Monitoring sedation status over time in ICU patients: reliability and validity of the Richmond Agitation-Sedation Scale (RASS). *JAMA.*, 2003 Jun 11, 289(22), 2983-91.

Hong, CM; Tosun, C; Kurland, DB; Gerzanich, V; Schreibman, D; Simard, JM. Biomarkers as outcome predictors in subarachnoid hemorrhage--a systematic review. *Biomarkers*, 2014 Mar, 19(2), 95-108.

Karnatovskaia, LV; Lee, AS; Festic, E; Kramer, CL; Freeman, WD. Effect of prolonged therapeutic hypothermia on intracranial pressure, organ function, and hospital outcomes among patients with aneurysmal subarachnoid hemorrhage. *Neurocrit Care.*, 2014 Dec, 21(3), 451-61.

Kim, SH; Lilot, M; Sidhu, KS; Rinehart, J; Yu, Z; Canales, C; Cannesson, M. Accuracy and precision of continuous noninvasive arterial pressure monitoring compared with invasive arterial pressure: a systematic review and meta-analysis. *Anesthesiology*, 2014 May, 120(5), 1080-97.

Kistka, H; Dewan, MC; Mocco, J. Evidence-based cerebral vasospasm surveillance. *Neurol Res Int.*, 2013, 2013, 256713.

Kurtz, P; Fitts, V; Sumer, Z; Jalon, H; Cooke, J; Kvetan, V; Mayer, SA. How does care differ for neurological patients admitted to a neurocritical care unit versus a general ICU? *Neurocrit Care.*, 2011 Dec, 15(3), 477-80. doi: 10.1007/s12028-011-9539-2.

Lantigua, H; Ortega-Gutierrez, S; Schmidt, JM; Lee, K; Badjatia, N; Agarwal, S; Claassen, J; Connolly, ES; Mayer, SA. Subarachnoid hemorrhage: who dies, and why? *Crit Care.*, 2015 Aug 31, 19, 309.

Lehman, LH; Saeed, M; Talmor, D; Mark, R; Malhotra, A. Methods of Blood Pressure Measurement in the ICU. *Crit Care Med.*, 2013 Jan, 41(1), 34–40.

Le Roux, P; Menon, DK; Citerio, G; Vespa, P; Bader, MK; Brophy, GM; Diringer, MN; Stocchetti, N; Videtta, W; Armonda, R; Badjatia, N; Böesel, J; Chesnut, R; Chou, S; Claassen, J; Czosnyka, M; De Georgia, M; Figaji, A; Fugate, J; Helbok, R; Horowitz, D; Hutchinson, P; Kumar, M; McNett, M; Miller, C; Naidech, A; Oddo, M; Olson, D; O'Phelan, K; Provencio, JJ; Puppo, C; Riker, R; Robertson, C; Schmidt, M; Taccone, F. Consensus summary statement of the International Multidisciplinary Consensus Conference on Multimodality Monitoring in Neurocritical Care: a statement for healthcare professionals from the Neurocritical Care Society and the European Society of Intensive Care Medicine. *Neurocrit Care.*, 2014 Dec, 21 Suppl 2, S1-26.

Lv, Y; Wang, D; Lei, J; Tan, G. Clinical observation of the time course of raised intracranial pressure after subarachnoid hemorrhage. *Neurol Sci.*, 2015 Jul, 36(7), 1203-10.

Mascia, L. Acute lung injury in patients with severe brain injury: a double hit model. *Neurocrit Care.*, 2009 Dec, 11(3), 417-26.

Miyata, K; Mikami, T; Asai, Y; Iihoshi, S; Mikuni, N; Narimatsu, E. Subarachnoid hemorrhage after resuscitation from out-of-hospital cardiac arrest. *J Stroke Cerebrovasc Dis.*, 2014 Mar, 23(3), 446-52.

Sarrafzadeh, AS; Haux, D; Lüdemann, L; Amthauer, H; Plotkin, M; Küchler, I; Unterberg, AW. Cerebral ischemia in aneurysmal subarachnoid hemorrhage: a correlative microdialysis-PET study. *Stroke*, 2004 Mar, 35(3), 638-43.

Selig, C; Riegger, C; Dirks, B; et al. Bispectral index and suppression ratio as an early predictor of unfavourable neurological outcome after cardiac arrest. *Resuscitation*, 2014, 85, 221-6.

Wachter, D; Christophis, P; Stein, M; Oertel, MF. Use of multimodal electrophysiological monitoring to predict outcome after subarachnoid hemorrhage? A prospective series. *J Neurosurg Sci.*, 2011 Sep, 55(3), 179-87.

Zweifel, C; Castellani, G; Czosnyka, M; Carrera, E; Brady, KM; Kirkpatrick, PJ; Pickard, JD; Smielewski, P. Continuous assessment of cerebral autoregulation with near-infrared spectroscopy in adults after subarachnoid hemorrhage. 2010 *Stroke*, 41(9), 1963–1968.

In: Spontaneous Subarachnoid Haemorrhage
Editors: Thomas Kapapa and Ralph König
ISBN: 978-1-63485-270-8

Chapter 14

NEUROPROTECTION: DCI, VASOSPASM, NIMODIPINE

Christian Heinen
Department of Neurosurgery, Evangelic Hospital Oldenburg,
Medical Campus University of Oldenburg, Germany

ABSTRACT

Cerebral posthaemorrhagic vasospasm and delayed cortical ischaemia are dreaded complications associated above all with aneurysmal subarachnoid haemorrhage. These phenomena are also observed during traumatic SAH or inflammatory CNS disease [1]. Mortality in relation to SAH is approx. 50% and includes patients who die on the spot and do not reach a hospital. The mortality rate in patients receiving hospital treatment is still 25% regardless of all diagnostic and therapeutic options [2]. Vasopasms and delayed cortical ischaemia are entities that should each be considered individually. The clinical significance is the subject of much discussion.

Keywords: neuroprotection, delayed cortical ischemia, cerebral vasospasm

INTRODUCTION

In a meta-analysis, Frontera et al. reported that symptomatic vasospasms (clinical findings with no changes on imaging) occurred in 16% of patients, delayed cortical ischaemia (DCI) (clinical findings WITH changes on imaging) in 21%, angiographic vasospasms in 31% and on TCD in 45% [3]. This stresses the fact that morphological findings do not necessarily have to have a clinical impact and that there must be mechanisms which extend beyond simple vasospasm.

It is therefore important to be clear about the terms and to distinguish one from another.

CEREBRAL VASOSPASM - CVS

CVS basically means the pathological constriction of the cerebral arteries following SAH. In the literature, varying and sometimes contradictory forms of CVS, the clinical implications of which vary considerably, are grouped together under this generic term. Vasospasms detected on *angiography*, i.e., a decrease in the vascular cross-section compared to previous images, were described as early as 1951 [4]. The incidence is specified as 60%-70%. However, this is not necessarily associated with clinical deterioration. In contrast, CVS is found on *transcranial Doppler/Duplex* (TCD), and occurs in approx. 50% of all SAH patients. A relative constriction of the vessels is thereby measured indirectly from a change in blood flow velocity according to Poiseuille's Law. The difficulty with the term CVS is that, as already mentioned, it offers no indication of the clinical impact and refers merely to the vasoconstriction itself, without allowing for the other pathological mechanisms.

DELAYED CORTICAL ISCHAEMIA - DCI

The term delayed cortical ischaemia (DCI) was therefore introduced. Firstly, it refers to new changes revealed by CCT/MRI images e.g., constriction of the vessels, and also to ischaemia or perfusion deficits that were not identifiable on the initial scans. Secondly, symptoms of clinical deterioration are recorded. These include new-onset aphasia, unilateral symptoms, deterioration of the GCS (Glasgow Coma Score) by 2 points, neglect, or apraxia. The changes should last at least one hour, not have a direct temporal relationship to aneurysm treatment, and not be attributable to other diseases (infection/electrolyte imbalance/cardiac events, etc.) [5]. In 20%-30% of patients, DCI appears to be responsible for the severe neurological damage that develops as a secondary complication. In approx. 7%-10% this can even prove fatal [6], regardless of any particular treatment. The term DCI is therefore more broadly defined and does not focus on vasospasm alone.

The following sections provide a summary of the possible components that contribute to the development of DCI.

PATHOMECHANISM

A number of pathomechanisms are proposed as contributory factors in DCI. How it develops precisely, however, is still unclear. Besides disrupted autoregulation of the arterial system, inflammatory processes are of particular relevance. Ultimately, there is a preponderance of vasoconstrictive and obstructive agents with at the same time a significant reduction in antagonistic vasodilators. Basically, there are different phases of ischaemia in SAH.

The *early phase ("early brain injury")* occurs during acute rupture as global ischaemia due to the acute rise in intracranial pressure (ICP) with a consecutive decrease in cerebral perfusion pressure (CPP), and spans the first 72 hours after the bleeding occurs. It is posited that the consequences of this early damage sometimes are only seen over the course [7]. Acute vasospasm in response to the haemorrhagic extravasate has been described [8]. The blood-brain barrier is permeated and autoregulation disrupted. During the *late phase*, a number of simultaneous processes takes place, leading to local structural change in the vascular wall with resulting intimal thickening and media proliferation [9].

In its physiological state **NO,** as a cGMP inducer, is an essential and potent vasodilator that is stored in pre- and postganglionic perivascular neurons.

However, NO has a high affinity to haemoglobin. The latter binds increasingly to NO during SAH decreasing signifantly NO-levels as a vasodilator. SAH also leads to neuron reduction with an emphasis on NO deficiency. *Endothelin-1* is the most potent vasoconstrictor known [10]. Increased concentrations are found both in the cerebrospinal fluid and in the plasma of SAH patients; clinically these closely correlate with the occurrence of CVS [11, 12]. Endothelin-1 usually appears in astrocytes, neurons, smooth muscle cells and the endothelium. As a result of activating leukocytes in the cerebrospinal fluid, SAH appears to increase the production and in turn the secretion of endothelin-1 [13]. Various degradation mechanisms release *free radicals*, which damage cell membranes in the endothelium, smooth muscle cells and in vasoregulatory neurons. Additional vasoconstrictive substances such as arachidonic acids may be released through these cascade with a dysregulated calcium influx being the consequence [14]. Moreover, the increased development of *microemboli* and *cortical spreading depression (CSD)* seems to play a part in the emergence of DCI. Cerebral ischaemia was found in 77% of post-mortem examinations without any angiographic evidence of vasospasms [15]. A combination of pathologically activated coagulation and simultaneously decreased fibrinolysis is believed to be responsible for the formation of *microemboli* [16].

CSD describes waves of depolarisation spreading through the grey matter.

This occurs spontaneously in SAH and lasts longer than the otherwise usual 5-15 minutes. In healthy individuals, vasoconstriction occurs shortly before CSD, followed by vasodilation during the CSD phase (spreading hyperperfusion) and a phase of reduced and delayed tissue perfusion during the recovery phase after the CSD wave [17]. However, the vascular reaction is altered in SAH patients. Therefore, the CSD can lead either to no change in the vascular width or to a pathological vasoconstriction known as *cortical spreading ischaemia* [18] without a relaxation phase. If CSD occur more and more frequently in quick succession, the affected areas of cortex cannot recover from the hypoperfusion. CSD occurs more often between day 5 and 7 post haemorrhage [19].

NEUROPROTECTION

Numerous strategies have arisen based on recent insights into the pathological mechanism. The therapeutic options that are actually available for treating or preventing DCI, however, are rather sobering. Despite all efforts, the calcium channel blocker nimodipine constitutes the drug with the only evidence to date of a significantly better outcome. An overview of the pharmacological and non-pharmacological options and their impact is provided in the following few paragraphs (see also Table 1 and 2).

Table 1. Overview substances and recommendation level

Substance	*Mechanism of action*	*Indication*	*American Stroke Association recommendation*
Ca^{++} blocker	Vasodilation/anti-inflammatory	Prevention and treatment of CVS/DCI	Yes
Mg^{++}	Vasodilation/(anti-inflammatory)	Prevention of CVS	No
Statins	Anti-inflammatory, improved endothelial function	Treatment of CVS	No
Anti-epileptics	Anticonvulsive/diminished cortical spreading depression	Treatment of convulsions	No
Aspirin	Platelet aggregation inhibition	Prevention of DCI	No
Glucocorticoids	Anti-inflammatory	Prevention of CVS	No
Enoxaparin	Antithrombotic	Prevention of DCI	No
Tirilazad	Membrane stabilisation	Treatment of CVS	No
Clazosentan	Vasodilation	Treatment of CVS	No

CVS: cerebral vasospasm DCI: delayed cerebral ischemia

Pharmacological

Nimodipine

Nimodipine is a dihydropyridine and therefore a selective Ca++ channel blocker. It binds to the voltage-dependent L-type Ca++ channels and appears to have an increased affinity to cerebral and renal vessels. In Europe both oral and intravenous pharmaceutical forms are available, whereas in the USA only oral administration is approved.

Intra-arterial administration via an intracranially placed microcatheter is also possible [20]. There have also been reports of intrathecal doses [21]. In comparative studies, the efficacy of intravenous and oral doses did not differ [22, 23]. Those studies that were able to demonstrate efficacy were based on oral intake [24]. It is important to mention that many of the nimodipine studies were carried out many years, sometimes decades ago, but the results are still valid in terms of clinical routine [24, 25]. The only larger-scale study to which reference is still made and which on meta-analysis suggests that nimodipine has a significantly better outcome, dates back to 1989 [26]!

Neuroprotection

The original assumption that the positive effect was derived merely from vasodilatation has more recently been revised. In contrast to other Ca++ channel blockers, nimodipine obviously has other neuroprotective properties, particularly after SAH. However, its exact mechanism of action has not yet been fully explained. Nimodipine plays a part in activating fibrinolysis, which may then attenuate the development of microthrombi [27]. It also prevents uncontrolled Ca++ influx into the neurons subsequent to an ischaemic event. This influx would normally lead to neuronal cell destruction [28]. In rat model nimodipine seemed also to attenuate CSD [29].

Intra-Arterial

Intra-arterial administration of nimodipine is considered in particular for refractory or rapidly recurring CVS and DCI [30, 31]. In addition to adverse drug reactions, the risks associated with the surgical procedure such as thrombosis, vascular perforations, air embolisms etc. must be taken into account [32].

Intrathecal

As early as 1982, Auer et al. described the local intrathecal use of nimodpine in the prevention of symptomatic vasospasm [33]. This idea was revisited over the course, whereby nimodipine was administered via lumbar drain and not locally as during clipping procedure [21].

However, the validity of the efficacy data is limited given that larger comparative studies are not available. Other Ca++ channel blockers have also been applied locally via an external ventricular drain, a catheter placed in the circle of Willis, or as pellets. There are no clear recommendations due to the lack of larger-scale randomised studies, however [34].

Adverse Reactions

The side effect profile of nimodipine is broad. Pulmonary arteriovenous shunts with consecutively impaired gas exchange, hypotension, thrombopenia, allergic reactions and gastroparesis can occur. Reciprocal interactions occur (according to the package leaflet from Bayer) with certain antibiotics (e.g., erythromycin, quinupristin/dalfopristin), HIV drugs (e.g., ritonavir), certain antimycotics (e.g., ketoconazole) and antidepressants (e.g., nefazodone, fluoxetine), antiepileptics (e.g., valproic acid).

Triple-H Therapy: Hypertension/Hypervolaemia/Haemodilution

The principle behind triple-H therapy is to maintain perfusion by increasing the arterial pressure and decreasing viscosity (according to Poiseuille's Law) in the case of vascular dysregulation [35]. This is based on the observation that SAH patients developed new neurological deficits in the event of hypotension. Responses to triple-H therapy were recorded as early as the 1950s [36]. This method was and remains widespread, although there is still no clear evidence of its effectiveness. Meta-analyses performed in 2004 and 2010 did not reveal advantage from either combined triple-H therapy or the individual components (hypervolaemia/hypertension only, etc.) [37]. In contrast, hypervolaemia would appear to result in more complications [38]. At present, euvolaemia and "mild hypertension" are therefore recommended [39].

Magnesium

Mg++ is a competitive blocker of voltage-dependent calcium channels. Its effect ranges from vasodilatation, inhibition of platelet aggregation, and improvement in erythrocyte elasticity, as far as stabilisation of the endothelium [34]. Other neuroprotective effects have been detected experimentally [40]. Interestingly, hypomagnesaemia occurs in approx. 50% of all SAH patients. It can be used as a predictor of DCI, particularly between day 2 and 12 post haemorrhage [41]. Despite the high expectations for Mg++, no evidence of a positive effect on the outcome has been forthcoming – large-scale studies (e.g., MASH-II study) notwithstanding [42]. There is no clear recommendation for routine use in SAH [39].

Statins

As stabilisers of the endothelium, platelet adhesion/aggregation inhibitors and anti-inflammatory agents, statins seem predestined for neuroprotection. However, neither meta-analyses nor a large-scale, multicentre, randomised, double-blind phase 3 study managed to identify a significant difference between simvastatin and a placebo [43-45]. Statins thus are not used routinely at present.

Endothelin-1 Receptor Antagonists

As already mentioned, endothelin-1 (ET-1) is the most potent vasoconstrictor known. The first study used the non-selective ET-inhibitor TAK-044 [46], without achieving any significant improvement. Subsequently, other study groups demonstrated an improvement in the angiographic vasospasm and the occurrence of delayed ischaemic neurological deficits (DIND) with the specific ET-1-inhibitor clazosentan. However, outcome was not more favourable [10]. Moreover, significant adverse effects such as pulmonary oedema, anaemia and hypotension [47] occured, and the subset of clipped patients showed a poorer response. The study (CONSCIOUS-2) was discontinued and the planned follow-up study, CONSCIOUS-3, was not even started [35].

Other Substance Classes

There are numerous other literature references concerning neuroprotection in SAH. Various substances such as corticosteroids, radical scavengers (tirilazad), aspirin, low-molecular-weight heparins, metalloproteinases, progesterone/oestrogen, antiepileptics and antifibrinolytics, have been studied for their suitability as neuroprotective agents in SAB [47-49]. But, none of them proved satisfactory.

NON-PHARMACOLOGICAL

Interventional

Intracerebral

Aside from the intra-arterial administration of nimodipine discussed above, balloon dilatation in the treatment of refractory symptomatic vasospasms also plays an important role. The best outcomes are achieved if treatment ensues within two hours after onset of the symptoms [50]. Because material from the coronary angiography had to be used in the initial phase, the material has improved considerably in the last few years. At the same time, growing expertise has helped to lower periprocedural complications and improve the results, even in the case of multiple treatments [51] (see Table 2).

Intra-Aortic Counterpulsation

As an adaptation of the treatment for cardiogenic shock, this method involves the intra-aortic insertion of a balloon proximal to the cerebral vessels. If the aortic valve closes, it is inflated so as to increase the diastolic cerebral arterial flow [50].

Hypothermia

Evidence was found that hypothermia has a positive effect on mean flow velocity in the middle cerebral artery in the case of both increased ICP and DCI. This is still to be confirmed by larger studies [52].

Stellate Ganglion Block (SGB)

The potential efficacy is based on the assumption that noradrenergic sympathetic innervation of the cerebral vessels originates largely from the superior cervical ganglion. Consequently, this system has a vasoconstrictive effect. Vasorelaxation is therefore achieved by blocking this ganglion. The technique is simple: infiltration at the transverse process of C6 using approx. 8-10 ml of a local anaesthetic. In spite of the vasodilation (measured indirectly from the TCD), autoregulation seems be preserved when blocking the stellate ganglion [53]. One study of clipped SAH patients (n = 15) revealed that both a clinical improvement and a drop in TCD flow rates were achieved [54]. Since larger studies have not yet been conducted, the role of such a concept cannot be reliably judged.

Table 2. Evidence level of measures in refractory cerebral vasospasm

	Administration	*Effect*	*Evidence level*
Hypertension	IV	MAP increase	B
Balloon angioplasty	IA (cerebral)	Mechanical dilatation	B
Drug-eluting angioplasty	IA (bolus/continuous)	Vasodilation/anti-inflammatory	C
Intra-aortic counterpulsation	IA extracerebral	Increased cerebral perfusion	C
Ca^{++} channel blockers	Intrathecal	Vasodilation/anti-inflammatory	D
NO	Intrathecal	Vasodilation	D
Hypothermia	Systemic		D
Stellate block	Stellate ganglion	Vasodilation	D

IV: intravenous MAP: middle arterial pressure IA: intra-arterial

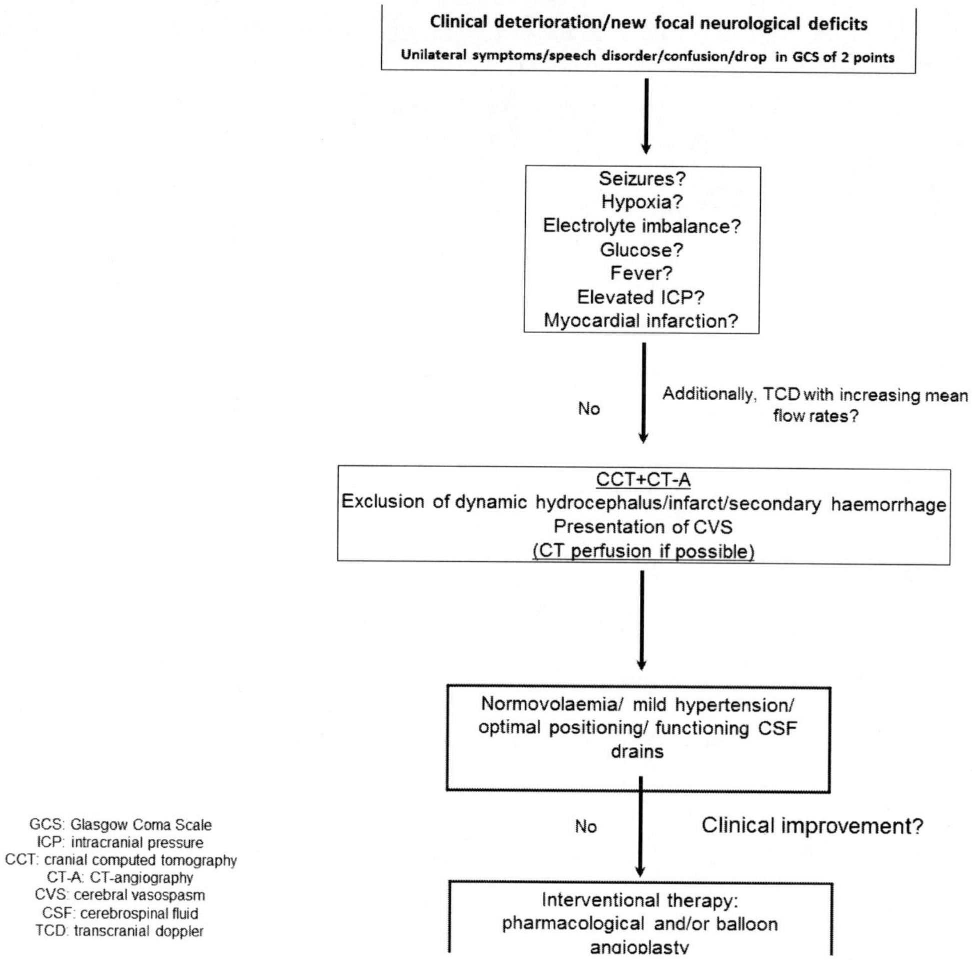

Figure 1 possible treatment algorithm.

Conclusion

There is no consistency in the terminology as regards CVS and DCI, meaning that vasospasm (on angiography/TCD), DIND and DCI are often used synonymously. DCI can also occur WITHOUT morphological changes, as various pathomechanisms occur simultaneously and do not necessarily lead to vasoconstriction. However, it is of utmost importance to recognize and treat these pathologies (see proposed treatment algorithm Figure 1). Despite intensive research at all levels, DCI therapy is still proving futile. Orally administered nimodipine is the only medicine to date that has exhibited a neuroprotective effect specifically in SAH. Hopefully, with growing knowledge of the pathophysiological background and translational studies, it will be possible to develop additional, effective treatment options. At the same time, it would be desirable to have reliable and easily detectable biomarkers for DCI with a view to establishing the diagnosis as well as monitoring treatment. Genetic factors that predispose patients to DCI may be the key to identifying and treating patients [55, 56] (Figure 1).

REFERENCES

[1] Eisenhut, M. Vasospasm in cerebral inflammation. *Int J Inflam. Hindawi Publishing Corporation*, 2014, 2014, 509707.

[2] van Gijn, J; Rinkel, GJ. Subarachnoid haemorrhage: diagnosis, causes and management. *Brain.*, 2001 Feb, 124(Pt 2), 249–78.

[3] Frontera, JA; Fernandez, A; Schmidt, JM; Claassen, J; Wartenberg, KE; Badjatia, N; et al. Defining Vasospasm After Subarachnoid Hemorrhage: What Is the Most Clinically Relevant Definition? *Stroke.*, 2009 May 22, 40(6), 1963–8.

[4] Ecker, A; Riemenschneider, PA. Arteriographic demonstration of spasm of the intracranial arteries, with special reference to saccular arterial aneurysms. *Journal of Neurosurgery.*, 1951 Nov, 8(6), 660–7.

[5] Vergouwen, MDI; Vermeulen, M; van Gijn, J; Rinkel, GJE; Wijdicks, EF; Muizelaar, JP; et al. Definition of Delayed Cerebral Ischemia After Aneurysmal Subarachnoid Hemorrhage as an Outcome Event in Clinical Trials and Observational Studies: Proposal of a Multidisciplinary Research Group. *Stroke.*, 2010 Sep 27, 41(10), 2391–5.

[6] Tjahjadi, M; König, R; Wirtz, CR; Woischneck, D; Kapapa, T. Cerebral Vasospasm and Health-Related Quality of Life After Subarachnoid Hemorrhage. World Neurosurgery. Elsevier Inc, 2013 Jul 8, 80(1-2), 113–20.

[7] Kusaka, G; Ishikawa, M; Nanda, A; Granger, DN; Zhang, JH. Signaling pathways for early brain injury after subarachnoid hemorrhage. *J Cereb Blood Flow Metab.*, 2004 Aug, 24(8), 916–25.

[8] Macdonald, RL; Pluta, RM; Zhang, JH. Cerebral vasospasm after subarachnoid hemorrhage: the emerging revolution. *Nat Clin Pract Neurol.*, 2007 May, 3(5), 256–63.

[9] Hughes, JT; Schianchi, PM. Cerebral artery spasm. A histological study at necropsy of the blood vessels in cases of subarachnoid hemorrhage. *Journal of Neurosurgery.*, 1978 Apr, 48(4), 515–25.

[10] Kramer, A; Fletcher, J. Do Endothelin-Receptor Antagonists Prevent Delayed Neurological Deficits and Poor Outcomes After Aneurysmal Subarachnoid Hemorrhage? *A Meta-Analysis. Stroke.* 2009 Sep 25, 40(10), 3403–6.

[11] Fassbender, K; Hodapp, B; Rossol, S; Bertsch, T; Schmeck, J; Schütt, S; et al. Endothelin-1 in subarachnoid hemorrhage: An acute-phase reactant produced by cerebrospinal fluid leukocytes. *Stroke.*, 2000 Dec, 31(12), 2971–5.

[12] Seifert, V; Löffler, BM; Zimmermann, M; Roux, S; Stolke, D. Endothelin concentrations in patients with aneurysmal subarachnoid hemorrhage. Correlation with cerebral vasospasm, delayed ischemic neurological deficits, and volume of hematoma. *Journal of Neurosurgery.*, 1995 Jan, 82(1), 55–62.

[13] Yakubu, MA; Leffler, CW. Regulation of ET-1 biosynthesis in cerebral microvascular endothelial cells by vasoactive agents and PKC. *Am J Physiol.*, 1999 Feb, 276(2 Pt 1), C300–5.

[14] Chaichana, KL; Pradilla, G; Huang, J; Tamargo, RJ. Role of inflammation (leukocyte-endothelial cell interactions) in vasospasm after subarachnoid hemorrhage. *World Neurosurgery.*, 2010 Jan, 73(1), 22–41.

[15] Neil-Dwyer, G; Lang, DA; Doshi, B; Gerber, CJ; Smith, PW. Delayed cerebral ischaemia: the pathological substrate. *Acta Neurochir (Wien).*, 1994, 131(1-2), 137–45.

[16] Hirashima, Y; Nakamura, S; Endo, S; Kuwayama, N; Naruse, Y; Takaku, A. Elevation of platelet activating factor, inflammatory cytokines, and coagulation factors in the internal jugular vein of patients with subarachnoid hemorrhage. *Neurochem Res.*, 1997 Oct, 22(10), 1249–55.

[17] Lauritzen, M; Dreier, JP; Fabricius, M; Hartings, JA; Graf, R; Strong, AJ. Clinical relevance of cortical spreading depression in neurological disorders: migraine; malignant stroke, subarachnoid and intracranial hemorrhage; and traumatic brain injury. *Journal of Cerebral Blood Flow and amp, Metabolism.* Nature Publishing Group, 2010 Nov 3, 31(1), 17–35.

[18] Dreier, JP; Major, S; Manning, A; Woitzik, J; Drenckhahn, C; Steinbrink, J; et al. Cortical spreading ischaemia is a novel process involved in ischaemic damage in patients with aneurysmal subarachnoid haemorrhage. *Brain.*, 2009 Jun 24, 132(7), 1866–81.

[19] Bosche, B; Graf, R; Ernestus, RI; Dohmen, C; Reithmeier, T; Brinker, G; et al. Recurrent spreading depolarizations after subarachnoid hemorrhage decreases oxygen availability in human cerebral cortex. Ann Neurol. Wiley Subscription Services, Inc., A Wiley Company, 2010 May, 67(5), 607–17.

[20] Doukas, A; Petridis, AK; Barth, H; Jansen, O; Maslehaty, H; Mehdorn, HM. Resistant vasospasm in subarachnoid hemorrhage treated with continuous intraarterial nimodipine infusion. *Acta Neurochir Suppl.* Vienna: Springer Vienna, 2011, 112(Chapter 16), 93–6.

[21] Hänggi, D; Beseoglu, K; Turowski, B; Steiger, HJ. Feasibility and safety of intrathecal nimodipine on posthaemorrhagic cerebral vasospasm refractory to medical and endovascular therapy. *Clinical Neurology and Neurosurgery.*, 2008 Sep, 110(8), 784–90.

[22] Kronvall, E; Undrén, P; Romner, B; Säveland, H; Cronqvist, M; Nilsson, OG. Nimodipine in aneurysmal subarachnoid hemorrhage: a randomized study of intravenous or peroral administration. *Journal of Neurosurgery.*, 2009 Jan, 110(1), 58–63.

[23] Soppi, V; Karamanakos, PN; Koivisto, T; Kurki, MI; Vanninen, R; Jaaskelainen, JE; et al. A randomized outcome study of enteral versus intravenous nimodipine in 171 patients after acute aneurysmal subarachnoid hemorrhage. *World Neurosurgery.*, 2012 Jul, 78(1-2), 101–9.

[24] Dorhout Mees SM, Rinkel GJ, Feigin VL, Algra A, van den Bergh WM, Vermeulen M, van Gijn J. Calcium antagonists for aneurysmal subarachnoid haemorrhage (Review). Cochrane Library; 2008 (2):1-42.Feigin, VL; Rinkel, GJ; Algra, A; Vermeulen, M; van Gijn, J. Calcium antagonists in patients with aneurysmal subarachnoid hemorrhage: a systematic review. *Neurology.*, 1998 Apr, 50(4), 876–83.

[25] Pickard, JD; Murray, GD; Illingworth, R; Shaw, MD; Teasdale, GM; Foy, PM; et al. Effect of oral nimodipine on cerebral infarction and outcome after subarachnoid haemorrhage: British aneurysm nimodipine trial. *BMJ. BMJ Group*, 1989 Mar 11, 298(6674), 636–42.

[26] Vergouwen, MDI; Vermeulen, M; de Haan, RJ; Levi, M; Roos, YB. Dihydropyridine calcium antagonists increase fibrinolytic activity: a systematic review. *J Cereb Blood Flow Metab.*, 2007 Jul, 27(7), 1293–308.

[27] Pisani, A; Calabresi, P; Tozzi, A; D'Angelo V; Bernardi G. L-type Ca2+ channel blockers attenuate electrical changes and Ca2+ rise induced by oxygen/glucose deprivation in cortical neurons. *Stroke.*, 1998 Jan, 29(1), 196–201–discussion202.

[28] Dreier, JP; Windmüller, O; Petzold, G; Lindauer, U; Einhäupl, KM; Dirnagl, U. Ischemia triggered by red blood cell products in the subarachnoid space is inhibited by nimodipine administration or moderate volume expansion/hemodilution in rats. *Neurosurgery.*, 2002 Dec, 51(6), 1457–65–discussion1465–7.

[29] Wolf, S; Martin, H; Landscheidt, JF; Rodiek, SO; Schürer, L; Lumenta, CB. Continuous Selective Intraarterial Infusion of Nimodipine for Therapy of Refractory Cerebral Vasospasm. *Neurocrit Care.*, 2009 Dec 22, 12(3), 346–51.

[30] Kim, JH; Park, IS; Park, KB; Kang, DH; Hwang, SH. Intraarterial Nimodipine Infusion to Treat Symptomatic Cerebral Vasospasm after Aneurysmal Subarachnoid Hemorrhage. *J Korean Neurosurg Soc.*, 2009, 46(3), 239.

[31] Tsurushima, H; Kamezaki, T; Nagatomo, Y; Hyodo, A; Nose, T. Complications associated with intraarterial administration of papaverine for vasospasm following subarachnoid hemorrhage--two case reports. *Neurol Med Chir (Tokyo).*, 2000 Feb, 40(2), 112–5.

[32] Auer, LM; Ito, Z; Suzuki, A; Ohta, H. Prevention of symptomatic vasospasm by topically applied nimodipine. *Acta Neurochir (Wien).*, 1982, 63(1-4), 297–302.

[33] Westermaier, T. Neuroprotective Treatment Strategies for Delayed Cerebral Ischemia after Subarachnoid Hemorrhage – Review of Literature and Future Prospects. *J Neurol Neurophysiol.*, 2013, 05(01), 1–8.

[34] Rowland, MJ; Hadjipavlou, G; Kelly, M; Westbrook, J; Pattinson, KTS. Delayed cerebral ischaemia after subarachnoid haemorrhage: looking beyond vasospasm. *Br J Anaesth.*, 2012 Aug 9, 109(3), 315–29.

[35] DENNY-BROWN, D. The treatment of recurrent cerebrovascular symptoms and the question of "vasospasm". *Med Clin North Am.*, 1951 Sep, 35(5), 1457–74.

[36] Dankbaar, JW; Slooter, AJ; Rinkel, GJ; Schaaf, ICVD. Effect of different components of triple-H therapy on cerebral perfusion in patients with aneurysmal subarachnoid haemorrhage: a systematic review. Crit Care. *BioMed Central Ltd*, 2010, 14(1), R23.

[37] Rinkel, GJE; Feigin, VL; Algra, A; van Gijn, J. Circulatory volume expansion therapy for aneurysmal subarachnoid haemorrhage. *Cochrane Database Syst Rev.*, 2004, (4), CD000483.

[38] Connolly, ES; Rabinstein, AA; Carhuapoma, JR; Derdeyn, CP; Dion, J; Higashida, RT; et al. Guidelines for the management of aneurysmal subarachnoid hemorrhage: a guideline for healthcare professionals from the American Heart Association/american Stroke Association. Stroke. Lippincott Williams and Wilkins, 2012, pp, 1711–37.

[39] Dong, JF; Cruz, MA; Aboulfatova, K; Martin, C; Choi, H; Bergeron, AL; et al. Magnesium maintains endothelial integrity; up-regulates proteolysis of ultra-large von Willebrand factor; and reduces platelet aggregation under flow conditions. *Thromb Haemost.*, 2008 Mar, 99(3), 586–93.

[40] van den Bergh, WM; Algra, A; van der Sprenkel, JWB; Tulleken, CAF; Rinkel, GJE. Hypomagnesemia after Aneurysmal Subarachnoid Hemorrhage. *Neurosurgery.*, 2003 Feb, 52(2), 276–82.

[41] MD, SMDM; MD, PAA; MD, PWPV; van Kooten, MDF; MD, HAK; MD, JB; et al. Magnesium for aneurysmal subarachnoid haemorrhage (MASH-2): a randomised placebo-controlled trial. *The Lancet. Elsevier Ltd*, 2012 Jul 7, 380(9836), 44–9.

[42] Dorhout Mees SM, Algra A, Vandertop WP, van Kooten F, Kuijsten HA, Boiten J, van Oostenbrugge RJ, Al-Shahi Salman R, Lavados PM, Rinkel GJ, van den Bergh WM; MASH-2 Study Group. Magnesium for aneurysmal subarachnoid haemorrhage (MASH-2): a randomised placebo-controlled trial. Lancet. 2012 Jul 7;380(9836):44-9Liu, J; Chen, Q. Effect of statins treatment for patients with aneurysmal subarachnoid hemorrhage: a systematic review and meta-analysis of observational studies and randomized controlled trials. *Int J Clin Exp Med.*, 2015, 8(5), 7198–208.

[43] FMedSci, PJK; MSc, CLT, PhD, CS, FRCS, PPJH, PhD, PGDM, Collaborators, FTS. Simvastatin in aneurysmal subarachnoid haemorrhage (STASH): a multicentre randomised phase 3 trial. *Lancet Neurol. Elsevier Ltd*, 2014 Jun 10, 13(7), 666–75.

[44] Shen, J; Pan, JW; Fan, ZX; Xiong, XX; Zhan, RY. Dissociation of vasospasm-related morbidity and outcomes in patients with aneurysmal subarachnoid hemorrhage treated with clazosentan: a meta-analysis of randomized controlled trials. *Journal of Neurosurgery.*, 2013 Jul, 119(1), 180–9.

[45] Kirkpatrick PJ, Turner CL, Smith C, Hutchinson PJ, Murray GD; STASH Collaborators. Simvastatin in aneurysmal subarachnoid haemorrhage (STASH): a multicentre randomised phase 3 trial. Lancet Neurol. 2014 Jul;13(7): 666-75.Behrouz, R; Sadat-Hosseiny, Z. Pharmacological Agents in Aneurysmal Subarachnoid Hemorrhage. *Clinical Neuropharmacology.*, 2015 May, 1–5.

[46] Mehta, V; Russin, J; Spirtos, A; He, S; Adamczyk, P; Amar, AP; et al. Matrix Metalloproteinases in Cerebral Vasospasm following Aneurysmal Subarachnoid Hemorrhage. *Neurology Research International.*, 2013, 2013(7), 1–4.

[47] Findlay, JM; Nisar, J; Darsaut, T. RÉSUMÉ. *Can J Neurol Sci.*, 2015 Sep 2, 1–18.

[48] Chalouhi, N; Tjoumakaris, S; Thakkar, V; Theofanis, T; Hammer, C; Hasan, D; et al. Endovascular management of cerebral vasospasm following aneurysm rupture: outcomes and predictors in 116 patients. *Clinical Neurology and Neurosurgery.*, 2014 Mar, 118, 26–31.

[49] Seule, M; Muroi, C; Sikorski, C; Hugelshofer, M; Winkler, K; Keller, E. Therapeutic Hypothermia Reduces Middle Cerebral Artery Flow Velocity in Patients with Severe Aneurysmal Subarachnoid Hemorrhage. *Neurocrit Care.*, 2013 Oct 17, 20(2), 255–62.

[50] Naidu, RK. A Review of the Stellate Ganglion Block/Cervical Sympathetic Block on the Prevention and Therapy of Cerebral Vasospasm After Subarachnoid Hemorrhage. ICU Director. SAGE Publications, 2013 Jul 19, 4(4), 161–5.

[51] Dash, H; Chouhan, R; Jain, V; Rath, G; Bithal, P; Suri, A. Stellate ganglion block for treatment of cerebral vasospasm in patients with aneurysmal subarachnoid hemorrhage - A preliminary study. *J Anaesth Clin Pharmacol.*, 2011, 27(4), 516–6.

[52] Rosalind Lai, PM; Du, R. Role of Genetic Polymorphisms in Predicting Delayed Cerebral Ischemia and Radiographic Vasospasm After Aneurysmal Subarachnoid Hemorrhage: A Meta-Analysis. *World Neurosurgery.*, 2015 Jun 11.

[53] Baumann, A; Devaux, Y; Audibert, G; Zhang, L; Bracard, S; Colnat-Coulbois, S; et al. Gene Expression Profile of Blood Cells for the Prediction of Delayed Cerebral Ischemia after Intracranial Aneurysm Rupture: A Pilot Study in Humans. Cerebrovasc Dis. Karger Publishers, 2013, 36(3), 236–42.

In: Spontaneous Subarachnoid Haemorrhage
Editors: Thomas Kapapa and Ralph König
ISBN: 978-1-63485-270-8

Chapter 15

ENDOVASCULAR TREATMENT OPTIONS FOR CEREBRAL VASOSPASM AFTER SPONTANEOUS SUBARACHNOID HAEMORRHAGE

Yigit Ozpeynirci and Bernd Schmitz
Section Neuroradiology, University of Ulm, Günzburg, Germany

ABSTRACT

When vasospasm is suspected in a patient with subarachnoid haemorrhage, medical treatment is usually the first choice. Unfortunately, vasospasm is often refractory to medical therapy and, moreover, the percentage of patients who cannot tolerate mainstream non-invasive treatment, usually due to cardiopulmonary complications, is not minute. Early endovascular treatment appears to be the best alternative for this group of patients.

Endovascular treatment of cerebral vasospasm is divided into two categories: chemical dilatation of the spasm by intra-arterial administration of vasoactive drugs, and transluminal balloon angioplasty of spastic segments. Flow augmentation strategies involving aortic obstruction with balloons are being actively investigated. However, they have not yet found a place in current practice.

Keywords: vasospasm, endovascular, angioplasty

GENERAL INDICATIONS FOR AND TIMING OF INVASIVE INTERVENTIONAL MANAGEMENT

In their guidelines, the American Heart Association (AHA) and American Stroke Association (ASA) consider endovascular therapy as reasonable in patients with symptomatic cerebral vasospasm (CV), recommending it in particular for those who do not rapidly respond to hypertensive therapy (Class IIa; Level of Evidence B) [1].

Endovascular intervention is often performed in patients who, despite intensive medical therapy, have a diminishing neurological status, develop sudden focal neurological deficits or in whom there is concern regarding complications from medical management. In many poor grade SAHs, however, routine clinical examination is not sensitive to acute changes in neurological status, since most of these patients are already comatose. The same applies to intubated and sedated patients. In these patients, the physician therefore has to rely on serial non-invasive imaging studies and it would be wise to treat moderate to severe CV revealed by such studies and confirmed by digital subtraction angiography (DSA).

Transcranial Doppler ultrasound (TCD) is an easy-to-perform bedside method which can be used on a daily basis during the vasospasm-sensitive phase to detect rising flow velocities. It is also helpful in the follow-up of patients after treatment.

CT angiography (CTA) supported by CT perfusion (CTP) is more sensitive than TCD in the detection of CV. CTP is able to illustrate the perfusion at tissue level and thus is sensitive to CV of both proximal and distal arteries. It is a very helpful in demonstrating delayed cerebral ischaemia (DCI) and impending infarction in intubated patients or patients with low Glasgow Coma Scores (GCS) [9] (Figure 1).

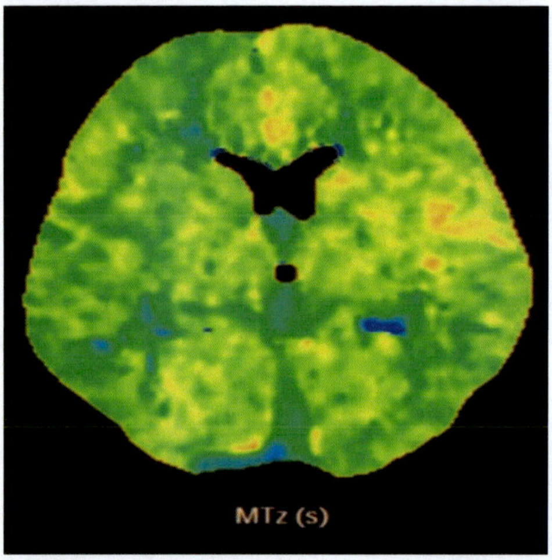

(A)

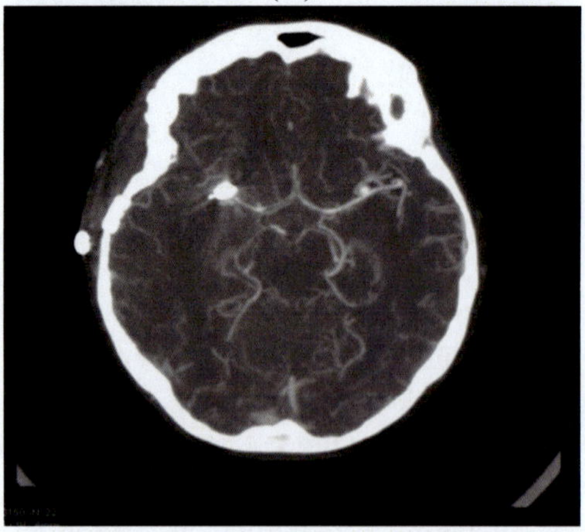

(B)

Figure 1. (Continued)

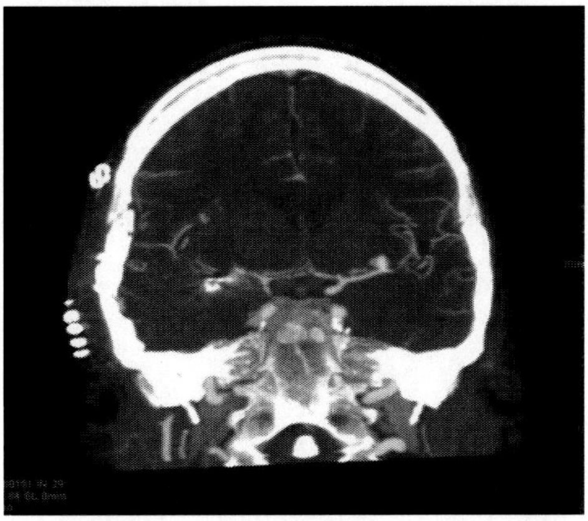

(C)

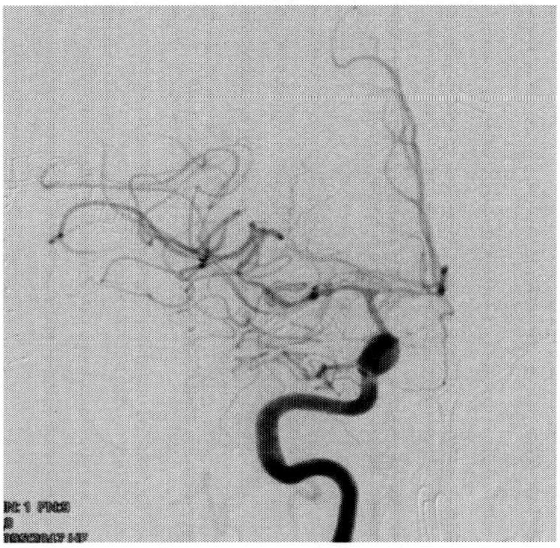

(D)

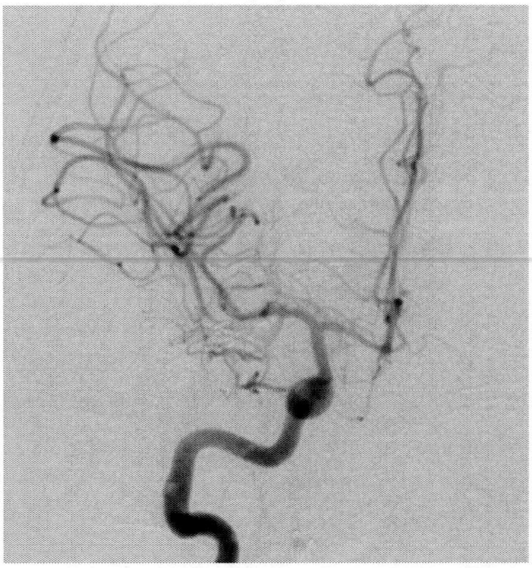

(E)

Figure 1. The Mean Transit Time (MTT) map (A) shows prolongation in both ACA territories and the right MCA territory without deficient perfusion on the CBV map (not shown). CTA demonstrates severe CV (B and C). DSA confirms the severe CV on the right (D). Control DSA 10 days after continuous IAIT with nimodipine reveals complete resolution of CV (E).

Angiographic findings of CV consist of decreased luminal calibre, increased cerebral circulation time and in severe cases retrograde filling of the affected vascular territory through leptomeningeal collaterals.

Studies suggest that there is a 2h time window after symptom onset in most patients during which endovascular therapy will be beneficial [2, 3, 4, 5, 6, 7, 8]. Thus it is reasonable to frequently check the neurological status of awake patients and assess the flow velocities of cerebral arteries via TCD in the patient with lower GCSs.

Endovascular Prophylaxis

As prophylactic transluminal balloon angioplasty (TBA) is related to very high mortality and has not been found to have a positive effect on outcome, and the therapeutic effects of all drugs administered IA are transient, CV prophylaxis is not recommended [1, 7].

Intra-Arterial Infusion Therapy (IAIT)

Several vasodilator agents have been infused intra-arterial (IA) through transarterial catheters to treat patients with CV. They include phosphodiesterase inhibitors (papaverine, milrinone and amrinone), calcium channel blockers (nimodipine, verapamil, nicardipine), protein kinase inhibitors (fasudil hydrochloride) and adenylyl cyclase activators (colforsin daropate hydrochloride) [5, 6]. The main effect is a temporary relaxation of smooth muscle cells in the vascular wall, causing vasodilatation.

There have been no randomised clinical trials to demonstrate the benefit of intra-arterial infusion therapy (IAIT) over medical therapy alone. The data is mostly based on large case series [10, 11, 12, 13, 14, 15, 16, 17, 18, 19, 20, 21, 22, 23]. Nimodipine is the most intensively studied, and only, drug approved by the US Food and Drug Administration for use in the treatment of CV. According to the studies. IA nimodipine is safe and effective in the treatment of CV. Angiographic improvement in up to 43% of interventions and clinical improvement in 76% of treated patients were achieved using IA nimodipine [12, 13, 23]. This so-called clinicoangiographic dissociation has been explained by the presumably neuroprotective effects of nimodipine.

The drugs can be injected through selective or superselective catheterisation. Superselective catheterisation would only be prudent where two circulations are unevenly affected distal to a bifurcation. However, in most patients only selective catheterisation would be enough to effectively treat CV and the risk of thrombus formation in a superselectively catheterised vasospastic artery is very high.

The methods involve either slow bolus administration of drug or prolonged infusions lasting approximately 30 to 120 min, or a combination of the two methods. Follow-up angiography is usually performed 10-15 minutes after the injection. A typical IA infusion dose of nimodipine per vessel is 1 to 2 mg over 10 to 30 minutes (total dose not exceeding 4 to 5 mg). If a significant effect is observed, the procedure can be ended and the patient returns to the intensive care unit for further follow-up. When required, multiple sessions have to be performed in order to achieve a better outcome. Some authors therefore prefer to leave the introducer sheath in the artery during the sensitive period to avoid multiple femoral punctures in case of recurrent CV. If a minor angiographic effect is seen, continuous infusion therapy could be considered. The catheter will be left in the artery and continuous infusion therapy initiated, starting from 2 hours and lasting up to 10 days. Depending on the duration of the therapy the infusion rates of nimodipine vary between 1 and 6 mg/h.

At our institution, we usually treat severe CV with IAIT via indwelling catheters. Mostly it takes 5-7 days to return the size of the cerebral arteries to normal, but we have had a few patients in whom the IA catheters remained *in situ* for 10 days without significant complications (Figures 2 and 3).

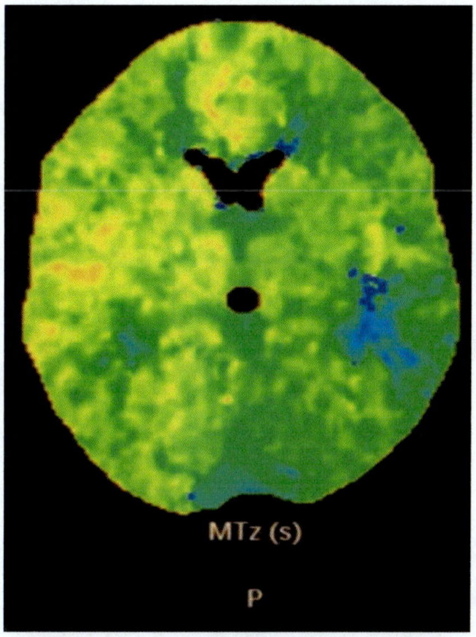

(A)

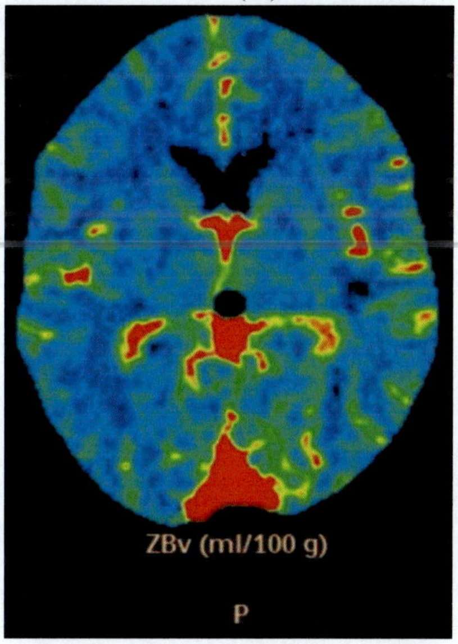

(B)

Figure 2. (Continued).

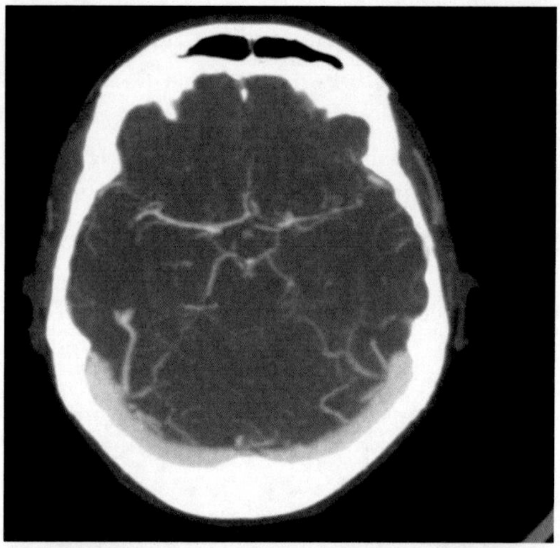

(C)

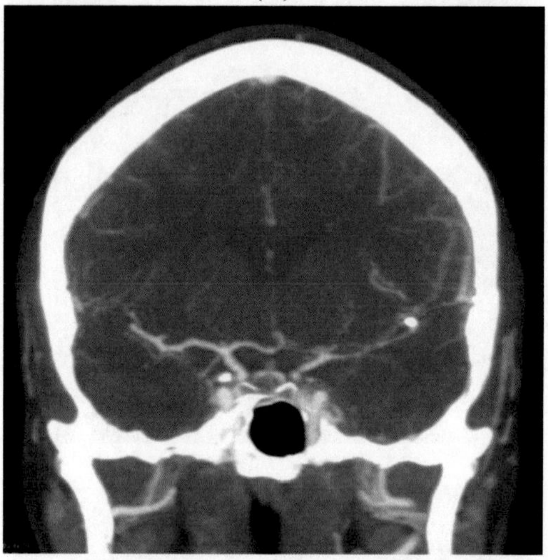

(D)

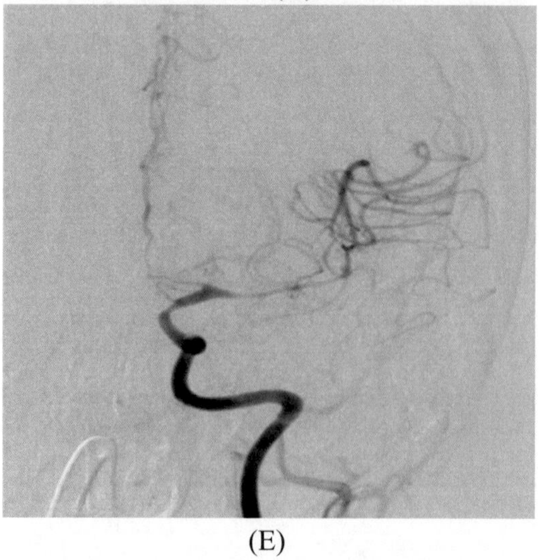

(E)

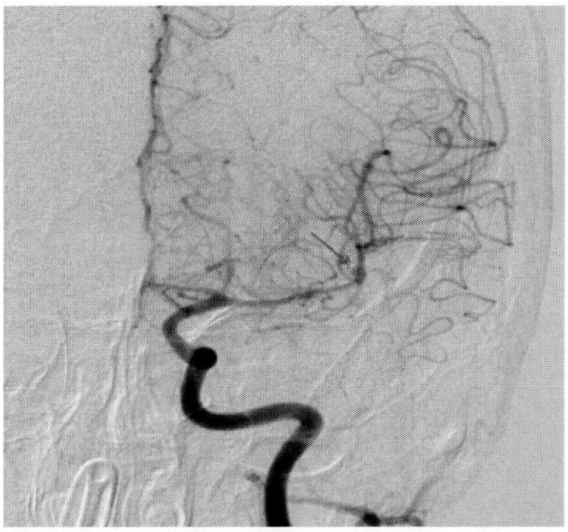

(F)

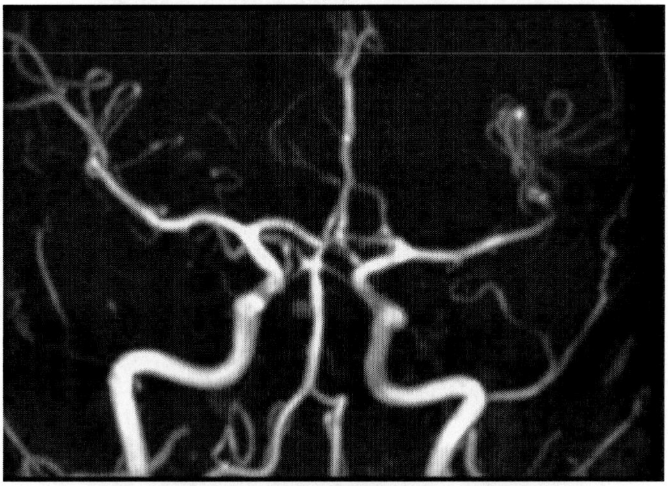

(G)

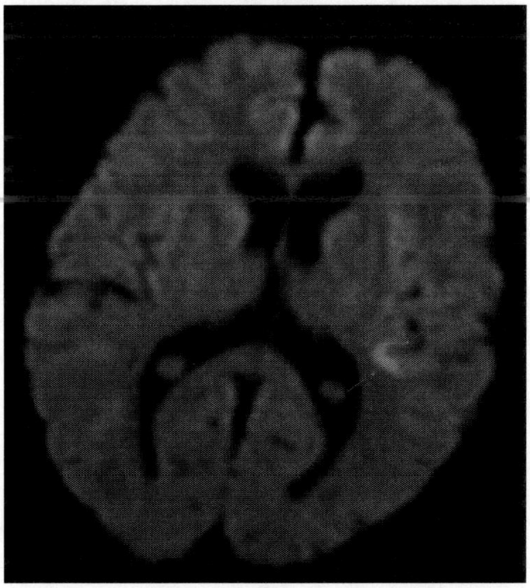

(H)

Figure 2. (Continued).

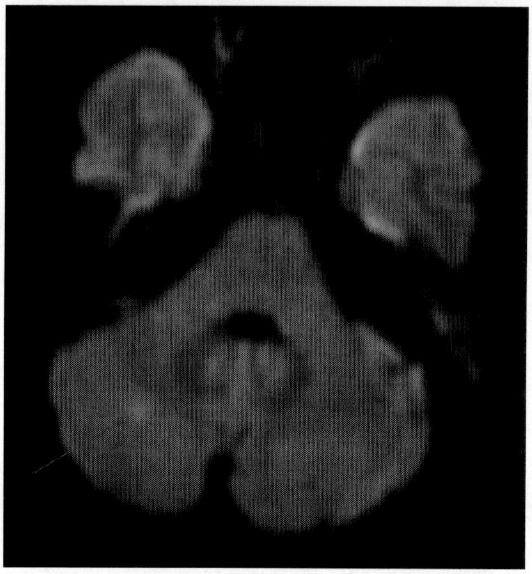

(I)

Figure 2. The Mean Transit Time (MTT) map (A) shows prolongation in the left MCA territory with deficient perfusion on the CBV map (B) in the posterior insula. CTA (C and D) and DSA (E) images confirm severe CV of the proximal and distal arteries on the left. DSA (F) performed after 8 days of continuous IAIT with nimodipine demonstrates significant regression of CV. The arrow indicates the ruptured and coiled aneurysm in the left MCA. MRA (G) 7 days after IAIT shows arteries of normal size. On DWI (arrows on H and I) the infarctions in the left posterior insula and right cerebellum are visible. No significant complications related to the treatment of CV.

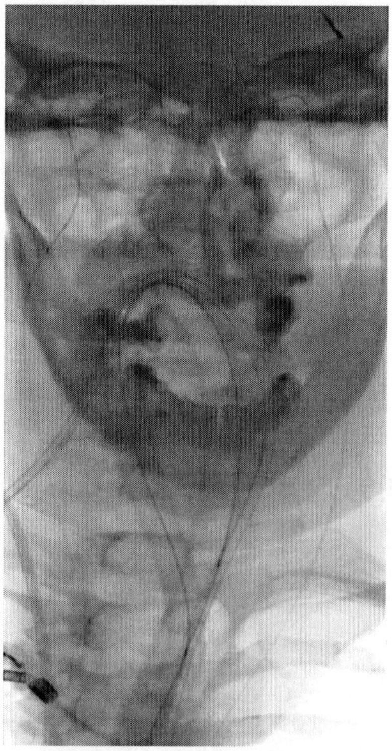

(A)

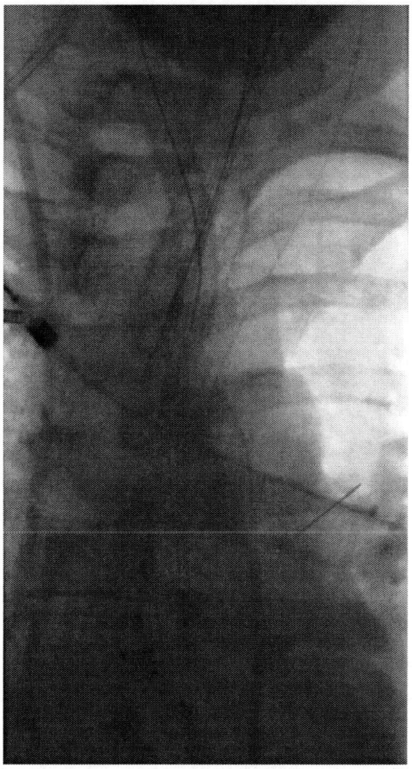

(B)

Figure 3. The distal markers of the indwelling microcatheters for continuous IAIT are illustrated (arrow on A). They lie in each petrous segment of the ICA. At B the distal tip of the guiding catheter can be seen in the descending aorta (arrow on B). The guiding catheter is usually placed at such a level to avoid injuring a vessel.

If no effect is observed, another therapy regimen should be considered.

The agents can be injected without danger to treat CV regardless of the vessel size and orientation. However, care should be taken when injecting Nimotop (Bayer, Leverkusen, Germany), since the solution contains 23.7vol% ethanol (alcohol) and interactions with alcohol-incompatible drugs can occur.

Verapamil and nicardipine are the next two drugs whose use is being increasingly reported in the literature [10, 14, 15].

Specific Considerations Regarding IAIT

Delayed onset of action, a transient therapeutic effect and the potential increase in intracranial pressure (ICP) are some of the disadvantages of IAIT. IA nimodipine may increase the ICP by extravasation of fluid into the interstitial space in the brain or decrease the blood pressure through systemic vasodilation. Both have the potential to lower the cerebral perfusion pressure (CPP) with subsequent ischaemia in especially delicate vasospastic areas. Therefore, direct monitoring of ICP is necessary for excluding such a risk.

In order to prolong the effects of IAIT and avoid multiple sessions, nimodipine can be infused continuously via indwelling arterial microcatheters placed in the internal carotid artery or vertebral artery. This therapy is especially useful in cases of severe proximal and distal CV [16, 18, 19, 20, 21, 22]. However, vessel wall dissection, catheter dislocation, thromboemboli and sepsis due to indwelling foreign material are risks which should be kept in mind (Figure 4). Aggressive measures to prevent thromboembolism should be undertaken which in turn could pose a problem in patients with severe SAH. At our institution, we usually give patients heparin and aspirin and routinely perform a Multiplate test (Roche, Basel, Switzerland) in each patient to exclude any unresponsiveness.

With a session-wise treatment strategy the delayed response to vasodilator infusion should be kept in mind before evaluating the therapeutic response and adjusting the drug dosage. Feng et al. demonstrated angiographic improvement when performing a control angiogram 10-15 minutes after treatment [14].

Transluminal Balloon Angioplasty (TBA)

TBA for CV is documented thoroughly in the literature [1, 3, 4, 5, 6, 7, 24, 25, 26, 27, 28]. TBA is currently performed with commercially available single and double-lumen over the wire balloon catheters. As with IAIT, TBA has never been investigated in a randomised controlled trial. Uncontrolled clinical case series have demonstrated its safety and technical efficacy, however. The technical efficacy of TBA for reversing CV ranges between 80% and 100%. Clinical success varies considerably, with reversal of DCI in 31% to 77% of patients [6, 7, 24, 25, 26, 27, 28]. Early treatment within 2 h from symptom onset makes a significant positive contribution toward clinical improvement.

When a balloon is inflated in the lumen of a spastic artery, it stretches and disrupts both the already contracted and degenerated muscle and the proliferative non-muscular components, mainly in the tunica media. It paralyses the vessel wall. Thus, the therapeutic effects of TBA are generally long-lasting and retreatment is rarely necessary.

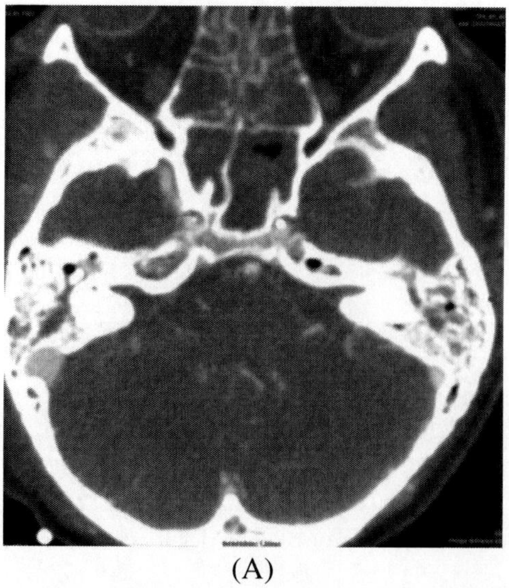

(A)

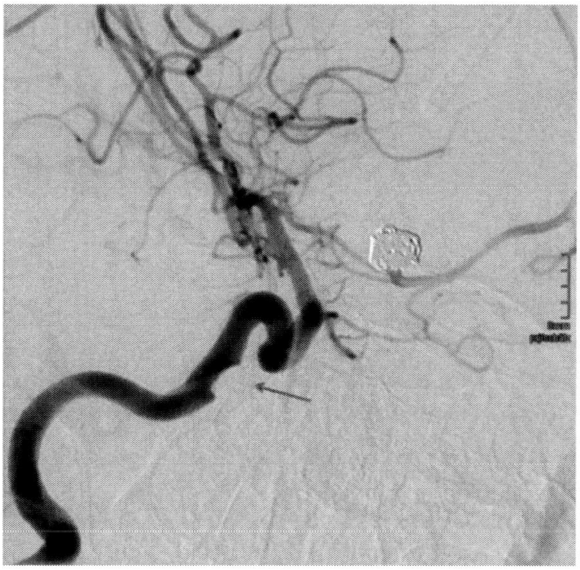

(B)

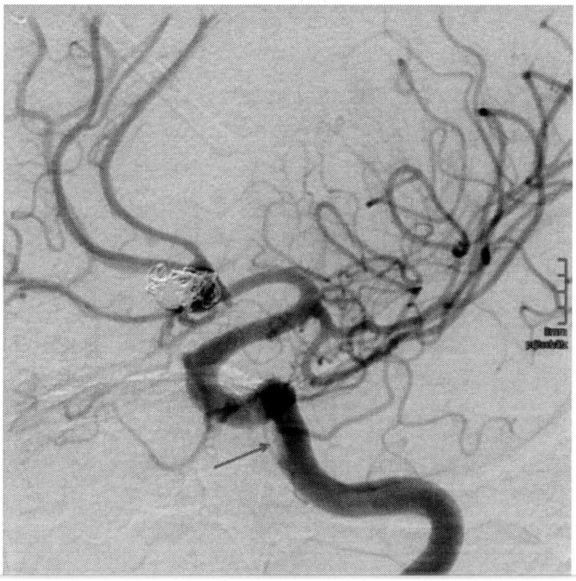

(C)

Figure 4. Thrombus formation in the internal carotid artery due to indwelling catheters without significant narrowing of the lumen. Arrows on CTA image (A) and on DSA images (B and C).

Many experts believe that an expanding balloon in a non-contracted vessel lumen would not achieve the same therapeutic effect. Therefore, many neurointerventionists choose to perform TBA before the initiation of IAIT when combined therapy is planned. With respect to catheterisation and introduction of a balloon catheter, however, it is sometimes necessary to prepare the target vessel with IAIT before TBA.

TBA has been graded as a Class IIb treatment with evidence level B according to guidelines published by the AHA and ASA [1].

SPECIFIC CONSIDERATIONS REGARDING TBA

TBA is usually limited to the proximal vessels of the circle of Willis with diameters greater than 2 mm. Distal balloon angioplasty is generally not recommended. Despite the recent advances in microcatheter technology, tortuous vessels and angioplasty of the anterior cerebral artery still remain technically challenging.

The rate of major complications is approx. 5%. TBA-related complications are vessel rupture, occlusion, dissection, distal embolism, reperfusion injury, displacement of surgical clips and rebleeding from uncontrolled aneurysms.

Prior to TBA, the anatomy of the target vessel before the spasm should be carefully reviewed in order to avoid overdilatation. In the absence of a baseline angiogram, it is often difficult to estimate the normal calibre of a spastic artery and dilatation of a hypoplastic or fenestrated artery may sometimes be encountered. This can be avoided by carefully scrutinising the available angiographic studies. When inflating the balloon, undersizing it to about 80% of the normal vessel diameter is advised. If planning multiple dilatations on a vessel, it is prudent to start distally and continue proximally in order to avoid crossing a fresh angioplasty site with the endovascular material (Figure 5). To avoid multiple dilatations, the balloon length should if possible correspond to the longest straight segment of the target vessel.

TBA is generally contraindicated if the patient has already developed a large infarction in the territory of the target vessel. The same principles of endovascular treatment for acute ischaemic stroke can be applied here. Attempts to restore tissue perfusion to a large infarcted area would increase the risk of reperfusion haemorrhage. Fatal cases of reperfusion haemorrhage have indeed been reported to occur up to 24 h after treating CV with TBA [29].

It is inadvisable to perform TBA adjacent to clipped ruptured aneurysms given that it has been associated with fatal rupture of the parent artery.

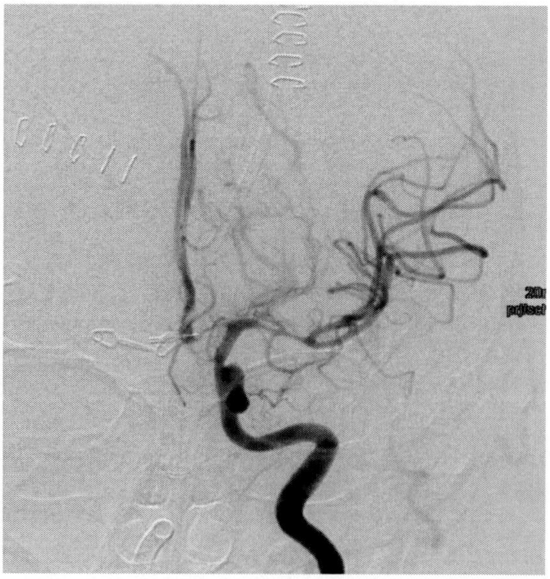

(A)

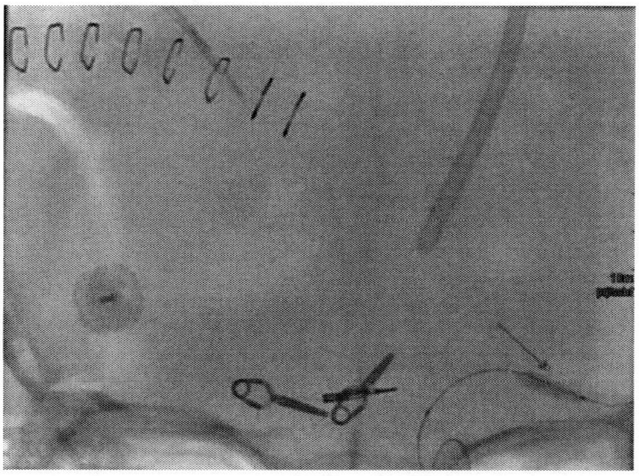

(B)

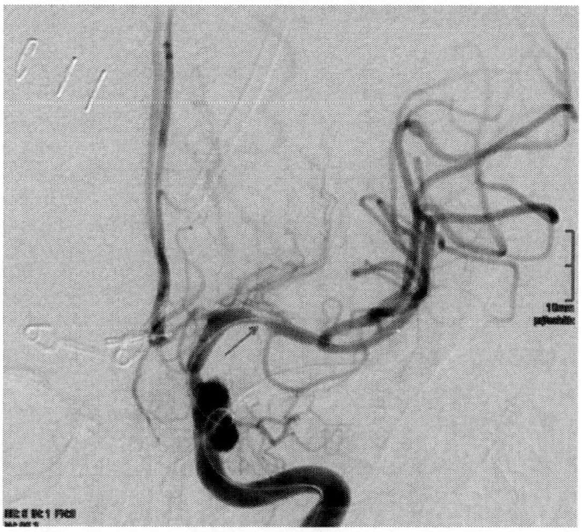

(C)

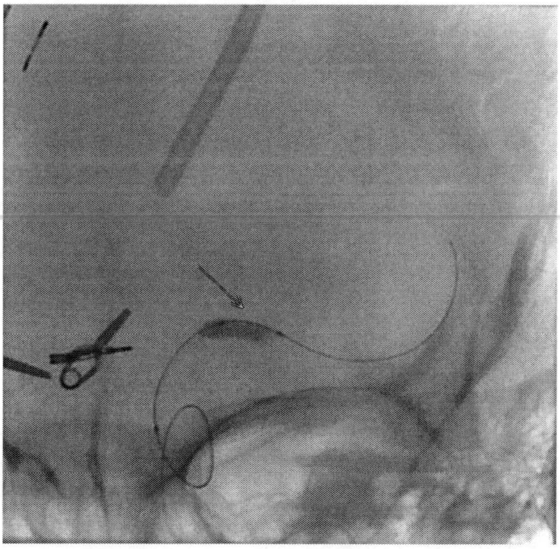

(D)

Figure 5. (Continued).

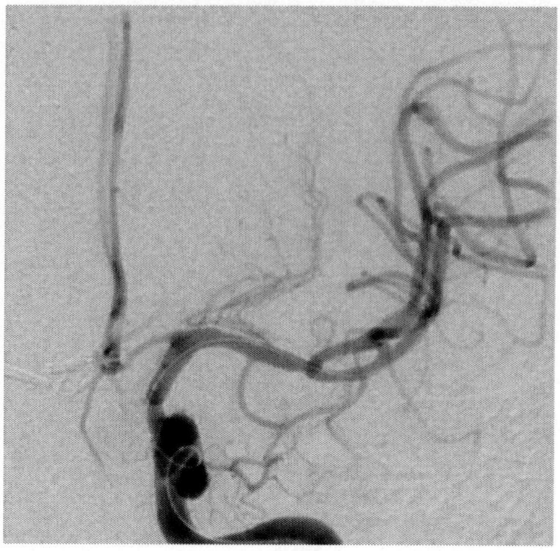

(E)

Figure 5. Severe CV of the proximal intracranial arteries (A). TBA performed from distal (C) to proximal. The inflated balloon can be seen (arrows on B and D). Control scan demonstrates good filling of the proximal MCA (E).

Permanent occlusion of the artery, endothelial injury inflicted by the balloon and other standard factors associated with any endovascular intervention mean that appropriate anticoagulation is necessary. Usually, bolus infusion of heparin at the beginning of the procedure followed by repeat doses according to the ACT level should suffice.

Although uncommon, vasospasm may also recur after angioplasty.

Brief Discussion and Wrap-Up

The endovascular therapy of CV consists of two different treatment modalities which can either be used separately or in a complementary fashion. IAIT procedures are generally used in the management of CV involving the distal arteries beyond the circle of Willis, whereas TBA is the treatment of choice for CV of the larger vessels.

IA administration of vasodilating drugs can be safely undertaken in awake patients. On the other hand, most interventionalists prefer to perform TBA on patients under general anaesthesia, because paralysis potentially lowers the risks of the procedure and offers better visibility of the balloon.

In cases of high-grade SAH and delayed presentation to the hospital, CV will often be encountered. If endovascular treatment is planned in such cases, CV can be managed in the same session with aneurysm embolisation [11, 30].

References

[1] Connolly E. S. Jr., Rabinstein A. A., Carhuapoma J. R., Derdeyn C. P., Dion J., Higashida R. T., Hoh B. L., Kirkness C. J., Naidech A. M., Ogilvy C. S., Patel A. B., Thompson B. G., Vespa P.; American Heart Association Stroke Council; Council on

Cardiovascular Radiology and Intervention; Council on Cardiovascular Nursing; Council on Cardiovascular Surgery and Anesthesia; Council on Clinical Cardiology. Guidelines for the management of aneurysmal subarachnoid hemorrhage: a guideline for healthcare professionals from the American Heart Association/American Stroke Association. *Stroke*. 2012;43(6): 1711-37.

[2] Hayashi K., Hirao T., Sakai N., Nagata I.; JR-NET2 Study Group. Current status of endovascular treatment for vasospasm following subarachnoid hemorrhage: analysis of JR-NET2. *Neurol Med Chir* (Tokyo). 2014;54(2):107-12.

[3] Keyrouz S. G., Diringer M. N. Clinical review: Prevention and therapy of vasospasm in subarachnoid hemorrhage. *Crit Care*. 2007;11(4):220.

[4] Athar M. K., Levine J. M. Treatment options for cerebral vasospasm in aneurysmal subarachnoid hemorrhage. *Neurotherapeutics*. 2012;9(1):37-43.

[5] Durrant J. C., Hinson H. E. Rescue therapy for refractory vasospasm after subarachnoid hemorrhage. *Curr Neurol Neurosci Rep*. 2015;15(2): 521.

[6] Dabus G., Nogueira R. G. Current options for the management of aneurysmal subarachnoid hemorrhage-induced cerebral vasospasm: a comprehensive review of the literature. *Interv Neurol*. 2013;2(1):30-51.

[7] Abruzzo T., Moran C., Blackham K. A., Eskey C. J., Lev R., Meyers P., Narayanan S., Prestigiacomo C. J. Invasive interventional management of post-hemorrhagic cerebral vasospasm in patients with aneurysmal subarachnoid hemorrhage. *J Neurointerv Surg*. 2012;4(3):169-77.

[8] Lylyk P., Vila J. F., Miranda C., Ferrario A., Romero R., Cohen J. E. Partial aortic obstruction improves cerebral perfusion and clinical symptoms in patients with symptomatic vasospasm. *Neurol Res*. 2005; 27:129-35.

[9] Cremers C. H., Vos P. C., van der Schaaf I. C., Velthuis B. K., Vergouwen M. D., Rinkel G. J., Dankbaar J. W. CT perfusion during delayed cerebral ischemia after subarachnoid hemorrhage: distinction between reversible ischemia and ischemia progressing to infarction. *Neuroradiology*. 2015.

[10] Nogueira R. G., Lev M. H., Roccatagliata L., Hirsch J. A., Gonzalez R. G., Ogilvy C. S., Halpern E. F., Rordorf G. A., Rabinov J. D., Pryor J. C. Intra-arterial nicardipine infusion improves CT perfusion-measured cerebral blood flow in patients with subarachnoid hemorrhage- induced vasospasm. *AJNR Am J Neuroradiol*. 2009;30(1): 160-4.

[11] Oran I., Cinar C. Continuous intra-arterial infusion of nimodipine during embolization of cerebral aneurysms associated with vasospasm. *AJNR Am J Neuroradiol*. 2008; 29(2):291-5.

[12] Hänggi D., Turowski B., Beseoglu K., Yong M., Steiger H. J. Intra-arterial nimodipine for severe cerebral vasospasm after aneurysmal subarachnoid hemorrhage: influence on clinical course and cerebral perfusion. *AJNR Am J Neuroradiol*. 2008;29(6):1053-60.

[13] Biondi A., Ricciardi G. K., Puybasset L., Abdennour L., Longo M., Chiras J., Van Effenterre R. Intra-arterial nimodipine for the treatment of symptomatic cerebral vasospasm after aneurysmal subarachnoid hemorrhage: preliminary results. *AJNR Am J Neuroradiol*. 2004;25(6): 1067-76.

[14] Feng L., Fitzsimmons B. F., Young W. L., Berman M. F., Lin E., Aagaard B. D., Duong H., Pile-Spellman J. Intraarterially administered verapamil as adjunct therapy

for cerebral vasospasm: safety and 2-year experience. *AJNR Am J Neuroradiol.* 2002; 23(8):1284-90.

[15] Sehy J. V., Holloway W. E., Lin S. P., Cross D. T. 3rd, Derdeyn C. P., Moran C. J. Improvement in angiographic cerebral vasospasm after intra-arterial verapamil administration. *AJNR Am J Neuroradiol.* 2010; 31(10):1923-8.

[16] Ott S., Jedlicka S., Wolf S., Peter M., Pudenz C., Merker P., Schürer L., Lumenta C. B. Continuous selective intra-arterial application of nimodipine in refractory cerebral vasospasm due to aneurysmal subarachnoid hemorrhage. *Biomed Res Int.* 2014;2014:970741.

[17] Cho W. S., Kang H. S., Kim J. E., Kwon O. K., Oh C. W., Son Y. J., Know B. J., Jung C., Hang M. H. Intra-arterial nimodipine infusion for cerebral vasospasm in patients with aneurysmal subarachnoid hemorrhage. *Interv Neuroradiol.* 2011;17(2):169-78.

[18] Doukas A., Petridis A. K., Barth H., Jansen O., Mehdorn H. M. Continuous intra-arterial infusion of nimodipine at the onset of resistant vasospasm in aneurysmal subarachnoidal haemorrhage. Technical report. *Neurol Res.* 2011;33(3):290-4.

[19] Mayer T. E., Dichgans M., Straube A., Birnbaum T., Müller-Schunk S., Hamann G. F., Schulte-Altedorneburg G. Continuous intra-arterial nimodipine for the treatment of cerebral vasospasm. *Cardiovasc Intervent Radiol.* 2008;31(6):1200-4.

[20] Doukas A., Petridis A. K., Barth H., Jansen O., Maslehaty H., Mehdorn H. M. Resistant vasospasm in subarachnoid haemorrhage treated with continuous intraarterial nimodipine infusion. *Acta Neurochir Suppl.* 2011;112:93-6.

[21] Wolf S., Martin H., Landscheidt J. F., Rodiek S. O., Schürer L., Lumenta C. B. Continuous selective intraarterial infusion of nimodipine for therapy of refractory cerebral vasospasm. *Neurocrit Care.* 2010; 12(3):346-51.

[22] Musahl C., Henkes H., Vajda Z., Coburger J., Hopf N. Continuous local intra-arterial nimodipine administration in severe symptomatic vasospasm after subarachnoid hemorrhage. *Neurosurgery.* 2011;68(6): 1541-7.

[23] Hui C., Lau K. P. Efficacy of intra-arterial nimodipine in the treatment of cerebral vasospasm complicating subarachnoid haemorrhage. *Clin Radiol.* 2005;60(9):1030-6.

[24] Santillan A., Knopman J., Zink W., Patsalides A., Gobin Y. P. Transluminal balloon angioplasty for symptomatic distal vasospasm refractory to medical therapy in patients with aneurysmal subarachnoid hemorrhage. *Neurosurgery.* 2011;69(1):95-102.

[25] Mortimer A. M., Steinfort B., Faulder K., Bradford C., Finfer S., Assaad N., Harrington T. The detrimental clinical impact of severe angiographic vasospasm may be diminished by maximal medical therapy and intensive endovascular treatment. *J Neurointerv Surg.* 2014 pii: neurintsurg-2014-011403.

[26] Mortimer A. M., Steinfort B., Faulder K., Erho T., Dexter M., Assaad N., Harrington T. Institution of sustained endovascular treatment prior to clinical deterioration in patients with severe angiographic vasospasm: A retrospective observational study of clinico-radiological outcomes. *J Neuroradiol.* 2015;42(3):176-83.

[27] Chalouhi N., Tjoumakaris S., Thakkar V., Theofanis T., Hammer C., Hasan D., Starke R. M., Wu C., Gonzalez L. F., Rosenwasser R., Jabbour P. Endovascular management of cerebral vasospasm following aneurysm rupture: outcomes and predictors in 116 patients. *Clin Neurol Neurosurg.* 2014;118:26-31.

[28] Heit J. J., Choudhri O., Marks M. P., Dodd R. L., Do H. M. Cerebral angioplasty using the Scepter XC dual lumen balloon for the treatment of vasospasm following intracranial aneurysm rupture. *J Neurointerv Surg.* 2015;7(1):56-61.

[29] Higashida R. T., Halbach V. V., Cahan L. D. et al. Transluminal angioplasty for treatment of intracranial arterial vasospasm. *J Neurosurg* 1989;71:648-53.

[30] Cho Y. D., Han M. H., Ahn J. H., Jung S. C., Kim C. H., Kang H. S., Kim J. E., Lim J. W. Simultaneous endovascular treatment of ruptured cerebral aneurysms and vasospasm. *Korean J Radiol.* 2015;16(1):180-7.

In: Spontaneous Subarachnoid Haemorrhage
Editors: Thomas Kapapa and Ralph König

ISBN: 978-1-63485-270-8

Chapter 16

CHRONIC HYDROCEPHALUS AFTER SUBARACHNOID HAEMORRHAGE

***Alexandra Huthmann*[*] *and Christoph A. Tschan*[†]**
Department of Neurosurgery, Ludmillenstift Meppen,
Meppen, Germany

ABSTRACT

Subarachnoid haemorrhage (SAH) causes acute and chronic hydrocephalus. Treatment strategies and alternatives are described from clinical point of view. Modern therapy strategies of chronic hydrocephalus in SAH will be discussed. Treatment methods and modern strategies in daily clinical routine for acute and chronic hydrocephalus in SAH are demonstrated. Ventricular drainage, lumbar drainage, endoscopic third ventriculostomy, intraventricular fibrinolysis and different shunting procedures are focused. Ventricular drainage is gold standard for treatment of acute hydrocephalus in SAH. Additional or exchange to lumbar drainage is discussed to prevent cerebral vasospasm and chronic hydrocephalus. In case of chronic hydrocephalus ventriculoperitoneal shunting is necessary. Different shunt types and valves are available. To prevent overdrainage, a gravitational valve can be added to the differential pressure valve. Adjustable shunt valves allow optimizing pressure level and individual needs. In SAH early CSF drainage can avoid chronic hydrocephalus. Early lumbar drainage may reduce onset of cerebral vasospasm. In case of ventriculoperitoneal shunting adjustable differential pressure valves are effective. The combination with gravitational valves prevents overdrainage.

Keywords: SAH, Ventricular Drain, Lumbar Drain, Ventriculoperitoneal Shunt, Gravitational Valve, Chronic Hydrocephalus

---

[*] Huthmann@Ludmillenstift.de.
[†] Tschan@Ludmillenstift.de.

The occurrence of disturbances in the circulation of cerebrospinal fluids (CSF) takes two forms: acute and chronic hydrocephalus [1]. The latter will be discussed in this chapter since the acute hydrocephalus was discussed in chapter nine.

The initial therapy of disturbances in the circulation of CSF after subarachnoid haemorrhage is often managed by placement of an external ventricular drainage to manipulate the amount of CSF within the ventricular system. For this procedure a frontal burr hole is placed in order to insert a draining catheter into the anterior horn of the lateral ventricle [2, 3, 4]. In most cases a silicon catheter with a perforated tip is used. Within several minutes after insertion, physiological levels of intracranial pressure can be achieved by this measure; often pressure relief is necessary to achieve optimal conditions for potential aneurysm treatment. An alternative to a silicon catheter is a steel needle (Duisburger Needle) that is introduced through a pre-inserted bolt [5]. In the absence of occlusions in the cerebrospinal fluid circulation, single or repeated lumbar punctures or placement of a lumbar silicon catheter (lumbar drainage, LD) [6, 7] for continuous CSF drainage can be performed. Furthermore the removal of blood from subarachnoid space with a lumbar drainage (LD) may decrease development of cerebral vasospasm [8, 9, 10, 11]. In both cases (ventricular drainage, LD) the silicon catheter will be connected to a sealed draining system (Figure1) [3]. According to the principles of communicating tubes and containers, the amount of cerebrospinal fluid drained, and consequently the intracranial pressure may be adjusted by manipulating the height of the drainage system relatively to the head, or more specific to the ventricles [12].

In our hospital we set up the pressure level of the container 10 cm above the foramen Monroi level (approximately the level of the external auditory canal). Monitoring of the CSF outflow should be documented and in case of over or underdrainage pressure level needs to be readjusted. Maximum outflow in adults should be round about 200 ml in 24 hours.

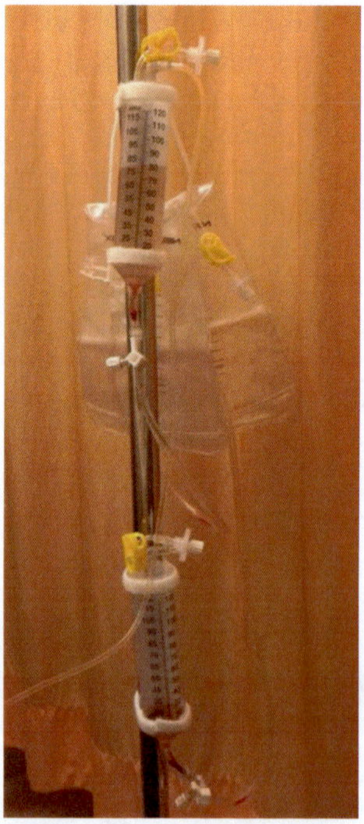

Figure 1. Sealed draining systems for ventricular and lumbal drain.

The ventricular drain allows ICP monitoring. For this a Statham reservoir (pressure measurement chamber e.g., same system for blood pressure monitoring) has to be added to the system. In some systems the measure unit is integrated. To measure the correct ICP, the drain has to be closed for a while in front of the container. Measurement in open systems or in case of overdrainage (slit ventricles) reveals wrong ICP values.

In case of severe intraventricular bleeding the drain can be occluded by clots. Sterile flushing is possible. Up to now there is no clear evidence for reducing the risk of chronic hydrocephalus development by using intraventricular fibrinolysis [13, 14].

Chronic hydrocephalus has an incidence of 25% to 37% [15, 16]. Unfortunately, the functionality of CSF circulation is not always restored with the resorption of subarachnoid blood. Additionally, it is quite difficult to identify a potential chronic hydrocephalus in progress by merely evaluating the imaging diagnostics while the drainage system is in function. One way to tackle this issue is by constant clinical and radiographic evaluation of the patient during gradual reduction of the CSF flow rate and subsequent removal of the catheter [17, 18, 19, 20, 21].

If follow up CT- or MRI-scans of the patient show an enlargement of the ventricular system with corresponding clinical deterioration, indicating a potential development of chronic hydrocephalus, a long-term treatment is indicated. A significantly higher rate for need of shunt-therapy was observed in older patients (> 65 years), poor initial neurological status and additional intraventricular haemorrhage [22, 23, 24].

CSF IL-6 values of $\geq$ 10,000 pg/ml in the early post-SAH period and assessment of S100B levels in CSF and serum may be useful as predictive parameters for shunt dependency in patients with hydrocephalus following aneurysmal SAH [25, 26].

The long-term treatment is commonly carried out by implantation of a ventriculoperitoneal shunt system (VP-shunt) [27]. Also the use of lamina terminalis fenestration and endoscopic third ventriculostomy is discussed, but both procedures remain to be of limited efficacy. Maybe ETV can be employed as a temporary intervention in certain conditions, such as during the waiting period for the clearance of CSF before inserting a VP-shunt or to treat an obstructive hydrocephalus in case of an additional intraventricular haemorrhage [28, 29, 30].

In our clinical routine CSF protein and cell count are used to decide the right moment for implantation of a VP-Shunt. CSF-Protein should be less than 1g to avoid valve obstruction and CSF samples should count less than 50 cells per µl and no microbiological activity.

The objective of the VP-shunt is to connect the ventricles with the peritoneal cavity (subcutaneously) to avoid excessive CSF accumulation in the ventricular system by draining according to the differential pressure gradient between the ventricle and the tip of the distal catheter.

Similar to the technique of implanting an external ventricular drainage, a common method to perform this task is to insert a silicon catheter with a multi-perforated proximal tip in one of the lateral ventricles (usually the right ventricle) through a frontal burr hole. This is connected within a few centimetres with a CSF-reservoir (Control Reservoir) and (a) pressure controlling valve(s). These parts are connected in turn with a distal silicon catheter that ends in the peritoneal cavity through subcutaneous tunnelling [31, 32].

The function of the CSF-reservoir (with unidirectional pump function) is to control the shunt's functionality and to access the CSF circulation if needed. To optimize the flow rate of the CSF, avoiding over- or underdrainage, adjustable differential pressure (DP) valves are used [33, 34, 35].

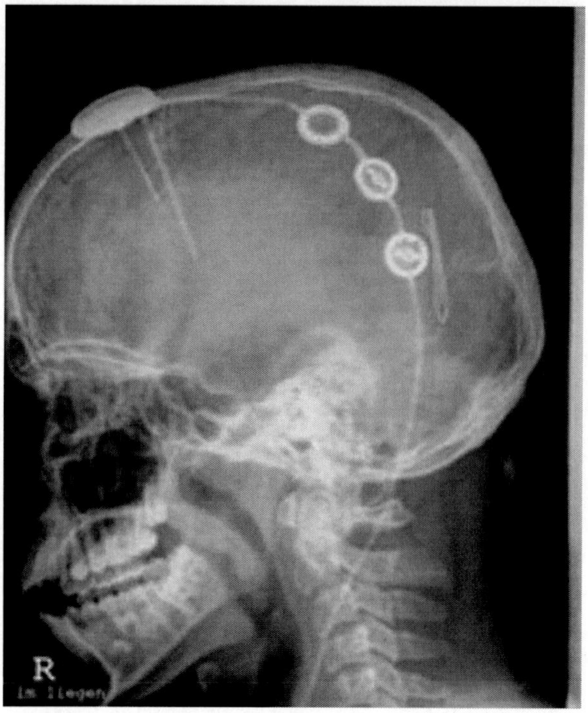

Figure 2. X-ray of the skull with implanted Miethke proSA®-Shunt system with upstream CSF Control-Reservoir, programmable differential pressure valve and programmable gravitational valve (Christoph Miethke GmbH and Co. KG, Aesculap AG, Germany) and telemetric ICP-probe (NEUROVENT®-P-tel, RAUMEDIC AG, Germany)

A common problem that mostly occurs during mobilization of shunted patients is overdrainage of CSF, which is poorly controlled by the DP valve. This led to the development of additional gravitational valves (Figure 2) that control flow in the upright position, eventually optimizing CSF flow in various postures, accounting for diurnal variations [36, 37, 38, 39]. Typical signs and symptoms of overdrainage include postural headaches in the upright position that are alleviated by lying down. A typical finding in radiographic scans of the brain (e.g., CT, MRI) is a pronounced reduction in the size of the ventricles (slit ventricles) or subdural hygroma.

Hydrocephalus might take weeks or even months after an instance of SAH to manifest itself, which is why a long-term intensive follow up of such patients is crucial [40, 41, 42]. For this reason diagnostic telemetric ICP-measurement and long-term monitoring are useful especially in difficult cases [43, 44].

References

[1] Germanwala AV, Huang J, Tamargo RJ. Hydrocephalus after aneurysmal subarachnoid hemorrhage. *Neurosurg. Clin. N. Am.* 2010 Apr;21(2): 263-70. Review.

[2] Huyette DR, Turnbow BJ, Kaufman C, Vaslow DF, Whiting BB, Oh MY. Accuracy of the freehand pass technique for ventriculostomy catheter placement: Retrospective assessment using computed tomography scans. *J. Neurosurg.* 2008;108: 88–91.

[3] Quinones-Hinojosa A. Philadelphia, PA: Saunders; 2012. Schmidek and Sweet Operative Neurosurgical Techniques: *Indications, Methods, and Result.*

[4] Muralidharan R. External ventricular drains: Management and complications. SurgNeurol Int. 2015; 6(Suppl 6): S271–S274.

[5] Meyer B, Schaller K, Rhode V, Hassler W. Percutaneous needle trephination. Experience in 200 cases. *Acta Neurochir.* (Wien). 1994;127(3-4): 232-5.

[6] Hoekema D, Schmidt RH, Ross I. Lumbar drainage for subarachnoid hemorrhage: technical considerations and safety analysis. *Neurocrit. Care.* 2007;7(1): 3-9.

[7] Ormond DR, Dressler A, Kim S, Ronecker J, Murali R. Lumbar drains may reduce the need for permanent CSF diversion in spontaneous subarachnoid haemorrhage. *Br. J. Neurosurg.* 2013 Apr;27(2): 171-4.

[8] Park S, Yang N, Seo E. The effectiveness of lumbar cerebrospinal fluid drainage to reduce the cerebral vasospasm after surgical clipping for aneurysmal subarachnoid hemorrhage. *J. Korean Neurosurg. Soc.* 2015 Mar;57(3): 167-73.

[9] de Aguiar PH, Barros I, Paiva BL, Simm RF. Removal of clots in subarachnoid space could reduce the vasospasm after subarachnoid hemorrhage. *Acta Neurochir. Suppl.* 2013;115: 91-3.

[10] Kwon OY, Kim YJ, Kim YJ, Cho CS, Lee SK, Cho MK. The Utility and Benefits of External Lumbar CSF Drainage after Endovascular Coiling on Aneurysmal Subarachnoid Hemorrhage. *J. Korean Neurosurg. Soc.* 2008 Jun;43(6): 281-7.

[11] Klimo P Jr, Kestle JR, MacDonald JD, Schmidt RH. Marked reduction of cerebral vasospasm with lumbar drainage of cerebrospinal fluid after subarachnoid hemorrhage. *J. Neurosurg.* 2004 Feb;100(2): 215-24.

[12] Bisnaire D, Robinson L. Accuracy of levelling intraventricular collection drainage systems. *J. Neurosci. Nurs.* 1997 Aug; 29(4): 261-8.

[13] Gerner ST, Kuramatsu JB, Abel H, Kloska SP, Lücking H, Eyüpoglu IY, Doerfler A, Schwab S, Huttner HB. Intraventricular fibrinolysis has no effects on shunt dependency and functional outcome in endovascular-treated aneurysmal SAH. *Neurocrit Care.* 2014 Dec;21(3): 435-43.

[14] Kramer AH, Fletcher JJ. Locally-administered intrathecal thrombolytics following aneurysmal subarachnoid hemorrhage: a systematic review and meta-analysis. *Neurocrit. Care.* 2011 Jun;14(3):489-99. doi: 10.1007/s12028-010-9429-z. Review.

[15] Yoshioka H, Inagawa T, Tokuda Y, Inokuchi F. Chronic hydrocephalus in elderly patients following subarachnoid hemorrhage. *Surg. Neurol.* 2000 Feb;53(2): 119-24; discussion 124-5.

[16] Yang TC, Chang CH, Liu YT, Chen YL, Tu PH, Chen HC. Predictors of shunt-dependent chronic hydrocephalus after aneurysmal subarachnoid haemorrhage. Eur Neurol. 2013;69(5):296-303. doi: 10.1159/ 000346119. *Epub* 2013 Feb 26.

[17] Zolal A, Juratli T, Dengl M, Ficici KH, Schackert G, Sobottka SB. Daily drained CSF volume is a predictor for shunt dependence - A retrospective study. *Clin. Neurol. Neurosurg.* 2015 Aug 28; 138:147-150.

[18] Lewis A, Kimberly WT. A retrospective analysis of cerebrospinal fluid drainage volume in subarachnoid hemorrhage and the need for early or late ventriculoperitoneal shunt placement. *J. Neurosurg. Sci.* 2014 Dec 17.

[19] Lewis A, Irvine H, Ogilvy C, Kimberly WT. Predictors for delayed ventriculoperitoneal shunt placement after external ventricular drain removal in patients with subarachnoid hemorrhage. *Br. J. Neurosurg.* 2015 Apr;29(2): 219-24.

[20] Lewis A, Taylor Kimberly W. Prediction of ventriculoperitoneal shunt placement based on type of failure during external ventricular drain wean. *Clin. Neurol. Neurosurg.* 2014 Oct;125: 109-13.

[21] Klopfenstein JD, Kim LJ, Feiz-Erfan I, Hott JS, Goslar P, Zabramski JM, SpetzlerRF.Comparison of rapid and gradual weaning from external ventricular drainage in patients with aneurysmal subarachnoid hemorrhage: a prospective randomized trial. *J. Neurosurg.* 2004 Feb;100(2): 225-9.

[22] Bae IS, Yi HJ, Choi KS, Chun HJ. Comparison of Incidence and Risk Factors for Shunt-dependent Hydrocephalus in Aneurysmal Subarachnoid Hemorrhage Patients. *J. Cerebrovasc. Endovasc. Neurosurg.* 2014 Jun;16(2): 78-84.

[23] Czorlich P, Ricklefs F, Reitz M, Vettorazzi E, Abboud T, Regelsberger J, Westphal M, Schmidt NO. Impact of intraventricular hemorrhage measured by Graeb and LeRoux score on case fatality risk and chronic hydrocephalus in aneurysmal subarachnoid hemorrhage. *Acta Neurochir.* (Wien). 2015 Mar;157(3): 409-15.

[24] Kwon JH, Sung SK, Song YJ, Choi HJ, Huh JT, Kim HD. Predisposing factors related to shunt-dependent chronic hydrocephalus after aneurysmal subarachnoid hemorrhage. *J. Korean Neurosurg. Soc.* 2008 Apr;43(4): 177-81.

[25] Wostrack M, Reeb T, Martin J, Kehl V, Shiban E, Preuss A, Ringel F, Meyer B, Ryang YM.Shunt-dependent hydrocephalus after aneurysmal subarachnoid hemorrhage: the role of intrathecal interleukin-6. *Neurocrit. Care.* 2014 Aug;21(1): 78-84.

[26] Brandner S, Xu Y, Schmidt C, Emtmann I, Buchfelder M, Kleindienst A. Shunt-dependent hydrocephalus following subarachnoid hemorrhage correlates with increased S100B levels in cerebrospinal fluid and serum. *Acta Neurochir. Suppl.* 2012;114:217-20.

[27] Kang S.Efficacy of lumbo-peritoneal versus ventriculo-peritoneal shunting for management of chronic hydrocephalus following aneurysmal subarachnoid haemorrhage. *Acta Neurochir.* (Wien). 2000;142(1): 45-9.

[28] Komotar RJ, Hahn DK, Kim GH, Starke RM, Garrett MC, Merkow MB, Otten ML, Sciacca RR, Connolly ES Jr. Efficacy of lamina terminalis fenestration in reducing shunt-dependent hydrocephalus following aneurysmal subarachnoid hemorrhage: a systematic review. Clinical article. *J. Neurosurg.* 2009 Jul;111(1): 147-54. Review.

[29] Fukuhara T, Shimizu T, Namba Y. Limited efficacy of endoscopic third ventriculostomy for hydrocephalus following aneurysmal subarachnoid hemorrhage. *Neurol. Med. Chir.* (Tokyo). 2009 Oct;49(10): 449-55.

[30] Obaid S, Weil AG, Rahme R, Bojanowski MW. Endoscopic third ventriculostomy for obstructive hydrocephalus due to intraventricular hemorrhage. *J. Neurol. Surg. A Cent. Eur. Neurosurg.* 2015 Mar;76(2):99-111. doi: 10.1055/s-0034-1382778. *Epub* 2014 Jul 21.

[31] Chalouhi N, Whiting A, Anderson EC, Witte S, Zanaty M, Tjoumakaris S, Gonzalez LF, Hasan D, Starke RM, Hann S, Ghobrial GM, Rosenwasser R, Jabbour P.

Comparison of techniques for ventriculoperitoneal shunting in 523 patients with subarachnoid hemorrhage. *J. Neurosurg.* 2014 Oct;121(4): 904-7.

[32] Greenberg MS. Handbook of Neurosurgery. 7th ed. New York: Thieme; 2010. *CSF diversionary procedures*; pp. 207–14.

[33] Lee L, King NK, Kumar D, Ng YP, Rao J, Ng H, Lee KK, Wang E, Ng I. Use of programmable versus nonprogrammable shunts in the management of hydrocephalus secondary to aneurysmal subarachnoid hemorrhage: a retrospective study with cost-benefit analysis. *J. Neurosurg.* 2014 Oct;121(4): 899-903.

[34] Kim KH, Yeo IS, Yi JS, Lee HJ, Yang JH, Lee IW. A pressure adjustment protocol for programmable valves. J Korean Neurosurg Soc. 2009 Oct;46(4):370-7. doi: 10.3340/jkns.2009.46.4.370. *Epub* 2009 Oct 31.

[35] Katano H, Karasawa K, Sugiyama N, Yamashita N, Ohkura A, Kamiya K. Clinical evaluation of shunt implantations using Sophy programmable pressure valves: comparison with Codman-Hakim programmable valves. *J. Clin. Neurosci.* 2003 Sep;10 (5): 557-61.

[36] Aschoff A, Kremer P, Benesch C, Fruh K, Klank A, Kunze S. Overdrainage and shunt technology. A critical comparison of programmable, hydrostatic and variable-resistance valves and flow-reducing devices. *Childs Nerv. Syst.* 1995 Apr;11(4): 193-202.

[37] Czosnyka Z, Czosnyka M, Richards HK, Pickard JD.Posture-related overdrainage: comparison of the performance of 10 hydrocephalus shunts in vitro. *Neurosurgery.* 1998 Feb;42(2): 327-33; discussion 333-4.

[38] Kehler U, Kiefer M, Eymann R, Wagner W, Tschan CA, Langer N, Rohde V, Ludwig HC, Gliemroth J, Meier U, Lemcke J, Thomale UW, Fritsch M, Krauss JK, Mirzayan MJ, Schuhmann M, Huthmann A. PROSAIKA: A prospective multicenter registry with the first programmable gravitational device for hydrocephalus shunting. *Clin. Neurol. Neurosurg.* 2015 Oct;137: 132-6.

[39] Tschan CA, Antes S, Huthmann A, Vulcu S, Oertel J, Wagner W. Overcoming CSF overdrainage with the adjustable gravitational valve proSA. ActaNeurochir (Wien). 2014 Apr;156(4): 767-76; discussion 776.

[40] Walcott BP, Iorgulescu JB, Stapleton CJ, Kamel H. Incidence, Timing, and Predictors of Delayed Shunting for Hydrocephalus After Aneurysmal Subarachnoid Hemorrhage. *Neurocrit. Care.* 2015 Aug;23(1): 54-8.

[41] Yang TC, Chang CH, Liu YT, Chen YL, Tu PH, Chen HC. Predictors of shunt-dependent chronic hydrocephalus after aneurysmal subarachnoid haemorrhage. *Eur. Neurol.* 2013;69(5): 296-303.

[42] Wang YM, Lin YJ, Chuang MJ, Lee TH, Tsai NW, Cheng BC, Lin WC, Su BY, Yang TM, Chang WN, Huang CC, Kung CT, Lee LH, Wang HC, Lu CH. Predictors and outcomes of shunt-dependent hydrocephalus in patients with aneurysmal sub-arachnoid hemorrhage. *BMC Surg.* 2012 Jul 5;12: 12.

[43] Antes S, Tschan CA, Kunze G, Ewert L, Zimmer A, Halfmann A, Oertel J.Clinical and radiological findings in long-term intracranial pressure monitoring. *Acta Neurochir.* (Wien). 2014 May;156(5): 1009-19; discussion 1019.

[44] First clinical results with a new telemetric intracranial pressure-monitoring system. Welschehold S, Schmalhausen E, Dodier P, Vulcu S, Oertel J, Wagner W, Tschan CA. *Neurosurgery.* 2012 Mar;70 (1 Suppl. Operative): 44-9; discussion 49.

In: Spontaneous Subarachnoid Haemorrhage
Editors: Thomas Kapapa and Ralph König
ISBN: 978-1-63485-270-8

Chapter 17

EPILEPTIC SEIZURES IN ASSOCIATION WITH SPONTANEOUS SUBARACHNOID HAEMORRHAGE

Sarah Jesse
Department of Neurology, University of Ulm,
Ulm, Germany

ABSTRACT

Epileptic tonic-clonic seizures in relation to spontaneous subarachnoid haemorrhage (SAH) should be classified into initial seizures within the first 24 h after SAH, early seizures during the first 14 days, and late onset then with symptomatic epilepsy, given that the therapeutic approach and prognosis are correlated to such clinical stratification. Since randomised controlled and double-blind clinical trials into the management of epileptic seizures with SAH are lacking, therapeutic recommendations can only be made based on the guidance of the Neurocritical Care Society and American Stroke Association.

Initial seizures related to the manifestation of bleeding occur in up to 21%. Anticonvulsant medication should be administered until treatment of the aneurysm, albeit for a maximum of three days, preferably with non-enzyme inducers so as to avoid drug interactions with nimodipine. The incidence of early seizures within the following 14 days does not appear to differ between patients undergoing surgery and those receiving endovascular treatment for ruptured aneurysms (10%-11%). If there are risk factors, such as multiple epileptic seizures or the existence of parenchymal defects, drug therapy should be administered for 3-6 months. The late onset of epileptic seizures post SAH accounts for 12% of the patient population and should, as with any symptomatic form of epilepsy, be managed long-term with anticonvulsants. Non-convulsive seizures and non-convulsive status epilepticus occur in 18% and 13% of cases, respectively, and should be considered in particular in quantitative disorders of consciousness as well as diagnosed with the help of an EEG.

After neurovascular events, epilepsy – with a prevalence of 0.5%-1% – is the second most commonly occurring neurological disorder. It has an incidence of 46 in 100,000 per year and increases with age, and mostly results from symptomatic conditions such as intracerebral/subarachnoid bleeding, ischaemia or neoplasias. Irrespective of whether epilepsy has been diagnosed, the lifetime prevalence in terms of a single epileptic seizure occurring in the normal population is > 10% [1].

In relation to spontaneous subarachnoid haemorrhage (SAH), (simple or complex) partial epileptic seizures generally occur, often with secondary generalisation. It is useful to differentiate between initial seizures within the first 24 h after SAH, early seizures during the first 14 days, and late onset then with symptomatic epilepsy, given that the therapeutic approach and prognosis are correlated to such clinical stratification.

INITIAL SEIZURE

In patients with SAH, 3%-21% initially exhibit tonic-clonic seizures at onset or within the first 24 hours of bleeding [2, 3], often if the patient is younger [4] as well as with a higher Fisher score, accompanied by localised cisternal, intraventricular or intraparenchymal bleeds [5]. The occurrence of these initial seizures is associated with a complicated stay in hospital and is often accompanied by further epileptic attacks, an increased rate of pneumonia, and delayed onset of cerebral ischaemia related to vasospasm [6]. Despite the higher risk of complications, the long-term prognosis of the patient does not appear to be adversely affected, particularly as after six months the functional outcome is no worse, mortality is not increased and the prevalence of epilepsy is no higher in those affected [6, 7]. Prophylactic anticonvulsant therapy at this stage is hotly debated, but would seem reasonable for spanning the period until treatment of the aneurysm [8] in light of the fact that the risk of rebleeding is known to be closely correlated with increased systolic blood pressure. Thus, further convulsive epileptic seizures in relation to an untreated aneurysm signify an indirect risk of secondary bleeding [9, 10], which itself is associated with a clinical outcome that is far worse [11]. As systematic studies into anticonvulsive therapy in this regard are still awaited, it is advisable – as recommended by the Guidelines of the Neurocritical Care Society and the American Stroke Association – to administer prophylactic drug therapy during the immediate posthaemorrhagic phase until surgical or endovascular treatment is carried out, albeit for a maximum of three days [12, 13].

EARLY SEIZURE

Epileptic seizures occurring within 14 days after the manifestation of SAH are referred to as early seizures. Data in the literature on ruptured aneurysms are inconsistent with respect to the periprocedural occurrence of epileptic seizures, which are reported at a rate of 13.6% and 8.3% for clipping versus coiling, respectively [14]; this relatively high incidence decreases over the subsequent five years to 9.6% and 6.4%, respectively. In this case younger age as well as a high Fischer or Hunt and Hess score, or delayed ischaemic complications, are also major risk factors/predictors for epilepsy [14, 15]. Contrary to these results, an international study in a total of more than 20,000 patients with spontaneous SAH detected no relevant difference as regards the occurrence of early seizures or epilepsy (10.0% versus 11.1%) between operation and intervention [16].

Postoperative prophylactic drug therapy is frequently administered despite the absence of prior epileptic seizures, but is also hotly debated in the light of recent study data. Randomised controlled trials into the safety and efficacy of anticonvulsant drugs for primary and secondary prophylaxis post SAH are lacking [17, 18]. Moreover, there are studies that have demonstrated an inferior outcome in those patients treated prophylactically with anticonvulsants [19, 20]. The literature available on this topic primarily addresses the use of phenytoin, and in rarer cases carbamazepine and phenobarbital. Apart from the typical side effects of the individual anticonvulsants in the treated populations, an increased number of neurological deficits was detected in particular on account of the higher incidence of ischaemia, possibly owing to the interaction between the given enzyme inducers and coadministration of nimodipine. Its plasma concentration is reduced by up to 70% due to induction of cytochrome p450 [21]. Few studies are available on levetiracetam, which compared to phenytoin does not trigger enzyme production; no difference in the outcome has been noted [22, 23], whilst tolerability with respect to side effects is improved overall [24].

In line with the recommendations of the Neurocritical Care Society (Guidelines 2011) and American Stroke Association (Guidelines 2012), therefore, it is in principle advisable to forgo prophylactic anticonvulsant therapy during the postoperative phase if there are no signs indicative of epileptic seizures. Administration of drug therapy for 3-6 months for early seizures, in the same way as for cerebral ischaemia, appears to be justified [25, 26] if epileptic seizures have already occurred and if, in particular, parenchymal damage has resulted from the SAH or secondary ischaemia [12, 13, 27, 28].

LATE SEIZURE

The long-term incidence of symptomatic epilepsy after spontaneous SAH is 8% during the first year post haemorrhage, and 12% during the subsequent five years. The probability of epilepsy occurring is associated with higher Hunt and Hess grades and with parenchymal damage [29, 30]. Additional risk factors appear to be early epileptic seizures [31] as well as a lower rating on the Glasgow Outcome Scale at hospital discharge [32]. With late-onset seizures carrying a higher risk of recurrence and usually being correlated with a parenchymal defect, a patient should be assumed to have symptomatic epilepsy that will then require treatment in accordance with the guidelines of the ILAE [1].

NON-CONVULSIVE SEIZURE

Non-convulsive seizures occur in 8%-18% of patients [33]. A number of studies that performed continuous EEG monitoring in SAH patients revealed an incidence of up to 18% for complex partial non-convulsive seizures and up to 13% for non-convulsive status epilepticus, which was associated with the increased age of the patients as well as higher mortality. Furthermore, delayed cerebral ischaemia could be predicted in one study based on specific EEG changes (reduced delta/alpha ratio, relative alpha variability and amplitude) [34]. As continuous EEG monitoring is not practicable in clinical routine, it certainly will not replace regular Doppler ultrasound in the detection of vasospasms. However, in patients with persistent disorders of consciousness – whether in terms of quantity or quality – an EEG should be performed to rule out non-convulsive seizures or non-convulsive status epilepticus.

Epileptic activity as a differential diagnosis in localised subarachnoid signal alterations on CT and MRI.

Both computed tomography (as the "gold standard" for early diagnosis of SAH) and magnetic resonance imaging permit detection of signal alterations in the subarachnoid space which in addition to SAH are also attributable on differential diagnosis to other conditions, such as an inflammatory exudate in meningitis, meningeal spread, hypertension-induced exudate associated with posterior reversible encephalopathy syndrome, cerebral amyloid angiography, cortical venous thrombosis or vascular malformation [35]. Further differential diagnoses include reversible cerebral vasokonstriction syndrome, hyperanticoagulation with vitamin K antagonists, and angiitis [36]. In association with renal failure, localised subarachnoid exudate can also appear on follow-up imaging after administration of a contrast agent [37]. Another important factor to be considered in the differential diagnosis of spontaneous SAH, as well as vasospasm-induced ischaemia, is localised cortical and also subarachnoid signal alteration in the event of protracted or frequent seizures as well as (non-convulsive) status epilepticus [38] (Figure1).

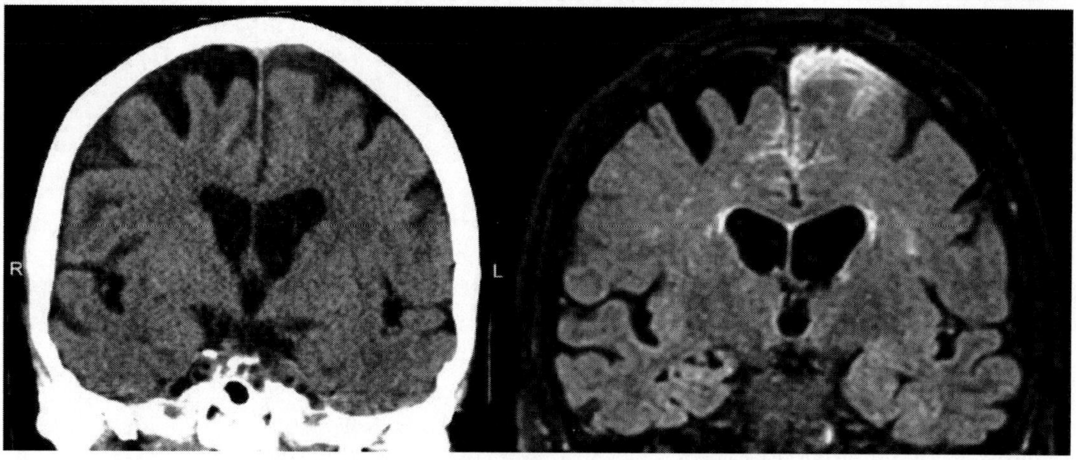

Figure 1. CT and MRI scans from a female patient with non-convulsive status epilepticus existing for several days. Evidence of localised subarachnoid hyperdensity/hyperintensity in the left upper frontal lobe consistent with protein-rich exudate. Courtesy of the Neuroradiological Department of Neurology, Rehabilitation Hospital Ulm, Ulm, Germany.

Summary of the major aspects of epileptic seizures in spontaneous SAH:

- Stratification of epileptic seizures into initial, early and late is reasonable given that treatment and prognosis are designed with these categories in mind.
- Since randomised controlled and double-blind clinical trials into the management of epileptic seizures with SAH are lacking, therapeutic recommendations can only be

made based on the guidance of the Neurocritical Care Society and American Stroke Association.

- Initial cases related to the manifestation of bleeding occur in up to 21% of SAH cases and are associated with a complex hospital stay. Anticonvulsant medication should be administered until treatment of the aneurysm, albeit for a maximum of three days, preferably with non-enzyme inducers so as to avoid drug interactions with nimodipine.
- The incidence of early seizures within the following 14 days does not appear to differ between patients undergoing surgery and those receiving endovascular treatment for ruptured aneurysms (10%-11%). If there are risk factors, such as multiple epileptic seizures or the existence of parenchymal defects, drug therapy should be administered for 3-6 months.
- The late onset of epileptic seizures post SAH accounts for 12% of the patient population and should, as with any symptomatic form of epilepsy, be managed long-term with anticonvulsants.
- Non-convulsive seizures and non-convulsive status epilepticus occur in 18% and 13% of cases, respectively, and should be considered in particular in quantitative disorders of consciousness as well as diagnosed with the help of an EEG.
- Subarachnoid signal alterations on CT and MRI can be indicative not only of SAH but also of other conditions, such as a protracted epileptic seizure or (non-convulsive) status epilepticus, and should be considered when deliberating the differential diagnosis.

REFERENCES

[1] Diener H-C, Weimar, C. Leitlinien für Diagnostik und Therapie in der Neurologie. Thieme-Verlag. 2012.

[2] Claassen J, Peery S, Kreiter KT, Hirsch LJ, Du EY, Connolly ES, et al. Predictors and clinical impact of epilepsy after subarachnoid hemorrhage. Neurology. 2003 Jan 28;60(2):208-14. PubMed. PMID: 12552032. *Epub* 2003/01/29. eng.

[3] Hasan D, Schonck RS, Avezaat CJ, Tanghe HL, van Gijn J, van der Lugt PJ. Epileptic seizures after subarachnoid hemorrhage. Annals of neurology. 1993 Mar;33(3):286-91. PubMed PMID: 8498812. *Epub* 1993/03/01. eng.

[4] Krishna H, Wani AA, Behari S, Banerji D, Chhabra DK, Jain VK. Intracranial aneurysms in patients 18 years of age or under, are they different from aneurysms in adult population? Acta neurochirurgica. 2005 May;147(5):469-76; discussion 76. PubMed PMID: 15812597. *Epub* 2005/04/07. eng.

[5] Guth JC, Gerard EE, Nemeth AJ, Liotta EM, Prabhakaran S, Naidech AM, et al. Subarachnoid extension of hemorrhage is associated with early seizures in primary intracerebral hemorrhage. Journal of stroke and cerebrovascular diseases : the official journal of National Stroke Association. 2014 Nov-Dec;23(10):2809-13.PubMed.PMID: 25194742. *Epub* 2014/09/10. eng.

[6] De Marchis GM, Pugin D, Lantigua H, Zammit C, Tadi P, Schmidt JM, et al. Tonic-clonic activity at subarachnoid hemorrhage onset: impact on complications and

outcome. PloS one. 2013;8(8):e71405. PubMed PMID: 23951155. Pubmed Central PMCID: 3741137. *Epub* 2013/08/21. eng.

[7] Fung C, Balmer M, Murek M, Z'Graggen WJ, Abu-Isa J, Ozdoba C, et al. Impact of early-onset seizures on grading and outcome in patients with subarachnoid hemorrhage. Journal of neurosurgery. 2015 Feb;122(2):408-13. PubMed PMID: 25479126. *Epub* 2014/12/06. eng.

[8] Lanzino G, D'Urso PI, Suarez J. Seizures and anticonvulsants after aneurysmal subarachnoid hemorrhage. Neurocritical care. 2011 Sep;15(2):247-56. PubMed PMID: 21751102. *Epub* 2011/07/14. eng.

[9] De Marchis GM, Lantigua H, Schmidt JM, Lord AS, Velander AJ, Fernandez A, et al. Impact of premorbid hypertension on haemorrhage severity and aneurysm rebleeding risk after subarachnoid haemorrhage. Journal of neurology, neurosurgery, and psychiatry. 2014 Jan;85(1):56-9. PubMed PMID: 23813741. *Epub* 2013/07/03. eng.

[10] Tang C, Zhang TS, Zhou LF. Risk factors for rebleeding of aneurysmal subarachnoid hemorrhage: a meta-analysis. PloS one. 2014;9(6):e99536. PubMed PMID: 24911172. Pubmed Central PMCID: 4049799. *Epub* 2014/06/10. eng.

[11] Park J, Woo H, Kang DH, Kim YS, Kim MY, Shin IH, et al. Formal protocol for emergency treatment of ruptured intracranial aneurysms to reduce in-hospital rebleeding and improve clinical outcomes. Journal of neurosurgery. 2015 Feb;122(2): 383-91. PubMed PMID: 25403841. *Epub* 2014/11/19. eng.

[12] Connolly ES, Jr., Rabinstein AA, Carhuapoma JR, Derdeyn CP, Dion J, Higashida RT, et al. Guidelines for the management of aneurysmal subarachnoid hemorrhage: a guideline for healthcare professionals from the American Heart Association/american Stroke Association. Stroke; a journal of cerebral circulation. 2012 Jun;43(6):1711-37. PubMed PMID: 22556195. *Epub* 2012/05/05. eng.

[13] Rowe AS, Goodwin H, Brophy GM, Bushwitz J, Castle A, Deen D, et al. Seizure prophylaxis in neurocritical care: a review of evidence-based support. Pharmacotherapy. 2014;34(4):396-409. PubMed PMID: 24277723. *Epub* 2013/11/28. eng.

[14] Hart Y, Sneade M, Birks J, Rischmiller J, Kerr R, Molyneux A. Epilepsy after subarachnoid hemorrhage: the frequency of seizures after clip occlusion or coil embolization of a ruptured cerebral aneurysm: results from the International Subarachnoid Aneurysm Trial. Journal of neurosurgery. 2011 Dec;115(6):1159-68. PubMed PMID: 21819189. *Epub* 2011/08/09. eng.

[15] Raper DM, Starke RM, Komotar RJ, Allan R, Connolly ES, Jr. Seizures after aneurysmal subarachnoid hemorrhage: a systematic review of outcomes. World neurosurgery. 2013 May-Jun;79(5-6):682-90. PubMed PMID: 23022642. *Epub* 2012/10/02. eng.

[16] Hoh BL, Nathoo S, Chi YY, Mocco J, Barker FG, 2nd. Incidence of seizures or epilepsy after clipping or coiling of ruptured and unruptured cerebral aneurysms in the nationwide inpatient sample database: 2002-2007. Neurosurgery. 2011 Sep;69(3):644-50; discussion 50. PubMed PMID: 21499155. *Epub* 2011/04/19. eng.

[17] Marigold R, Gunther A, Tiwari D, Kwan J. Antiepileptic drugs for the primary and secondary prevention of seizures after subarachnoid haemorrhage. The Cochrane database of systematic reviews. 2013;6:CD008710. PubMed PMID: 23740537. Epub 2013/06/07. eng.

[18] Rhoney DH, Tipps LB, Murry KR, Basham MC, Michael DB, Coplin WM. Anticonvulsant prophylaxis and timing of seizures after aneurysmal subarachnoid hemorrhage. Neurology. 2000 Jul 25;55(2):258-65. PubMed PMID: 10908901. *Epub* 2000/07/26. eng.

[19] Naidech AM, Kreiter KT, Janjua N, Ostapkovich N, Parra A, Commichau C, et al. Phenytoin exposure is associated with functional and cognitive disability after subarachnoid hemorrhage. Stroke; a journal of cerebral circulation. 2005 Mar;36(3): 583-7. PubMed PMID: 15662039. *Epub* 2005/01/22. eng.

[20] Rosengart AJ, Huo JD, Tolentino J, Novakovic RL, Frank JI, Goldenberg FD, et al. Outcome in patients with subarachnoid hemorrhage treated with antiepileptic drugs. Journal of neurosurgery. 2007 Aug;107(2):253-60. PubMed PMID: 17695377. *Epub* 2007/08/19. eng.

[21] Tartara A, Galimberti CA, Manni R, Parietti L, Zucca C, Baasch H, et al. Differential effects of valproic acid and enzyme-inducing anticonvulsants on nimodipine pharmacokinetics in epileptic patients. British journal of clinical pharmacology. 1991 Sep;32(3):335-40. PubMed PMID: 1777370. Pubmed Central PMCID: 1368527. *Epub* 1991/09/01. eng.

[22] Milligan TA, Hurwitz S, Bromfield EB. Efficacy and tolerability of levetiracetam versus phenytoin after supratentorial neurosurgery. Neurology. 2008 Aug 26;71(9):665-9. PubMed PMID: 18725591. *Epub* 2008/08/30. eng.

[23] Murphy-Human T, Welch E, Zipfel G, Diringer MN, Dhar R. Comparison of short-duration levetiracetam with extended-course phenytoin for seizure prophylaxis after subarachnoid hemorrhage. World neurosurgery. 2011 Feb;75(2):269-74. PubMed PMID: 21492729. *Epub* 2011/04/16. eng.

[24] Karamchandani RR, Fletcher JJ, Pandey AS, Rajajee V. Incidence of delayed seizures, delayed cerebral ischemia and poor outcome with the use of levetiracetam versus phenytoin after aneurysmal subarachnoid hemorrhage. Journal of clinical neuroscience : official journal of the Neurosurgical Society of Australasia. 2014 Sep;21(9):1507-13. PubMed PMID: 24919470. *Epub* 2014/06/13. eng.

[25] Kwan J, Wood E. Antiepileptic drugs for the primary and secondary prevention of seizures after stroke. The Cochrane database of systematic reviews. 2010 (1):CD005398. PubMed PMID: 20091574. *Epub* 2010/01/22. eng.

[26] Leung H, Man CB, Hui AC, Kwan P, Wong KS. Prognosticating acute symptomatic seizures using two different seizure outcomes. Epilepsia. 2010 Aug;51(8):1570-9. PubMed PMID: 20002147. *Epub* 2009/12/17. eng.

[27] Diringer MN, Bleck TP, Claude Hemphill J, 3rd, Menon D, Shutter L, Vespa P, et al. Critical care management of patients following aneurysmal subarachnoid hemorrhage: recommendations from the Neurocritical Care Society's Multidisciplinary Consensus Conference. Neurocritical care. 2011 Sep;15(2):211-40. PubMed PMID: 21773873. *Epub* 2011/07/21. eng.

[28] Ibrahim GM, Fallah A, Macdonald RL. Clinical, laboratory, and radiographic predictors of the occurrence of seizures following aneurysmal subarachnoid hemorrhage. Journal of neurosurgery. 2013 Aug;119(2):347-52. PubMed PMID: 23581590. *Epub* 2013/04/16. eng.

[29] Grunwald IQ, Kuhn AL, Schmitt AJ, Balami JS. Aneurysmal SAH: current management and complications associated with treatment and disease. The Journal

of invasive cardiology. 2014 Jan;26(1):30-7. PubMed PMID: 24402809. *Epub* 2014/01/10. eng.

[30] Huttunen J, Kurki MI, von Und Zu Fraunberg M, Koivisto T, Ronkainen A, Rinne J, et al. Epilepsy after aneurysmal subarachnoid hemorrhage: A population-based, long-term follow-up study. Neurology. 2015 Jun 2;84(22):2229-37. PubMed PMID: 25948726. *Epub* 2015/05/08. eng.

[31] Serafini A, Gigli GL, Gregoraci G, Janes F, Cancelli I, Novello S, et al. Are Early Seizures Predictive of Epilepsy after a Stroke? Results of a Population-Based Study. Neuroepidemiology. 2015 Jul 28;45(1):50-8. PubMed PMID: 26227564. *Epub* 2015/08/01. Eng.

[32] Buczacki SJ, Kirkpatrick PJ, Seeley HM, Hutchinson PJ. Late epilepsy following open surgery for aneurysmal subarachnoid haemorrhage. Journal of neurology, neurosurgery, and psychiatry. 2004 Nov;75(11):1620-2. PubMed PMID: 15489400. Pubmed Central PMCID: 1738819. *Epub* 2004/10/19. eng.

[33] Gilmore E, Choi HA, Hirsch LJ, Claassen J. Seizures and CNS hemorrhage: spontaneous intracerebral and aneurysmal subarachnoid hemorrhage. The neurologist. 2010 May;16(3):165-75. PubMed PMID: 20445426. *Epub* 2010/05/07. eng.

[34] Kondziella D, Friberg CK, Wellwood I, Reiffurth C, Fabricius M, Dreier JP. Continuous EEG monitoring in aneurysmal subarachnoid hemorrhage: a systematic review. Neurocritical care. 2015 Jun;22(3):450-61. PubMed PMID: 25277888. *Epub* 2014/10/04. eng.

[35] Cucchiara B, Sinson G, Kasner SE, Chalela JA. Pseudo-subarachnoid hemorrhage: report of three cases and review of the literature. Neurocritical care. 2004;1(3):371-4. PubMed PMID: 16174937. *Epub* 2005/09/22. eng.

[36] Renou P, Tourdias T, Fleury O, Debruxelles S, Rouanet F, Sibon I. Atraumatic nonaneurysmal sulcal subarachnoid hemorrhages: a diagnostic workup based on a case series. Cerebrovasc Dis. 2012;34(2):147-52. PubMed PMID: 22890017. *Epub* 2012/08/15. eng.

[37] Morris JM, Miller GM. Increased signal in the subarachnoid space on fluid-attenuated inversion recovery imaging associated with the clearance dynamics of gadolinium chelate: a potential diagnostic pitfall. AJNR American journal of neuroradiology. 2007 Nov-Dec;28(10):1964-7. PubMed PMID: 17893215. *Epub* 2007/09/26. eng.

[38] Villalobos-Chavez F, Rodriguez-Uranga JJ, Sanz-Fernandez G. [Sequential changes in magnetic resonance in a limbic status epilepticus]. Revista de neurologia. 2005 Mar 16-31;40(6): 354-7. PubMed PMID: 15795872. *Epub* 2005/03/30. Cambios secuenciales en la resonancia magnetica en estado epileptico limbico. spa.

In: Spontaneous Subarachnoid Haemorrhage
Editors: Thomas Kapapa and Ralph König
ISBN: 978-1-63485-270-8

Chapter 18

NEUROREHABILITATION AFTER SUBARACHNOID HAEMORRHAGE

Martin Schorl and Michael Hartwich
Early Neurological/Neurosurgical Rehabilitation,
Asklepios Schlossbergklinik Bad König,
Bad König, Germany

ABSTRACT

Neurorehabilitation after subarachnoid haemorrhage (SAH) is of major importance in all patients surviving the acute stage of their illness but remaining disabled. Neurorehabilitation aims at regaining self control in the activities of daily living in severely affected patients or the return to the workplace in moderate affected patients.

This chapter describes the German Phase model for neurorehabilitation after central nervous damage in general and focuses on the patients severely affected after SAH. Severely affected patients after central nervous system damage are treated by early neurological and neurosurgical rehabilitation as the link between acute care and rehabilitation. Early neurological and neurosurgical rehabilitation becomes increasingly specialized, nowadays integrating intensive care treatment modalities and rehabilitation. The aim was to minimise the need to return patients from early rehabilitation back to the emergency department and facilitate integrated rehabilitation treatment with accompanying treatment of the typical complications. For this to happen, a combination of multidisciplinary emergency and rehabilitative measures are usually needed which, depending on the respective medical situation, can be carried out in varying degrees of intensity and dominance.

The interdisciplinary approach of early neurological and neurosurgical rehabilitation is discussed in detail concerning the characteristics of the patients treated, the setting, the multidisciplinary treatment concept including the medical and therapeutic staff and the diagnostic equipment required.

Special aspects of neurorehabilitation after SAH are discussed in detail. Data concerning outcome are presented. Overall, they show the benefit of early neurological and neurosurgical rehabilitation both from the patient's and the society's perspective.

Keywords: neurorehabilitation, German phase model of neurorehabilitation, early neurological rehabilitation, early neurosurgical rehabilitation, interdisciplinary neurorehabilitation

Development of Neurorehabilitation and Legal Regulations

Early rehabilitation after stroke has proven superior to late rehabilitation [20]. Rehabilitation should therefore be commenced at the earliest opportunity in the acute phase during initial treatment so as to increase the chances of rehabilitation and not to lose any valuable time [4]. Since 2001, therefore, social law in Germany has included an entitlement to rehabilitation services during acute inpatient care (Section 27 of Social Security Code (SGB) IX).

However, the phase model for the rehabilitation of individuals with severe and very severe brain damage was inaugurated as early as 1995 by the Bundesarbeitsgemeinschaft Rehabilitation (BAR) [Federal Rehabilitation Council] [4]. The Bundesarbeitsgemeinschaft Rehabilitation is an amalgamation of different health insurance providers (umbrella organisations for health insurance, accident insurance, annuity insurance) with the participation of the Medical Review Board of the Statutory Health Insurance Funds, representatives of the federal states, medical societies and medical experts.

The aim of the phase model was to create an integrated treatment and rehabilitation chain targeted to the needs of patients and accounting for both medical and rehabilitative requirements.

Table 1. Phase model for neurorehabilitation of individuals with severe brain injury in Germany

Phase	*Definition*
A	Acute care including surgery, neurosurgery, interventional neuroradiology, neurointensive care.
B	Early post-acute rehabilitation treatment; intensive care facilities must be provided, may include mechanical ventilation.
C	Continuing rehabilitation. Vital signs are stable and the patient is able to participate actively in therapy, but requires some medical care. Partly dependent in activities of daily living (ADL).
D	Follow-up rehabilitation. Patients are mostly independent in ADL; medical therapies aimed at returning to work, may be performed on an outpatient rehabilitation basis.
E	Occupational retraining or reintegration.
F	Function-preserving nursing care and therapies for patients with disorders of consciousness or persistent, severe disabilities (e.g., occupational therapy, physiotherapy, oral tract therapy), either in specialized nursing homes or at home, sometimes with home ventilation therapy.

In this phase model, a distinction is made (Table 1) between an acute phase and several subsequent rehabilitation phases: ideally, once primary acute hospital treatment (Phase A) is complete, the patient initially receives care under Phase B (known as "early neurological rehabilitation"), then Phase C (continuing rehabilitation), and finally Phase D (follow-up rehabilitation). One or more of the above-mentioned phases can be skipped depending on the level of care required by the patient or the degree of independence achieved.

Occupational reintegration or retraining can take place in Phase E. If after early rehabilitation (Phase B) the level of independence is not sufficient to move on to the subsequent rehabilitation phases, out-of-hospital nursing care is introduced while continuing with the treatment programme (Phase F). The aim here is to at least maintain the level that has been achieved and avoid secondary complications.

With the introduction of a new hospital billing system (G-DRG) in 2001, early neurological rehabilitation is now predominantly funded through flat rates per case, which are based on the one hand on medical diagnoses and on the other hand on reimbursement-relevant procedures. The complex flat rate for "early neurological rehabilitation" (known as OPS 8-552) [7] can only be billed if certain qualitative structural and quantitative requirements are fulfilled. Therefore, among other things, at least 300 treatment minutes per patient per day must be provided and weekly team meetings with standardised assessments carried out.

In contrast to developments in other countries, where rehabilitation teams attend to severely affected patients during anaesthesiological and neurological/neurosurgical treatment (outreach rehabilitation), specialist clinics have been established in Germany that have the necessary medical and rehabilitative expertise along with the staff and equipment required to also deal with patients in critical condition who are still in need of intensive care immediately after undergoing emergency treatment. This enables rehabilitative approaches to be integrated into the treatment programme at the earliest opportunity.

As a result of neurorehabilitation becoming increasingly specialised in its position as the link between the acute disciplines of neurology and neurosurgery as well as rehabilitation, attempts have been made to introduce an additional qualification in neurorehabilitation or the separate title of specialist for neurorehabilitation into basic and advanced training. Relevant initiatives are also afoot internationally within the framework of the European Federation for NeuroRehabilitation (EFNR).

Early Neurological Rehabilitation/ Phase B According to the Phase Model

General Aspects

Patients

Among all patients in early neurological and neurosurgical rehabilitation, patients post subarachnoid haemorrhage (SAH) account for 7.5% to 28% [9, 12, 18] of total patient numbers depending on the specialisation of the hospital.

Patients in early neurological and neurosurgical rehabilitation are typically medically unstable over a lengthy period of time and may have a variety of complications ([3], Table 2). On the one hand, these are pre-existing comorbidities involving other organ systems, and on the other hand complications in the central and peripheral nervous system. A distinction is essentially made here between direct nervous system complications (e.g., epilepsy, critical illness polyneuropathy, hydrocephalus, sinking skin flap syndrome after decompressive craniectomy) or the impact of the symptoms of neurological damage on other organ systems (e.g., pneumonia following neurogenic dysphagia, electrolyte imbalance and arrhythmia as a result of central endocrine insufficiencies, intestinal motility disorders with vomiting as a result of autonomous functional disorders of the peripheral nervous system).

Table 2. Typical medical complications in early neurological/neurosurgical rehabilitation

Organ system	*Symptom*	
Central and peripheral nervous system	Meningitis/ventriculitis	
	Epileptic seizure	
	Convulsive and non-convulsive status epilepticus	
	Critical-illness polyneuropathy	
	Neurogenic dysphagia	
	Malresorptive hydrocephalus	
	Shunt dysfunction, shunt infection	
	Sinking skin flap syndrome	
Endocrine system	Diabetes insipidus	
	Cerebral salt-wasting syndrome	
	Syndrome of inappopriate ADH secretion	
	Electrolyte disorders	
	Acquired anterior pituitary insufficiency	
Vegetative system	Sympathicotonic dysregulation	Tachycardia
		Arterial hypertension
		Hyperhidrosis
		Tachypnoea
		Hyperthermia
	Gastrointestinal dysregulation	Vomiting
		Pylorospasm
		Reflux
		Diarrhoea
Cardiopulmonary system	Cardiac arrhythmias	
	Heart failure	
	Endocarditis	
	Takotsubo cardiomyopathy	
	Pneumonia	
	Bronchial obstruction	
	Thrombosis, pulmonary embolism	
	Pneumothorax	
	Pleural effusion	
	Pleuritis	
Gastrointestinal system	Gallstones, gallbladder sludge	
	Cholestasis	
	Cholecystitis	
	Hyperammonaemia	
	Gastritis, ventricular ulcer, duodenal ulcer	

Organ system	*Symptom*
	Ascites
	Peritonitis
Genitourinary system	Urinary tract infection
	Renal failure
	Nephrolithiasis
	Haematuria
	Incontinence
Musculoskeletal system	Heterotopic ossification
Bacteria requiring isolation	MRSA, 3-MRGN, 4-MRGN, clostridia, VRE
Pre-existing diseases	Cancer
	Coronary heart disease
	Bronchial asthma
	Mental illnesses
	Infectious diseases (hepatitis, HIV)
	Parkinson's disease, Parkinson's syndrome, multiple sclerosis
	Inflammatory bowel diseases
Medication	Sedative effects (e.g., antidepressants, antiepileptics)
	Interactions
	Proconvulsive effects (e.g., theophylline, anti-infectives, activating substances)

The BAR defined the task of early rehabilitation, among other things, as "the medical diagnosis and curative medical treatment of underlying diseases and comorbidities from neurological damage" [4, point 3.1.3., page 10] and mentioned explicitly that "management of life-threatening complications and any complications occurring during mobilisation must be possible" [4, point 3.1.3., page 10].

The aim was thus to minimise the need to return patients from early rehabilitation back to the emergency department and facilitate integrated rehabilitation treatment with accompanying treatment of the typical complications. For this to happen, a combination of multidisciplinary emergency and rehabilitative measures are usually needed which, depending on the respective medical situation, can be carried out in varying degrees of intensity and dominance. Significant overarching tasks in early neurological and neurosurgical rehabilitation involve the continuation of the curative medical efforts initiated as part of acute treatment, support in the remission of CNS/PNS damage by promoting neuroplasticity (basal objectives: improved vigilance, cooperation, ability to communicate), implementation of compensatory and adaptive measures that reduce the need for assistance and increase quality of life, evaluation of the potential for rehabilitation, and the organisation of further care [3]. Ideally, patients can be transferred to continuing rehabilitation phases (Phase C) if there is a corresponding improvement in independence.

Nowadays, patients are transferred to early neurological and neurosurgical rehabilitation immediately on completion of neurological, neurosurgical, or interventional neuroradiological acute medical care. At such a time, many patients are still under analgosedation and mechanical ventilation, and often still have cerebrospinal fluid drains in situ. Medically speaking, the main objectives at this early phase are medical stabilisation, weaning from ventilation, tapering off the analgosedation and achieving an adequate rehabilitative capacity. Initial, mostly passive rehabilitation measures run parallel to this. Ideally, as treatment progresses, intensive care takes a back seat in favour of rehabilitation that takes an increasingly active approach.

To this end, drugs that influence the level of consciousness and stabilise the circulation must be tapered off. As vigilance improves, sympathicotonic dysregulation of the autonomic nervous system often comes to the fore which, given the tendency for tachycardia and hypertension to develop, can be detrimental to early mobilisation and, as a result of hyperhidrosis, can lead to fluid losses and electrolyte imbalances. Nursing care (e.g., from the concept of basal stimulation) and positioning concepts are incorporated in the multidisciplinary approach alongside drug therapies. To make patient mobilisation easier, formulations of substances administered via enteral feeding tube are to be preferred for drug treatment in contrast to substances requiring intravenous application. As a result, changes in medication must also be undertaken frequently during the initial phase.

In the event of severe damage to the central nervous system, or as a result of critical illness polyneuropathy often occurring as a complication in up to 69% [27], there is often evidence of neurogenic dysphagia. After appropriate diagnostic testing, usually involving endoscopy, this will necessitate the insertion, at least temporarily, of a tracheostoma for protection against aspiration as well as percutaneous feeding tubes. The improvement in swallowing function with the aim of decannulation in the tracheotomised patient is also one of the primary objectives of early neurological rehabilitation, which is why swallowing rehabilitation is initiated as a multidisciplinary approach from the time of admission onwards.

Setting

Appropriate equipment and staffing are indispensable to the above-mentioned diagnostic and therapeutic activities, as an accompaniment to intensive care treatment, if the patient is not to be subjected to the stresses of being transferred. The aim is to offer patients "one-stop" care. Otherwise, rehabilitation would in the worst-case scenario be repeatedly interrupted. Early neurological and neurosurgical rehabilitation is therefore carried out predominantly in specially dedicated clinics that in some cases also offer subsequent rehabilitation phases (see below), more rarely as a functional facility affiliated with acute hospitals. Early neurological and neurosurgical rehabilitation is to a large extent characterised by interdisciplinarity – not only from a medical point of view, but also from the perspective of nursing and therapy.

Multidisciplinary Treatment Concept

Early neurological and neurosurgical rehabilitation is carried out under the supervision of a neurologist and/or neurosurgeon with at least three years of experience in neurorehabilitation. Depending on (intensive care) orientation and equipment, as well as the available diagnostic and therapeutic services, the medical team usually consists not only of neurologists, but also physicians, general practitioners, rehabilitation and intensive care specialists. Since transfers to neurosurgery constitute the second most frequent type of transfer alongside transfers to internal medicine [30], some facilities do now employ neurosurgeons or collaborate with neurosurgical clinics in order to offer elective secondary surgical procedures in-house alongside rehabilitation. Expertise in neuroradiology is usually provided via links with (neuro) radiology practices or centres, where teleradiological concepts are increasingly ensuring widespread availability and results of high quality.

Care staff receive basic and advanced training both in intensive care and neurorehabilitation. This combination is of particular importance since patients should benefit as early as possible from neurorehabilitative nursing while on intensive care, and rehabilitative care has huge significance in neurorehabilitation beyond basic care and treatment. This results primarily from the fact that in severely affected patients a number of rehabilitative aspects are viewed within the context of activities of daily living. Catalogues of nursing services have been defined on this basis [11].

The primary objective in physiotherapy is initially to achieve early mobilisation and train the circulation with the aim of sufficient cardiopulmonary capacity and stability in the autonomic nervous system in readiness for the subsequent rehabilitation steps. At the early phase, close coordination with the intensive care specialists and the therapists' own expertise in intensive and respiratory medicine are always essential aspects that can help to interpret the reactions of patients. The purpose of early mobilisation is also to achieve the best possible physiological muscle tone, facilitate first movements, develop targeted motor skills and incorporate them into activities of daily living, and improve postural control. An essential basis for improving motor skills on the one hand, and achieving progress in terms of dysphagia, level of consciousness and environmental interaction on the other, is verticalisation. Later on in the process of neurorehabilitation, the focus is then on change in position, transfers to a wheelchair, wheelchair locomotion and walking. In the case of very severely affected patients, efforts to influence pathologically affected muscle tone come to the fore.

In many early rehabilitation clinics, the therapeutic focus of occupational therapy is not only on motor rehabilitation of the upper extremities so as to restore the hand motor skills to a sufficient degree in everyday and professional life, but also dysphagia therapy, including tracheal cannula management and the reinstatement of an oral diet. This also requires specialist knowledge in respiratory therapy, instrumental diagnosis of dysphagia and close coordination with other therapeutic areas that frequently complement each other in their approaches to the problem (nursing, speech therapy).

The primary task of neuropsychology in early neurological and neurosurgical rehabilitation is on the one hand to diagnose and assess disorders of consciousness with regard to interpreting basic approaches of interaction and developing early communication methods for and with patients, and on the other hand to diagnose and treat the characteristic neuropsychological symptoms and syndromes. Supporting relatives is also very important, as is the advice and guidance of the therapeutic team in case of patients with mental (e.g., depression with suicidal tendency) or neuropsychological (e.g., organic brain syndrome with restlessness, aggressiveness and behaviour that is harmful to the self or others) disorders. Neuropsychology is often the discipline where first-line diagnosis and treatment of aphasic disorders are undertaken in the process of developing methods of communication.

Besides the diagnosis and treatment of aphasia and dysarthria, which are frequently limited in early neurological rehabilitation by concurrent neurocognitive deficits, the diagnosis and treatment of dysphagia is a further area of expertise covered by speech therapy.

Table 3 provides an overview of the respective treatment modalities.

Table 3. Overview of Therapeutic Treatments in Phase B

Nursing therapy 4-6 hr/d	• Diagnostics: Skin conditions, position tolerance, primary behavior observation, assessment of endurance • Basal stimulation: activating "guided" basic care, initiation of cooperation in mini-sequences in the ADL • Relaxing therapies in agitated phases: bathing, positions, communication, reduction of sedating medication
Physiotherapy 1-2 hr/d	• Diagnostics: muscular tone, joint flexibility, pathalogical movements • Prophylactic treatment to prevent complications: against contractures, pneumonia • Mobilisation (even if patients are on respiratortherapy): "Pilot"-seat, bed edge, wheel chair, improvement of circulatory endurance, initiation of first position and support reactions • Respiration therapy: assistance in weaning of respirator, secretion control • Multimodal stimulation for improvement of perception • Reduction of pathologically increased muscle tone: functional positioning, modified neurophysiologically orientated treatment procedures, casting • Regain of mobility: transfer and wheelchair training, treadmill training, balance training, walking with and without auxiliary devices
Occupational therapy 1-2 hr/d	• Diagnostics: swallowing function, secretion control, assessment of aspiration risk • Facio-oral tract (FOT) therapy: improvement of swallowing reflex, weaning from tracheal tube after successful weaning from the respirator, management of tracheal tube • Improvement of hand function: Reduction of pathological muscle tone, establishing first and functional movements, expansion of usage in actitivies of daily living, e.g., constraint induced movement therapy (CIMT), improvement of fine motor skills, reduction of apraxia and ataxia • Training of abilities in activities of daily living: bathing, clothing, eating • Improvement of multimodal perception • Adaption of auxiliary devices • Neurocognitive training: planning strategies, attention, memory
Neuropsychology 2-3 hr/wk	• Diagnostics: assessment of level of consciousness using standardized behavioral observation, scales and screenings • Recommendations for interaction with the patient • Daily scheduling based on endurance • Establishing communication: communication code, communication training • Family counseling
Speech therapy (complementary or as needed)	• Diagnostics: Different types of aphasia, dysarthria, swallowing disorders, evaluation of aspiration risk • Establishing communication communication code, auxiliary devices, communication training, compensation strategies • Facio-oral-tract-(FOT)-therapy • Training and improvement of swallowing and eating, compensation strategies • Management of tracheal tubes
Music therapy (as needed)	• Diagnostics: attempt to create musical contact in cases of severe disturbed consciousness • Establishing communication: relaxing or animating musical stimulation, musical communication code

In addition to these standard therapies, a variety of other treatments (e.g., music therapy, art therapy, animal-assisted therapy, physical therapy) are used in different combinations. Increasingly, modern (e.g., robot-assisted locomotion therapy) and evidence-based (e.g., constrained induced movement therapy) therapies find their way into early rehabilitation, sometimes adapted specifically to the patients.

The complexity of injury patterns in patients on the one hand and the variety of specialist disciplines involved in the treatment on the other hand rely on clear and thorough communication on the part of all those involved, and a flexible approach to planning with targeted selection and implementation of treatment. Regular interdisciplinary team meetings every week are therefore an opportunity to exchange information, focus on objectives and mutually agree on the treatment plan. Multidisciplinary treatment concepts (e.g., botulinum toxin injection into the salivary glands for reducing the amount of saliva in pseudohypersalivation with risk of aspiration following reduced swallowing frequency, thereby facilitating dysphagia therapy and extending tracheal cannula unblocking times) and concurrent programmes from various disciplines (e.g., physiotherapy for mobilisation into a sitting position and speech therapy for managing dysphagia in the achieved sitting position) are characteristic of the early neurological and neurosurgical rehabilitation activities that rely on considerable staff input.

Specific Aspects in Patients Post Subarachnoid Haemorrhage (SAH)

A few specific aspects must be considered in the neurorehabilitation of patients after SAH. These concern firstly the underlying condition, and secondly the characteristic symptoms and typical additional complications.

With regard to the underlying condition, the extent to which untreated, partially treated or fully treated aneurysms are to be given follow-up treatment and monitored must be agreed specifically with the neurosurgeons or neuroradiologists providing initial treatment. The modern interventional neuroradiological treatment procedures sometimes mean that anticoagulant therapy is necessary. This must be considered with respect to competing comorbidities and planning of the necessary secondary interventions (placement of percutaneous feeding tubes, elective neurosurgical secondary interventions). On the other hand, the anticoagulant therapy required for internal comorbidities can be hampered or prove impossible if the placement of a cerebrospinal fluid drain has to be performed repeatedly. As a result of the often early transfer of patients to early neurological and neurosurgical rehabilitation, vasospasm therapy or prophylaxis is also occasionally shifted to early rehabilitation, meaning that appropriate expertise and options for instrumental diagnosis must be available.

As occlusive hydrocephalus is initially common, and communicating hydrocephalus is not uncommon over the course, particularly in severe SAH, the diagnosis of hydrocephalus and indication for shunt placement is the preserve of early neurological and neurosurgical rehabilitation and must be closely coordinated with the neurosurgeon. Frequently, these patients are also transferred to early neurological and neurosurgical rehabilitation with cerebrospinal fluid drains still in situ. Handling these drains and weaning are also typically the responsibility of early rehabilitation.

The identification of absolute (e.g., occlusion) or relative (incorrect valve setting) shunt dysfunction in patients with implanted shunts is another issue to be managed as part of neurorehabilitative treatment. Clinically, these patients can usually only be assessed inadequately with regard to shunt dysfunction, as the symptoms of shunt dysfunction and primary damage overlap [5], are frequently only subtle, and merely cause the course of rehabilitation to stagnate [5]. Imaging procedures do not often sufficiently distinguish between shunt dysfunction and the consequences of the primary damage [5]. In recent years, there has been increased use of a gravitational unit ("shunt assistant") combined with the shunt valve as a means of preventing overdrainage when the body is in the upright position. However, in patients who are predominantly bedridden they can lead to a relative shunt dysfunction due to underdrainage [14] and should therefore not be implanted in this patient group.

With the increasing use of decompressive hemicraniectomy as the treatment of last resort in treatment-resistant increased intracranial pressure with accompanying intracerebral haemorrhage and vasospastic infarctions, the diagnosis of a sinking skin flap syndrome [1, 24, 31] that may lastingly impair neurorehabilitation [24] and identification of the need for cranioplasty is very important. After cranioplasty it is essential to promptly diagnose as well as introduce appropriate treatment for complications such as aseptic bone necrosis following autologous cranioplasty with a risk of bone resorption or a sinking bone syndrome [8].

Epileptic seizures are a well-known consequence of focal brain damage. In the differential diagnosis of disorders of consciousness as a result of primary damage, non-convulsive status is of particular significance. The preferred antiepileptics for treatment of symptomatic epilepsy are those that do not impair consciousness, have as little interaction potential as possible, and can be administered easily via a feeding tube. Given the difficulties of differential diagnosis in the case of disorders of consciousness (e.g., valproate-induced encephalopathy) and the potential of pharmacological interactions with loss of effectiveness (e.g., when administering the antibiotic meropenem, which is frequently used in intensive care), valproic acid should not be used as first-line treatment in these patients, which is in contrast to common therapy guidelines in epilepsy. In our own experience, lacosamide also leads to encephalopathy-type conditions time and again. In patients dependent on tube feeding, phenytoin is obsolete, as an effective drug level cannot be achieved [30, own experience].

Organic brain syndromes (OBS) with pronounced drive disorders are not unusual after SAH due to aneurysms commonly being found in the anterior communicating artery or the A1 and proximal A2 segment of the anterior cerebral artery [2]. Not uncommonly, like other neuropsychological symptoms, OBS are also crucial to the functional outcome [19] and can hinder rehabilitation. With regard to attempts at drug treatment, the differentiation of reactive depression, malresorptive hydrocephalus, a symptomatic sleep apnoea syndrome, endocrine problems and a non-convulsive status from organic brain syndromes with reduced drive is important. In the first instance, drug treatment to improve drive is attempted with amantadine, and also levodopa, drive-stimulating antidepressants, and more rarely with amphetamines. Our experience with modafinil is good, especially with simultaneously impaired vigilance. It is worth remembering that, apart from amantadine, the use of medication is beyond any approved indication and the relevant medicolegal aspects of off-label use should be considered. Amnestic syndromes are hardly accessible with drug therapy and require intensive neuropsychological treatment with development of compensation strategies and if necessary accommodation in a special setting (contained area).

At a rate of 47.5%, endocrine disorders of superordinate hypothalamic-pituitary hormone production occur more frequently after SAH than after traumatic brain injury (27.5%) [21]. Interestingly, the occurrence does not correlate with the severity of the subarachnoid haemorrhage [21]. They more often affect only one endocrine axis in isolation, and less often several at once [22]. Frequency figures fluctuate between 5.4% and 57.5% depending on the test procedures and their timing [22]. An essential problem results from a lack of reliable reference values for endocrine disorders in the early phase following brain damage.

Corticotropic insufficiency is of particular relevance to early neurological and neurosurgical rehabilitation, as it is aside from somatotropic insufficiency the most frequent insufficiency [22], often sidesteps routine laboratory tests (compared to thyrotropic insufficiency), is often difficult to diagnose on a clinical level as a result of the often unspecific or ambiguous symptoms, but in stressful situations (infections, operations) can even result in life-threatening Addisonian crisis. Furthermore, corticotropic insufficiency is usually only a relative one, with normal or borderline basal cortisol levels. Often, significantly higher substitution doses than usual are needed [26]. Other endocrine disorders in the form of diabetes insipidus (up to 3% [22]), syndrome of inappropriate ADH secretion or cerebral salt-wasting syndrome may occur.

As time goes on, spasticity frequently develops as a consequence of focal brain damage from concurrent bleeding or vasospastic infarctions, or herniation in severely affected patients. This often requires further therapy such as botulinum toxin injections, joint mobilisation under anaesthetic and corrective cast treatment in addition to the basic measure of physiotherapy. Systemic antispastic agents should preferably be avoided because of frequently occurring cognitive and gastrointestinal side effects with at the same time a mostly inadequate effect on severe spasticity, even at high doses. In contrast, experience with intrathecal baclofen therapy is positive [30; own experience]. Appropriate multimodal therapy in the case of severe spasticity requires, time and again, a combination of all therapeutic aspects and options and is ideally only to be performed in the early neurological and neurosurgical rehabilitation setting.

Critical illness polyneuropathy (CIP) often develops over the further course and is of particular significance in the rehabilitation process. It has additional negative implications in terms of the patient's motor skills, often leads to neurogenic dysphagia, reduces physical resilience and prolongs the process of weaning off ventilation in a highly significant way [27]. Because the symptoms of central nervous and peripheral nervous damage overlap, the clinical diagnosis of CIP in patients post SAH is unreliable [13]. Using a standardised electrophysiological test, the incidence of critical illness polyneuropathy as a concomitant condition was found to be 69% in patients in early neurological and neurosurgical rehabilitation [27].

Haemorrhaging in the vitreous body of the eye (Terson syndrome) is not uncommon after subarachnoid haemorrhage. The reported incidence fluctuates between 12% and 50% [6, 10]. The resulting visual disturbances often have a lasting negative impact on rehabilitation, as they are often recognised only late on in patients whose communication is impaired. Especially in this condition, ocular ultrasound is a simple and safe screening method.

Other complications often emerge at the interface with other medical disciplines (e.g., neurourology in the case of neurogenic bladder disorders, psychiatry in the case of depression, cardiology in the case of stress-induced cardiomyopathy [Takotsubo cardiomyopathy] or unspecific ECG changes, pulmonology in the case of neurogenic pulmonary oedema, gastroenterology in the case of gastrointestinal motility disorders with gastroparesis, reflux and vomiting, infectiology in the case of central fever, etc.).

In addition, complications that develop with other diseases but are not typically associated with SAH can also occur of course during the rehabilitation of SAH patients (Table 2). Given that infections are a frequent complication, clinically-orientated, moderate antibiotic treatment is essential in view of the increasing problem of multidrug-resistant pathogens firstly to adequately treat the infection, and secondly to minimise the selection of multidrug-resistant pathogens. Eradication is often impossible in neurological rehabilitation due to various factors (e.g., long-term placement of cannulae, broad spectrum antibiotics often necessary, multiple antibiotic pre-treatments in long-term intensive therapy and ventilation, incontinence, limited cooperativeness). The necessary isolation limits rehabilitation options, and the chances of successful rehabilitation are therefore reduced. Therefore, in the case of elevated body temperature it is appropriate to differentiate between bacterial infection and a central fever.

Finally, it is worth mentioning that many pharmacological approaches constitute off-label use in accordance with current regulatory provisions. Alongside the increased need for a clear indication, additional information and accurate documentation occasionally off-label use brings with it problems in relation to the reimbursement of the costs for expensive treatments (e.g., botulinum toxin) since health insurers can deny payment in this context.

Outcomes of Early Neurological/Neurosurgical Rehabilitation

The individual federal states are responsible for defining health policy in Germany. Germany-wide data are therefore scarce or can only be compared to a limited extent due to distinctions between the states. To illustrate the outcomes, the data from the Quality Assurance Institute in Hessen and data from our own hospital (also located in Hessen) are presented and compared. With six million inhabitants, Hessen is the fifth largest federal state in Germany. All stroke patients and thus all patients with SAH are registered by the acute hospitals as a compulsory measure with the Hessen Quality Assurance Institute. As early neurological and neurosurgical rehabilitation is also assigned to the acute hospital sector according to social legislation (Section 39 SGB V), comprehensive data are also available on this topic.

In 2013, 487 patients with SAH were admitted to acute hospitals in Hessen. The mean inpatient stay for acute hospital treatment for all patients with SAH was 15.7 days (standard deviation: $\pm$10.9 days). 259 out of 487 (53.2%) patients were ventilated. The mean duration of ventilation was 13.3 days (standard deviation: $\pm$12.6 days). Concerning the duration of ventilation it should be noted that some of the patients (especially the more severely affected) were transferred to early neurological and neurosurgical rehabilitation in a ventilated state and therefore were excluded in the above mentioned analysis.

Table 4 illustrates the functional outcome at the end of acute treatment, classified according to the modified Rankin Scale.

Throughout Hessen, 175 out of 487 (35.9%) patients post SAH were transferred to early neurological and neurosurgical rehabilitation. Table 5 compares the relevant characteristics of the patients in Hessen and at our own hospital.

Table 4. Functional outcome at the end of acute treatment (n = 487) based on the modified Rankin Scale

Scale	*Definition*	*Number of patients*	*%*
0	No symptoms	68	14.0
1	Symptoms with no relevant functional impairment	89	18.3
2	Mild functional impairment	30	6.2
3	Moderate functional impairment	39	8.0
4	Moderately severe functional impairment	57	11.7
5	Severe functional impairment	120	24.6
6	Death	84	17.2

Table 5. Comparison of relevant characteristics in all early rehabilitation patients post SAH in Hesse and our own hospital

Item	*Hessen*	*Bad König*
Patient number	175	46
Age [years] *	57.9 ± 11.9	56.2 ± 11.2
Age [years] **	57	53
Ratio men/women [n]	61/114	13/33
Ratio men/women [%]	34.9/65.1	28.3/71.7
Interval event – admission [days] *	45.7 ± 50.3	38.2 ± 46.4
Interval event – admission [days] **	28	23
Number of ventilated patients [n]	64/175	31/46
Number of ventilated patients [%]	36.6	67.4
Duration of ventilation [days] *	16.2 ± 21	10.4 ± 7.7
Duration of ventilation [days] **	11.5	8.5
Weaning ratio [n]	37/41	25/29
Weaning ratio [%]	90.2%	86.2%
Decannulation rate [n]	46/70	28/41
Decannulation rate [%]	65.7	68.3
Length of stay [days] *	52.6 ± 116.1	74.5 ± 71.6
Length of stay [days] **	38	37

*Mean ± standard deviation, **median, n = number

Table 6. Early Rehabilitation Barthel Index compared between the start and end of early neurological/neurosurgical rehabilitation

Population	*Hesse, total (n = 175)*						*Bad König (n = 46)*					
*Item **	*Admission*		*Discharge*		*Difference***		*Admission*		*Discharge*		*Difference***	
	n	%	*n*	%	*n*	%	*n*	%	*n*	%	*n*	%
Disorder requiring intensive medical monitoring	67	38.3	11	17.4	56/67	-83.6	36	78.3	8	17.4	28/36	-77.8
Tracheostoma requiring aspiration	70	40.0	24	28.3	46/70	-65.7	41	89.1	13	28.3	28/41	-68.3
Permanent/intermittent ventilation	41	23.4	4	9.7	37/41	-90.3	29	63.0	4	8.7	25/29	-86.2
Impaired orientation requiring supervision	44	25.1	21	30.4	23/44	-52.3	32	69.6	14	30.4	18/32	-56.3
Behavioural disorder requiring supervision	38	21.7	11	15.2	27/38	-71.1	23	50.0	7	15.2	16/23	-69.6
Severely impaired communication	85	48.6	48	37.0	37/85	-43.5	40	87.0	17	37.0	23/40	-57.5
Swallowing disorder requiring supervision	101	57.7	49	32.6	52/101	-51.5	43	93.5	15	32.6	28/43	-65.1

* Multiple answers possible, ** discharge vs admission

In Germany, the Barthel Index [15] was established as a standard tool for assessing functional independence, although it was originally designed for patients with quadri-/paraplegia and has some methodological weaknesses. Because of the severity of the damage and the resulting lack of independence, patients in early neurological and neurosurgical rehabilitation are not represented by the Barthel Index, or only late on in the course of the disease owing to the so-called floor effect. Therefore, in Germany, the Early Rehabilitation Barthel Index [23] was introduced to illustrate typical early rehabilitation items which better describe the severity of a patient's condition. Improvements in these items are therefore more appropriate than the Barthel Index for elucidating the advances in early rehabilitative treatment (Table 6).

Length of Acute Hospital Stay (for Patients Transferred to Early Neurological/ Neurosurgical Rehabilitation)

The length of stay for primary acute hospital treatment until transfer to early neurological and neurosurgical rehabilitation was 45.7 ± 50.3 days (median 28 days) in Hessen as a whole and 38.2 ± 46.4 days (median 23 days) at our clinic, and thus can be easily compared against an earlier 2005 overview of unselected diseases with a latency of transfer to early neurological and neurosurgical rehabilitation treatment of 47.0 ± 90.2 days (median 27 days) [28]. As this value also includes diseases (cerebral infarction, hypoxia) that are typically associated with shorter acute hospital stays compared to SAH and traumatic brain injury, it can be assumed that the length of acute hospital stay for patients with SAH admitted to early neurological and neurosurgical rehabilitation has slightly decreased in acute medicine in the last ten years.

Percentage of Ventilated Patients Admitted to Early Neurological and Neurosurgical Rehabilitation

The percentage of patients admitted to early neurological and neurosurgical rehabilitation still in a ventilated state (unselected diseases) was 16.6% in 2002 [12] and 18.4% in 2005 [28]. An increase can be established in this regard, as the Hessen-wide percentage of 36.6% among all the SAH patients admitted to early rehabilitation shows (Table 5). The rate at early rehabilitation facilities with a strong intensive care focus is even higher - 61.4% [9] and at our own clinic 67.4% (Table 5).

The further development in early neurological and neurosurgical rehabilitation in relation to intensive care content and procedures facilitates the tendency towards shorter acute medical stays and eases the burden on intensive neurosurgical or anaesthesiological units caring for patients with SAH.

Weaning

Published weaning rates from early neurological and neurosurgical rehabilitation (unselected diseases) in Germany are 68.3% [17], 69.8% [16], 78% [3] and 90.5%, respectively [25]. The weaning rate for patients with SAH is between 86.2% and 90.2% (Table 5). The median duration of weaning was 11.5 and 8.5 days, respectively (Table 5). These values demonstrate that in early neurological and neurosurgical rehabilitation there is now a high level of expertise in respiratory medicine and that patients requiring ventilation after SAH have very good chances of being successfully weaned despite often running the gamut of possible complications.

Decannulation Rates

Even with successful weaning, many patients in early neurological and neurosurgical rehabilitation remain dependent on a tracheostoma, as neurogenic dysphagia frequently develops which due to the associated risk of aspiration can mean that a blocked tracheal cannula is needed. The percentage of tracheotomised patients in the last few years in early neurological and neurosurgical rehabilitation has increased from 40% [28] in an unselected population of patients to up to 89% in patients with SAH (Table 6). Decannulation rates of 65.7% and 68.3%, respectively, (Table 5) indicate that under intensive swallowing rehabilitation over two thirds of patients with SAH can be weaned from the tracheal cannula, even if severely affected.

Length of Stay in Early Neurological/Neurosurgical Rehabilitation

The average length of stay in early neurological/neurosurgical rehabilitation for patients after SAH in 2013 was 62.6 $\pm$ 116.1 days (median 38 days) in Hessen as a whole and 74.5 + 71.6 days (median 37 days) at our own clinic. These values are highly consistent with those of other studies [3, 12, 18] in patients after SAH. Since 2002 there has been a gradual decrease in the lengths of stay for unselected patients, including patients post SAH, from 57 days in 2002 [12] to 37 and 38 days (Table 5) for SAH patients, in whom furthermore the course tends to be more fraught with complications. Alongside the increasing complexity and modalities of intensive therapy (e.g., ventilation), must also be considered. The reduction in the length of stay is most likely caused by the change in the billing system to flat rates per case and an increasingly restrictive attitude on the part of health insurers towards paying for the respective services.

Typical Early Rehabilitation Issues

Based on Schönle's Early Rehabilitation Barthel Index [23], Table 6 details the improvements in the respective items over the course of early rehabilitation therapy, which range from 43%-90% in Hessen as a whole and 56%-86% at our own clinic. It demonstrates that early neurological and neurosurgical rehabilitation, both in relation to medical stabilisation (e.g., termination of intensive care, weaning off ventilation, weaning off tracheostoma) and in relation to increased quality of life (e.g., improvement of swallowing disorders) and the establishment of conditions for further rehabilitation therapy or outpatient care (e.g., reducing orientation and behavioural disorders requiring supervision), constitutes a significant contribution in the care chain for patients after subarachnoid haemorrhage.

Transfer Rate in Subsequent Rehabilitation Phases

The reported transfer rates from early neurological and neurosurgical rehabilitation to subsequent rehabilitation phases are between 33.4% [28], 39.5% [18] and 55.4% [3] for unselected patient groups and 42.9% for patients post SAH [12]. However, agreements at the federal state level on phase transition should be considered here, meaning that the comparability of these figures is limited. At our own clinic, a comparable value of 43.5% is achieved (Table 7), whereas in Hessen as a whole it is somewhat lower (Table 7).

Table 7. Discharge from early neurological/neurosurgical rehabilitation

Population	*Hesse, total (n = 175)*		*Bad König (n = 46)*	
Goal of transfer	*n*	*%*	*n*	*%*
Home with non-professional assistance	6	3.4	2	4.4
Home with professional assistance	12	6.9	5	10.9
Inpatient rehabilitation (Phase C/D)	45	25.7	20	43.5
Alternative early rehabilitation	26	14.9	1	2.2
Transfer to acute hospital (subsequent readmission)	42 (28)	24.0	6 (4)	13.0
Care home	37	21.1	9	19.6
Deceased	7	4.0	3	8.7

Table 8. Functional outcome at the end of early neurological/neurosurgical rehabilitation based on the modified Rankin Scale

Population		*Hessen, total (n = 175)*		*Bad König (n = 46)*	
Score	*Definition*	*n*	*%*	*n*	*%*
0	No symptoms	3	1.7	0	0
1	Symptoms with no relevant functional deficit	2	1.1	0	0
2	Mild functional deficit	11	6.3	6	13.0
3	Moderate functional deficit	24	13.7	5	10.9
4	Moderately severe functional deficit	58	33.1	13	28.3
5	Severe functional deficit	72	41.1	19	41.3
6	Death	5	2.9	3	6.5

Transfer Rate in Care Facilities

The reported percentage of patients transferred to care facilities from early neurological and neurosurgical rehabilitation is between 16.2% [3] and 18.2% [18] in unselected patient groups and 21.9% in patients post SAH [12]. The rates in Hessen as a whole and at our own clinic are comparable at 21.1% and 19.6%, respectively (Table 7).

Return Transfer Rate in acute Care Hospitals

The rate of return transfer from early neurological and neurosurgical rehabilitation is between 11.4% [28] and 27.6% [18] and ensues primarily as a result of internal or neurosurgical complications [30]. Evaluation of the data from 2013 reveals a retransfer rate in Hessen as a whole of 24% and 13% at our own clinic, where an appropriate team of staff and equipment for intensive care are in place (Table 7). This is readily comparable with earlier data for patients after SAH at 10.5% [12]. With an appropriate intensive care setting, retransfers are almost exclusively limited to elective neurosurgical secondary interventions [our own data]. This shows that it is possible, with an appropriately designed early neurological and neurosurgical rehabilitation concept, to guarantee "one-stop" treatment and minimise transfers which can be stressful to patients and to some extent put them at risk.

Functional Outcome at the End of Early Neurological and Neurosurgical Rehabilitation

The modified Ranking Scale (mRS) is a frequently used instrument for evaluating the outcome after stroke. To some degree it must be stressed from our own experience that external evaluation scales are highly problematic in the evaluation of outcome or even quality of life. Usually a score of 1-3 on the mRS scale is rated as a good outcome. A good 20% of patients after SAH therefore achieve a good outcome from early neurological and neurosurgical rehabilitation, both in Hessen as a whole and at our own clinic. This value, though apparently low, must be viewed from the angle of initial disease severity: only severely and very severely affected patients after SAH are admitted to early neurological and neurosurgical rehabilitation, bypassing more mildly affected patients who enter later phases of rehabilitation or at best remain asymptomatic.

CONTINUING REHABILITATION (PHASE C)

Phase C is the link between early neurological/neurosurgical (Phase B) and follow-up rehabilitation (Phase D). Those treated are patients who can already actively participate in the programme but must still receive curative medical treatment and require a lot of nursing attention [4, point 3.2., page 12].

The patients must meet the entry criteria for Phase C [4, point 3.2.1., page 12]:

- Alertness, able to comply with simple commands, sufficient ability to actively participate in the treatment measures of 30 minutes each
- Ability to communicate and interact
- Mobilised in a wheelchair for 2-4 hours at a time
- Vital signs and autonomic nervous system stable with no need for intensive medical supervision/treatment
- No further need for ventilation
- Comorbidities must not hinder mobilisation
- No danger to self/others and no severe disturbances to social behaviour in small groups

However, in contrast to rehabilitation during follow-up (Phase D), the patients to a large extent still depend on assistance in activities of daily living. The overriding aim of continuing rehabilitation is to improve independence in activities of daily living (ADL) and to restore the basic function of the nervous system through to the full capacity to act. Moreover, the further rehabilitation potential and long-term prospects should be clarified, a long-term treatment plan established, and continued care planned and introduced [4, point 3.2.2., page 13].

FOLLOW-UP REHABILITATION (PHASE D)

With growing independence in activities of daily living, but persistent motor deficits and mental disturbances that frequently interfere in working life and the daily routine, follow-up rehabilitation (Phase D) can begin upon achieving a Barthel Index score of approx. 65-70 points [29], indicating a general ability and willingness to cooperate as well as the capacity to act and learn. The main aim of Phase D is to achieve complete independence in everyday life and ideally facilitate the professional reintegration of those patients of working age.

PRESERVATIVE NON-HOSPITAL NURSING CARE (PHASE F)

If motor deficits in particular should limit activities of daily living, preservative non-hospital nursing care (Phase F) while continuing treatments on an outpatient basis is indicated. This nursing care can be carried out both at home and also in an institutional setting, such as in care homes or specialist nursing homes with treatments adapted to the patient's condition.

ACKNOWLEDGMENTS

The authors wish to thank Dr. med. B. Misselwitz, MPH, Head of the Institute of Quality Assurance Hessen at the Hessische Krankenhausgesellschaft e. V., Frankfurter Strasse 10 – 14, 65760 Eschborn for providing the data used in this article.

REFERENCES

[1] Annan, M; De Toffol, B; Hommet, C; Mondon, K. Sinking skin flap syndrome (or syndrome of the trephined): a review. *Br J Neurosurg*, 2015, 29, 314-318.

[2] Bader, P. Vaskuläre Erkrankungen. In: Müller F, Walther E, Herzog J, editors. Praktische Neurorehabilitation. 1. Aufl., Stuttgart: Kohlhammer, 2014. 35-42.

[3] Bertram, M; Brandt, T. Neurologisch-neurochirurgische Frührehabilitation. *Nervenarzt*, 2007, 78, 1160-1174.

[4] Bundesarbeitsgemeinschaft für Rehabilitation (BAR). Empfehlungen zur neurologischen Rehabilitation von Patienten mit schweren und schwersten Hirnschädigungen in den Phasen B und C. *Frankfurt: Bundesarbeitsgemeinschaft für Rehabilitation*, 1995.

[5] Chen, Z; Song, W; Du, J; Li, G; Yang, Y; Ling, F. Rehabilitation of patients with chronic normal-pressure hydrocephalus after aneurysmal hemorrhage benefits from ventricularperitoneal shunt. *Top Stroke Rehabil*, 2009, 16, 330-338.

[6] Czorlich, P; Burkhardt, T; Knospe, V; Richard, G; Vettorazzi, E; Wagenfeld, L; et al. Ocular ultrasound as an easy applicable tool for detection of Terson's syndrome after aneurysmal subarachnoid hemorrhage. *PLoS ONE*, 9(12), e114907. doi:10.1371/ journal. pone. 0114907.

[7] Deutsches Institut für Medizinische Dokumentation und Information (DIMDI), im Auftrag des Bundesministeriums für Gesundheit unter Beteiligung der Arbeitsgruppe OPS des Kuratoriums für Fragen der Klassifikation im Gesundheitswesen (KKG), (Hrsg.). OPS Version 2015 - Systematisches Verzeichnis. Operationen- und

Prozedurenschlüssel – Internationale Klassifikation der Prozeduren in der Medizin. Köln: Deutscher Ärzteverlag; 2014. p 426. https:// www.dimdi.de/static/de/klassi/ops/kodesuche/onlinefassungen/opshtml2015/block-8-55...8-60.htm,Zugriffam28.06. 2015.

[8] Di Rienzo, A; Iacoangeli, M; Alvaro, L; Colasanti, R; Dobran, M; Di Somma, LGM; et al. The sinking bone syndrome? *Neurol Med Chir*, 2013, 53, 329-335.

[9] Eifert, B; Maurer-Karattup, P; Schorl, M. Integration of intensive care treatment and neurorehabilitation in patients with disorders of consciousness: a program description and case report. *Arch Phys Med Rehabil*, 2013, 94, 1924-1933. DOI: 10.1016/j-apmr.2013.03.030.

[10] Hassan, A; Lanzino, G; Wijdicks, EF; Rabinstein, AA; Flemming, KD. Terson's syndrome. *Neurocrit Care*, 2011, 15, 554-558.

[11] Hagen, T; Bennefeld, H; Diepolder, V; Haase, I; Leidner, O; Miosge, W; et al. Entwicklung eines Kataloges pflegetherapeutischer Maßnahmen in der neurologischen Frühehabilitation (Phase B). *Neurol Rehabil*, 2007, 13, 151-158.

[12] Hoffmann, B; Karbe, H; Krusch, C; Müller, B; Pause, M; Prosiegel, M; et al. Patientencharakteristika in der neurologisch/neurochirurgischen Frührehabilitation (Phase B): Eine multizentrische Erfassung im Jahr 2002 in Deutschland. *Akt Neurol*, 2006, 33, 287-296.

[13] Hund, EF; Fogel, W; Krieger, D; De Geogia, M; Hacke, W. Critical illness polyneuropathy: clinical findings and outcomes of a frequent cause of neuromuscular weaning failure. *Crit Care Med*, 1996, 24, 1328-1333.

[14] Kaestner, S; Kruschat, T; Nitzsche, N; Deinsberger, W. Gravitational shunt units may cause under-drainage in bedridden patients. *Acta Neurochirurgica*, 2009, 151, 217-221.

[15] Mahoney, FI; Barthel, D. Functional evaluation: The Barthel Index. *Md State Med J*, 1965, 14, 56-61.

[16] Oehmichen, F; Ketter, G; Mertl-Rötzer, M; Platz, T; Puschendorf, W; Rollnik, JD. Beatmungsentwöhnung in neurologischen Weaningzentren. *Nervenarzt*, 2012, 83, 1300-1307.

[17] Rollnik, JD; Berlinghof, K; Lenz, O; Bertomeu, AM. Beatmung in der neurologischen Frührehabilitation. *Akt Neurol*, 2010, 7, 316-318.

[18] Rollnik, JD; Janosch, U. Current trends in the length of stay in neurological early rehabilitation. *Dtsch Ärztebl Int*, 2010, 107 (16), 286-292.

[19] Saciri, BM; Kos, N. Aneurysmal subarachnoidal haemorrhage: outcomes of early rehabilitation after surgical repair of ruptured intracranial aneurysms. *JNNP*, 2002, 72, 334-337.

[20] Salter, K; Jutai, J; Hartley, M; Foley, N; Bhogal, S; Bayona, N; et al. Impact of early vs delayed admission to rehabilitation on functional outcomes in persons with stroke. *J Rehab Med*, 2006, 38, 113-117.

[21] Schneider, HJ; Kreitschmann-Andermahr, I; Ghigo, E; Stalla, GK; Agha, A. Hypothalamo-pituitary dysfunction following traumatic brain injury and aneurysmal subarachnoid hemorrhage. *JAMA*, 2007, 298, 1429-1438.

[22] Schneider, M; von Rosen, F. Neuroendokrinologie. In: Müller F, Walther E, Herzog J, editors. Praktische Neurorehabilitation. *1. Aufl., Stuttgart, Kohlhammer*, 2014. 300-305.

[23] Schönle, PW. Der Frühreha-Barthelindex (FBI) – eine frührehabilitationsorientierte Erweiterung des Barthelindex. *Rehabilitation*, 1995, 4, 69-73.

[24] Schorl, M. Sinking Skin Flap Syndrome (SSFS) – Clinical Spectrum and Impact on Rehabilitation. *Cent Eur Neurosurg*, 2009, 70, 68-72.

[25] Schorl, M; Eifert, B. Weaning in der neurologischen Frührehabilitation: individuelles Vorgehen führt zu hohen Erfolgsquoten (Poster). 28. *Arbeitstagung für Neurologische Intensiv- und Notfallmedizin (ANIM), Leipzig*, 12.01.-15.01.2011.

[26] Schorl, M; Flechsenhaar, D; Guthier, M; Imöhl, L; Hartwich, M. Ungewöhnliche Ursache rezidivierender Vigilanzminderungen bis zum Koma bei kompliziertem Verlauf nach Subarachnoidalblutung bei Ruptur eines Aneurysmas der A. communicans anterior (Poster). *Arbeitstagung Neurolointensivmedizin (ANIM)*, Berlin, 29.-31.01.2015.

[27] Schorl, M; Valerius-Kukula, S-J; Kemmer, TP. Critical-illness-polyneuropathy as sequelae of severe neurological illness: incidence and impact on ventilator therapy and rehabilitation. *Neurorehabilitation*, 2013, 32, 149-156. DOI: 10.3233/NRE-130832.

[28] Spranger, M; Hoffmann, B; Karbe, H; Krusch, C; Müller, B; Pause, M; et al. Der Stellenwert der neurologisch-neurochirurgischen Frührehabilitation in der Versorgungskette von Patienten mit schweren neurologischen Erkrankungen. *Neurol Rehabil*, 2005, 11, 317-322.

[29] Stier-Jarmer, M; Koenig, E; Stucki, G. Strukturen der neurologischen Frührehabilitation (Phase B) in Deutschland. *Phys Med Rehab Kuror*, 2002, 12, 260-271.

[30] Von Wedel-Parlow, FK; Gehring, K; Kutzner, M. Neurologische Frührehabilitation. In: Frommelt P, Lösslein H, editors. Neurorehabilitation. *Berlin, Heidelberg: Springer*, 2010. 501-556.

[31] Yamaura, A; Makino, H. Neurological deficits in the presence of the sinking skin flap following decompressive craniectomy. *Neurol Med Chir*, 1977, 17, 43-53.

In: Spontaneous Subarachnoid Haemorrhage
Editors: Thomas Kapapa and Ralph König
ISBN: 978-1-63485-270-8

Chapter 19

Cognitive Plasticity After Spontaneous Subarachnoid Haemorrhage

Christine Brand
Department of Neurosurgery, University of Ulm, Ulm, Germany

Abstract

Patients who suffer spontaneous subarachnoid haemorrhage (SAH) often find themselves in the full swing of life, not only personally but also professionally. It is a radical event that has a dramatic effect on a patient's physical and psychological well-being. More than 50% of all SAH patients describe cognitive deficits that have a negative impact on quality of life. The exact causes of cognitive deficits are not yet known. However, patients develop everyday strategies with which to compensate for these deficits, such as writing themselves notes. One of the most reported impaired functions is working memory, irrespective of the time at which they were examined. Never the less, the ability of the brain to restore or compensate for functions that have been lost plays a very important role following spontaneous SAH. It is essential to the success of rehabilitation, as well as the social and professional reintegration of the patient to identify cognitive deficits and to train them.

Keywords: SAH, cognitive plasticity, quality of life, rehabilitation, cognitive deficits

Patients who suffer spontaneous subarachnoid haemorrhage (SAH) often find themselves in the full swing of life, not only personally but also professionally. It is a radical event that has a dramatic effect on a patient's physical and psychological well-being and thus has a negative impact on quality of life [1, 2]. Patients who outwardly appear to have achieved a good therapeutic outcome, implying that they have no obvious disorders such as palsy or speech defects, are often still burdened by less noticeable deficits. Such deficits are immediately apparent to patients themselves, of course, as well as to their family [3]. Patients very often describe deficits in terms of working memory, concentration and attention [4]. Conversations involving a number of people prove difficult to follow. Professionally they become less resilient, finding that their working lives are more of a strain than before the haemorrhage. Co-workers and superiors expect the same level of input from the patient, who is no longer written off sick and has no noticeable signs of illness. Cognitive deficits also lead to potential conflicts at home. Patients feel misunderstood and often become emotionally withdrawn.

After spending approx. two to four weeks under critical neurosurgical care, patients with spontaneous SAH are transferred for neurological follow-up treatment, which as a rule lasts three weeks. Following the inpatient stay, the patient is discharged to the care of his or her family doctor. In Germany, referral to a neuropsychologist is not current practice. Under normal circumstances, the patient undergoes gradual professional reintegration so as to resume work as before. In reality, this proves successful in only very few cases. Success is dependent firstly on the severity of the residual deficits, secondly on the demands of the patient's acquired skill.

The nature and intensity of cognitive deficits after spontaneous SAH have now been studied thoroughly [5-7]. Potential patient- and therapy-related influential factors have been described [7]. The progress over time, the potential for recovery, and with it plasticity, have been illustrated by diverse studies [5, 8, 9]. There is only speculation, however, as to the exact causes or pathogenesis. Awareness of the nature and scope, as well as the possible chances of improvement in the cognitive deficits, is essential for establishing a therapeutic basis for rehabilitation. Long-term morbidity can thus be minimised and at best prevented. The aim, however, should be to avoid cognitive deficits by administering optimised therapy. To achieve this, however, the causes must be known. Patient-related factors cannot be influenced by the treating physicians in the emergency department.

The aim of treating spontaneous SAH in the acute phase as well as later on during rehabilitation should therefore be to minimise the patient's cognitive deficits so as to prevent long-term morbidity.

SPECTRUM OF COGNITIVE DEFICITS FOLLOWING SPONTANEOUS SUBARACHNOID HAEMORRHAGE

More than 50% of all SAH patients describe cognitive deficits [1, 4, 7, 10, 11] that have a negative impact on quality of life. In the clinical routine, patients most often describe concentration-related deficits [4]. Difficulty concentrating is apparent not only during activities of daily living, but also at work. Diverse studies have examined the ability to concentrate following spontaneous SAH. Relevant concentration disorders were found in 11%-13% of the SAH patients studied [8, 12, 13]. Impaired memory, especially working memory, is the disorder that is most noticeable to the majority of patients after spontaneous SAH. Patients develop everyday strategies with which to compensate for these deficits, such as writing themselves notes. Various studies have reported working memory deficits in 28%-71% of all SAB patients, irrespective of the time at which they were examined [4, 7, 12, 14, 15]. Professionally, impaired concentration and memory deficits prove to be the biggest hurdle. Another area that can be affected is the speed of information processing, an issue that has been found in 31%-65% of those affected [4, 7, 16]. In addition to the domains already mentioned, executive functions can also be impaired in SAH patients.

PLASTICITY AFTER SPONTANEOUS SUBARACHNOID HAEMORRHAGE

The ability of the brain to restore or compensate for functions that have been lost plays a very important role following spontaneous SAH. It is essential to the success of rehabilitation, as well as the social and professional reintegration of the patient. With today's ever-diminishing resources, the purpose and necessity for long inpatient stays, and thus costly inpatient rehabilitation programmes delivered by specially trained personnel, are called into question. Studies have been conducted to examine patients at varying times after spontaneous SAH in order to determine whether cognitive deficits have the potential to improve. It was demonstrated that skills in relation to speech comprehension, numeracy, verbal memory, attention, concentration and also executive functions do potentially improve [7, 8, 14]. The information processing rate appears to be a predictor for plasticity. The extent of the potential recovery depends on the severity of the bleeding and its localisation [17], as well as on patient-associated factors such as school education or age of the patient [7], and so cannot be influenced by the physician. Cognitive deficits can still improve even months after occurrence of the haemorrhage [7, 8, 16]. In practice this implies that one period of rehabilitation lasting several weeks is not sufficient. Specific, specialised outpatient follow-up care from a neuropsychologist is appropriate and necessary if an optimum outcome is to be achieved. This appears to be the only way to guarantee the best possible professional reintegration of the patient. Social integration could likewise be positively influenced in this manner. Long-term morbidity could thus be sustainably reduced.

FACTORS INFLUENCING COGNITIVE DEFICITS

To optimise therapy in the emergency department and create the best conditions for subsequent rehabilitation, the factors that influence cognitive performance and the quality of life of patients with spontaneous SAH have been examined [18-20]. In doing so, it is useful to divide these factors into two categories: patient-related and treatment-related factors. In the emergency setting, physicians cannot influence patient-related factors. School education, profession, laterality, pre-existing cardiac diseases, obesity, hyperlipidaemia, diabetes mellitus and nicotine abuse all appear to have a significant influence on the therapeutic outcome. Treatment-related factors are the primary focus of the attending physician. Some studies have looked at whether coiling or clipping of a ruptured aneurysm offers a better treatment outcome. The type of treatment does not appear to influence the cognitive treatment outcome, however [8]. Various conventional classification systems have been considered as potential prognostic tools. None could ultimately live up to expectations. Neither the Fisher score, which describes the extent of the bleeding based on diagnostic imaging, nor the Hunt and Hess scale, which documents the initial clinical condition, permitted a satisfactory estimation to be made of the treatment outcome [21]. Another popular system for grading the clinical condition is the Glasgow Outcome Score, though it does not describe the presence of cognitive deficits. The localisation of the aneurysm also appears, moreover, to have no impact on the existence of cognitive deficits [8, 22, 23].

Possible Causes of Cognitive Deficits, Therapeutic Strategies and Prospects

The exact causes of cognitive deficits are not yet known. Theories abound, however. It stands to reason that the bleeding itself is the cause of all evil [22]. On the one hand the haemorrhage causes localised damage, as well as deficits theoretically due to the effects of the bleeding. These include impaired CSF circulation, vasospasms and ischaemia. Or is the acute rise in intracranial pressure following rupture of the aneurysm responsible for the cognitive deficits [7]? It appears at least to explain why focal lesions also influence cognitive areas suspected to exist in other regions of the brain. From another angle, numerous functions such as memory may not be focussed on just one area of the brain. This subject certainly needs to be examined more closely.

In conclusion, it should be stated at least that cognitive deficits often develop in patients with spontaneous SAH and negatively influence quality of life in the long term. As a result, long-term morbidity increases. Cognitive deficits can be treated specifically by means of rehabilitation therapy. There is still a chance after several months that these deficits will improve. Outpatient follow-up care from a neuropsychologist subsequent to initial inpatient rehabilitation is therefore beneficial to the patient.

References

[1] Kapapa T. Lebensqualität nach spontaner Subarachnoidalblutung- Analyse klinischer Variablen, welche die gesundheitsbezogene Lebensqualität nach spontaner Subarachnoidalblutung beeinflussen. *Neurologie und Rehabilitation*. 2005:21-8.

[2] Tjahjadi M, Heinen, C., König, R., Rickels, R., Wirtz, C.R., Woischneck, D., Kapapa, T. Health-related quality of life after spontaneous subarachnoid hemorrhage measured in a recent patient population. World Neurosurg. 2013;79:296-307. *Epub* 2012 Oct 6.

[3] Kapapa T, Woischneck, D., Tjahjadi, M. Long-term health-relates quality of life after spontaneous nontraumatic subarachnoid hemorrhage: self and proxy reports in a 10-year period. *World Neurosurg*. 2014;81:105-9. Epub 2012 Oct 6.

[4] Hutter BO, Gilsbach JM, Kreitschmann I. Quality of life and cognitive deficits after subarachnoid haemorrhage. *British journal of neurosurgery*. 1995;9(4): 465-75. PubMed PMID: 1.

[5] McKenna P, Willison JR, Phil B, Lowe D, Neil-Dwyer G. Cognitive outcome and quality of life one year after subarachnoid haemorrhage. *Neurosurgery*. 1989 Mar;24(3):361-7. PubMed PMID: 4.

[6] Madureira S, Canhao P, Guerreiro M, Ferro JM. Cognitive and emotional consequences of perimesencephalic subarachnoid hemorrhage. *Journal of neurology*. 2000 Nov;247(11):862-7. PubMed PMID: 16.

[7] Brand C, Alber, B., Fladung, A.K., Knauer, K., König, R., Oechsner, A. Schneider, I.L., Tumani, H., Widder, B. Wirtz, C.R., Woischneck, D., Kapapa T. Cognitive performance following spontaneous subarachnoid haemorrhage versus other forms of intracranial haemorrhage. *Br. J. Neurosurg*. 2014;28:68-80.

[8] Haug T, Sorteberg A, Sorteberg W, Lindegaard KF, Lundar T, Finset A. Cognitive outcome after aneurysmal subarachnoid hemorrhage: time course of recovery and relationship to clinical, radiological, and management parameters. *Neurosurgery.* 2007 Apr;60(4):649-56; discussion 56-7. PubMed PMID: 17415201. Epub 2007/04/07. eng.

[9] Hop JW, Rinkel GJ, Algra A, van Gijn J. Changes in functional outcome and quality of life in patients and caregivers after aneurysmal subarachnoid hemorrhage. *J. Neurosurg.* 2001 Dec;95(6): 957-63. PubMed PMID: 11765839.

[10] Kreiter KT, Copeland D, Bernardini GL, Bates JE, Peery S, Claassen J, et al. Predictors of cognitive dysfunction after subarachnoid hemorrhage. *Stroke.* 2002;33:200-9.

[11] Mayer SA, Kreiter KT, Copeland D, Bernardini GL, Bates JE, Peery S, et al. Global and domain-specific cognitive impairment and outcome after subarachnoid hemorrhage. *Neurology.* 2002 Dec 10;59(11):1750-8. PubMed PMID: 12473764. Epub 2002/12/11. eng.

[12] Hutter BO, Gilsbach JM. Which neuropsychological deficits are hidden behind a good outcome (Glasgow = I) after aneurysmal subarachnoid hemorrhage? *Neurosurgery.* 1993 Dec;33(6):999-1005; discussion -6. PubMed PMID: 8134014.

[13] Hutter BO, Gilsbach JM. Early neuropsychological sequelae of aneurysm surgery and subarachnoid haemorrhage. *Acta Neurochirurgica.* 1996;138(12):1370-8; discussion 8-9. PubMed PMID: 14.

[14] Al- Khindi T, Loch Macdonald R, Schweizer TA. Cognitive and functional outcome after aneurysmal subarachnoid hemorrhage. *Stroke.* 2010;41: 519-36.

[15] Hutter BO, Gilsbach JM. Das Aachener Lebensqualitätsinventar für Patienten mit Hirnschädigung: Entwicklung und methodische Gütekriterien. Möllers HJ, Engel RR, Hoff P (Hrsg) Befunderhebnung in der Psychiatrie: Lebensqualität, Negativsymptomatik und andere aktuelle Entwicklungen *Springer*, Wien New York. 1996:83-101.

[16] Egge A, Waterloo K, Sjoholm H, Ingebrigtsen T, Forsdahl S, Jacobsen EA, et al. Outcome 1 year after aneurysmal subarachnoid hemorrhage: relation between cognitive performance and neuroimaging. *Acta Neurol. Scand.* 2005 Aug;112(2):76-80. PubMed PMID: 16008531. Epub 2005/07/13. eng.

[17] Kwen PL, Pullicino, P, Krenzer, R. Reversible impairment in cognition and midbrain hematoma. *J. Neuroimaging.* 1998;8:54-5.

[18] Tidswell P, Dias PS, Sagar HJ, Mayes AR, Battersby RD. Cognitive outcome after aneurysm rupture: relationship to aneurysm site and perioperative complications. *Neurology.* 1995 May;45(5): 875-82. PubMed PMID: 7746400.

[19] Wermer MJH, Kool H, Albrecht KW, Rinkel GJE. Subarachnoid hemorrhage treated with clipping: long term effects on employment, relationships, personality and mood. *Neurosurgery.* 2007;60:91-8.

[20] Kapapa T, Tjahjadi, M., König, R., Wirtz, C.R., Woischneck, D. Which clinical variable influences health-realated quality of life the most after spontaneous subarachnoid hemorrhage? Hund and Hess scale, Fishe score, World Federation of Neurosurgeons score, Brussels coma score, and Glasgow coma score compared. *World Neurosurg.* 2013;80: 853-8. Epub 2012 Sep 25.

[21] Cedzich C, Roth A. Neurological and psychosocial outcome after subarachnoid haemorrhage, and the hunt and hess scale as a predictor of clinical outcome. *Zentralblatt fur Neurochirurgie.* 2005 Aug;66(3):112-8. PubMed PMID: 18.

[22] Hutter BO, Kreitschmann-Andermahr I, Mayfrank L, Rohde V, Spetzger U, Gilsbach JM. Functional outcome after aneurysmal subarachnoid hemorrhage. *Acta Neurochir. Suppl.* 1999;72:157-74. PubMed PMID: 10337421. Epub 1999/05/25. eng.

[23] Ahola K, Vilkki, J., Servo, A. Frontal tests do not detect frontal infarctions after ruptured intracranial aneurysm. *Brain Cogn*. 1996;31: 1-16.

In: Spontaneous Subarachnoid Haemorrhage
Editors: Thomas Kapapa and Ralph König
ISBN: 978-1-63485-270-8

Chapter 20

HEALTH-RELATED QUALITY OF LIFE FOLLOWING SPONTANEOUS SUBARACHNOID HAEMORRHAGE AS AN ASSESSMENT CRITERION FOR THERAPEUTIC OUTCOME

Thomas Kapapa
Department of Neurosurgery, University of Ulm,
Ulm, Germany

ABSTRACT

Health-related quality of life serves as a supplement to the clinical criteria for determining the outcome of therapy. The lack of a higher-level definition for the term quality of life, however, is still problematic, but there is a general consensus on the individual approach and understanding as to what the term entails. The aim of this chapter is to make it clear that a good or very good clinical treatment outcome is not to be regarded as equivalent to good or very good quality of life. The subjective perception and attitude of the patient towards his or her personal situation after the haemorrhage are equally important when it comes to evaluating the treatment outcome. The individual assessment of the treatment outcome also very much depends on the expectations and experience of the patient. This should be taken into account when determining the said outcome.

Keywords: Outcome; rehabilitation; cognition, reintegration

Aristotle: “We are what we repeatedly do. Excellence, then, is not an act, but a habit!” But what happens when external or internal factors prevent us from continuing to do what we normally do so well? When is something new to be regarded as a habit? This rather philosophical approach in dealing with quality of life often cannot be reconciled with the concept of health-related quality of life. This is due on the one hand to the context within which quality of life needs to be understood. Terms such as lust for life, vitality, courage and trials of life are used synonymously. There are core intellectual elements such as political philosophy, social philosophy, environmental philosophy and medical ethics that deal with the term quality of life. Time, in the context of the here and now as well as transition, is another important factor for determining quality of life. All the differences described here lead us to surmise that there is no all-encompassing definition for quality of life.

The author sees the approach to quality of life in the medical context as a means of optimising patient care. To the author, health-related quality of life represents a collection of criteria reflected by objectives, values and principles, such as the certainty and length of life and a defined level of health, the freedom to seize opportunities, or personal and social recognition. Yet to the author health-related quality of life also inevitably includes criteria with alternative approaches to quality of life, such as the existence of economic conditions for achieving an ideal situation as expected by a society or self-imposed goals [1-3]. With this theory in mind, clinical endpoints are to be understood in the context of subjective satisfaction, psychosocial interaction and forward-looking behaviour [4].

The advances in the treatment of this complex condition, already described in this book, are so effective that mortality now accounts for only roughly a third of patients after one month. Results from the 1960s came to far more inferior conclusions, namely that approx. 33% of patients died before reaching a hospital and 27% of patients died during treatment [5, 6]. The Glasgow Outcome Scale and Modified Rankin Scale are the methods most commonly used for assessing the treatment outcome [7-9]. Not only is the rate of those surviving spontaneous subarachnoid haemorrhage increasing, but also the number of patients with a good treatment outcome [10]. The outcome of treating spontaneous subarachnoid haemorrhage is often described as “good”, “moderate”, or “poor”. There has been a clear improvement in the survival rate to almost 50% of patients classified in line with general criteria as having a “good” or “very good” outcome from such an event [11-14]. These categories are consistent mostly with functional neurological deficits. Little consideration is given in these ratings to psychological, cognitive and social components. The quality of life of many patients, despite their physical well-being, may still be impaired [3, 15]. It is not unusual to find that such disorders are caused by neuropsychological and cognitive deficits [15-17]. It is generally agreed that spontaneous subarachnoid haemorrhage has a considerable impact on quality of life [14].

The treatment outcome has a more lasting and profound impact than the patient’s condition at discharge alone. It must be judged in the context of the patient’s normal family life, routine social ties and social participation, as well as usual physical and mental achievements. Clinical parameters do not suffice to describe this situation. It has long been known that a disease can alter the conditions and thus the quality of life over an extended period of time [18]. Accordingly, health-related quality of life can be judged as 1) quality of personal situation, 2) satisfaction with personal situation, or 3) a combination of both [18]. Hence, the clinical treatment outcome is always an integrated part of the individual personal situation. To gain an insight into such a situation, health-related quality of life is useful. It is an illustration of the disease, the clinical outcome of treatment and the personal situation. It places the “patient” above the “disease” as the objective, and also establishes a connection between the two. This provides the opportunity to compare rational health indications, objective clinical ratings and progress against the patient’s subjective views and treatment outcomes.

The prevailing method for measuring quality of life is the questionnaire or interview. Various quality-of-life questionnaires are available for collating information universally on general characteristics, or specifically on disease-related characteristics [3, 14]. At present, there is no quality-of-life tool for the neurological/neurosurgical field that combines the objective and subjective indicators for satisfaction related to spontaneous subarachnoid haemorrhage.

Physical performance and role identity, i.e., the behavioural expectations (and behavioural codes) placed by others on the respective role holders, such as mother, father, employee, comforter, etc., are most affected by spontaneous subarachnoid haemorrhage and are reported in up to 60% of patients with diminished quality of life [19, 20]. Anxiety and depression are described by more than half of the patients with impaired quality of life [19, 20]. Both have a considerable influence on psychosocial interaction in the community. This is reflected in diminished vitality (43%) and emotions (40%) [19], and affects the ability to work. The ability of a patient to function socially after suffering spontaneous subarachnoid haemorrhage is influenced if physical identity as well as mental and emotional health are impaired [21]. A restriction to the quality of life after spontaneous subarachnoid haemorrhage may go unnoticed and untreated for a long time [2]. This situation is also unaffected by an improvement in residual physical deficits [22].

Descriptions of how the quality of life is influenced by clinical factors are inconsistent [14, 23]. The parameters most commonly reported, however, are age, sex, residual physical factors, neurological status on admission and Glasgow Outcome Score [14, 19, 22-29]. In this regard better scores are attained with the clinical factors, along with better results in terms of health-related quality of life. The Hunt and Hess Score and Fisher Score are seldom described as influential [27, 30].

In summary, it is evident that spontaneous subarachnoid haemorrhage has a lasting, negative impact on health-related quality of life. Such an influence is multifactorial, affecting several aspects of quality of life yet primarily the physical and emotional domains. Similarly, certain roles are affected which prove difficult to rehabilitate following critical care. It makes sense to document health-related quality of life three to six months after reintegrating the patient into his or her daily life. It is at this point that the implications of the haemorrhage can be evaluated and the therapeutic outcome can be further improved. Treatment of impaired health-related quality of life signals an improvement in the overall treatment outcome. Treatment is interdisciplinary, involving physical and occupational therapists, neuropsychologists and psychologists, and if necessary specialists in psychosomatic medicine and psychiatry, as well as social workers. It also engages the patient's entire family and circle of friends. If the improvement in the purely physical and clinical criteria of the treatment outcome following spontaneous subarachnoid haemorrhage comes to a standstill due to the fact e.g., that no new clips or coils, no new minimally invasive approach, and no new treatment for delayed cerebral ischaemia or hydrocephalus is forthcoming, another way in which to further enhance the treatment outcome is to define, document and instigate therapy with a view to health-related quality of life.

REFERENCES

[1] Kapapa T, Tjahjadi M, Konig R, Wirtz CR, Woischneck D. Which clinical variable influences health-related quality of life the most after spontaneous subarachnoid hemorrhage? Hunt and Hess scale, Fisher score, World Federation of Neurosurgeons score, Brussels coma score, and Glasgow coma score compared. *World Neurosurgery*. 2013 Dec;80(6):853-8. PubMed PMID: 23022643.

[2] Kapapa T, Woischneck D, Tjahjadi M. Long-term health-related quality of life after spontaneous nontraumatic subarachnoid hemorrhage: self and proxy reports in a 10-year period. *World neurosurgery*. 2014 Jan;81(1):105-9. PubMed PMID: 23046914.

[3] Tjahjadi M, Heinen C, Konig R, Rickels E, Wirtz CR, Woischneck D, et al. Health-related quality of life after spontaneous subarachnoid hemorrhage measured in a recent patient population. *World Neurosurgery*. 2013 Feb;79(2):296-307. PubMed PMID: 23046917.

[4] Kapapa T, König K, Heissler H, Ly MP, Zumkeller M, Schneekloth C, et al. [Health-related quality of life as an addendum to clinical criteria of outcome measurement in neurosurgery]. *Neurol. Rehabil.* 2006; 12(1):37-41.

[5] Locksley HB. Natural history of subarachnoid hemorrhage, intracranial aneurysms and arteriovenous malformations. *Journal of Neurosurgery*. 1966 Sep;25(3):321-68. PubMed PMID: 5921326.

[6] Locksley HB. Natural history of subarachnoid hemorrhage, intracranial aneurysms and arteriovenous malformations. Based on 6368 cases in the cooperative study. *Journal of Neurosurgery*. 1966 Aug;25(2):219-39. PubMed PMID: 5911370.

[7] Jennett B, Bond M. Assessment of outcome after severe brain damage. *Lancet*. 1975 Mar 1;1(7905):480-4. PubMed PMID: 46957.

[8] Rankin J. Cerebral vascular accidents in patients over the age of 60. II. Prognosis. *Scottish medical journal*. 1957 May;2(5):200-15. PubMed PMID: 13432835.

[9] van Swieten JC, Koudstaal PJ, Visser MC, Schouten HJ, van Gijn J. Interobserver agreement for the assessment of handicap in stroke patients. Stroke: *a Journal of Cerebral Circulation*. 1988 May;19(5):604-7. PubMed PMID: 3363593.

[10] Seule MA, Stienen MN, Cadosch D, Fournier JY, Lussmann R, Hildebrandt G, et al. [Aneurysmal subarachnoid hemorrhage - therapy and complications]. Anasthesiol Intensivmed Notfallmed Schmerzther. 2010 Jan;45(1):8-17. PubMed PMID: 20091471. Epub 2010/01/22. Aneurysmatische Subarachnoidalblutung - Diagnostik und Therapie zerebraler und systemischer Komplikationen. ger.

[11] Mocco J, Ransom ER, Komotar RJ, Sergot PB, Ostapkovich N, Schmidt JM, et al. Long-term domain-specific improvement following poor grade aneurysmal subarachnoid hemorrhage. *Journal of Neurology*. 2006 Oct;253(10):1278-84. PubMed PMID: 17063319.

[12] Mocco J, Zacharia BE, Komotar RJ, Connolly ES, Jr. A review of current and future medical therapies for cerebral vasospasm following aneurysmal subarachnoid hemorrhage. *Neurosurgical Focus*. 2006;21(3):E9. PubMed PMID: 17029348.

[13] Mocco J, Ransom ER, Komotar RJ, Schmidt JM, Sciacca RR, Mayer SA, et al. Preoperative prediction of long-term outcome in poor-grade aneurysmal subarachnoid

hemorrhage. Neurosurgery. 2006 Sep;59(3):529-38; discussion -38. PubMed PMID: 16955034.

[14] Passier PE, Visser-Meily JM, Rinkel GJ, Lindeman E, Post MW. Determinants of health-related quality of life after aneurysmal subarachnoid hemorrhage: a systematic review. Quality of Life Research: *An International Journal of Quality of Life Aspects of Treatment, Care and Rehabilitationan.* 2013 Jun; 22(5): 1027-43. PubMed PMID: 22956388.

[15] Brand C, Alber B, Fladung AK, Knauer K, Konig R, Oechsner A, et al. Cognitive performance following spontaneous subarachnoid haemorrhage versus other forms of intracranial haemorrhage. *British Journal of Neurosurgery.* 2014 Jan;28(1):68-80. PubMed PMID: 23879444.

[16] Hutter BO, Gilsbach JM. Which neuropsychological deficits are hidden behind a good outcome (Glasgow = I) after aneurysmal subarachnoid hemorrhage? Neurosurgery. 1993 Dec;33(6):999-1006. PubMed PMID: 8134014.

[17] Hutter BO, Gilsbach JM, Kreitschmann I. Quality of life and cognitive deficits after subarachnoid haemorrhage. *Br. J. Neurosurg.* 1995;9(4):465-75. PubMed PMID: 7576273.

[18] Felce D, Perry J. Quality of life: its definition and measurement. Research in developmental disabilities. 1995 Jan-Feb;16(1):51-74. PubMed PMID: 7701092.

[19] Katati MJ, Santiago-Ramajo S, Perez-Garcia M, Meersmans-Sanchez Jofre M, Vilar-Lopez R, Coin-Mejias MA, et al. Description of quality of life and its predictors in patients with aneurysmal subarachnoid hemorrhage. Cerebrovasc Dis. 2007;24(1):66-73. PubMed PMID: 17519546. Epub 2007/05/24. eng.

[20] Hackett ML, Anderson CS. Health outcomes 1 year after subarachnoid hemorrhage: An international population-based study. The Australian Cooperative Research on Subarachnoid Hemorrhage Study Group. Neurology. 2000 Sep 12;55(5):658-62. PubMed PMID: 10980729. *Epub* 2000/09/12. eng.

[21] van der Schaaf IC, Brilstra EH, Rinkel GJ, Bossuyt PM, van Gijn J. Quality of life, anxiety, and depression in patients with an untreated intracranial aneurysm or arteriovenous malformation. Stroke. 2002 Feb;33(2):440-3. PubMed PMID: 11823649. *Epub* 2002/02/02. eng.

[22] Hop JW, Rinkel GJ, Algra A, van Gijn J. Changes in functional outcome and quality of life in patients and caregivers after aneurysmal subarachnoid hemorrhage. *J. Neurosurg.* 2001 Dec;95(6):957-63. PubMed PMID: 11765839.

[23] Noble AJ, Schenk T. Which variables help explain the poor health-related quality of life after subarachnoid hemorrhage? A meta-analysis. *Neurosurgery.* 2010 Apr;66(4):772-83. PubMed PMID: 20190663. Epub 2010/03/02. eng.

[24] Agazzi S, de Tribolet N, Uske A, Regli L. Quality of life after aneurysmal subarachnoid hemorrhage in the elderly. Cerebrovasc Dis. 2004;18(2):174-5. PubMed PMID: 15256793. *Epub* 2004/07/17. eng.

[25] Cedzich C, Roth A. Neurological and psychosocial outcome after subarachnoid haemorrhage, and the Hunt and Hess scale as a predictor of clinical outcome. Zentralbl Neurochir. 2005 Aug;66(3):112-8. PubMed PMID: 16116553. *Epub* 2005/08/24. eng.

[26] Hutter BO, Kreitschmann-Andermahr I, Gilsbach JM. Health-related quality of life after aneurysmal subarachnoid hemorrhage: impacts of bleeding severity, computerized

tomography findings, surgery, vasospasm, and neurological grade. J Neurosurg. 2001 Feb;94(2):241-51. PubMed PMID: 11213961. *Epub* 2001/02/24. eng.

[27] Hutter BO, Kreitschmann-Andermahr I, Mayfrank L, Rohde V, Spetzger U, Gilsbach JM. Functional outcome after aneurysmal subarachnoid hemorrhage. *Acta Neurochir. Suppl.* 1999;72:157-74. PubMed PMID: 10337421.

[28] Visser-Meily JM, Rhebergen ML, Rinkel GJ, van Zandvoort MJ, Post MW. Long-term health-related quality of life after aneurysmal subarachnoid hemorrhage: relationship with psychological symptoms and personality characteristics. Stroke. 2009 Apr;40(4): 1526-9. PubMed PMID: 19095984. *Epub* 2008/12/20. eng.

[29] Wik KE, Lindegaard KF, Brunborg B, Bjork IT, Ruland C. [Life following acute subarachnoid haemorrhage]. Tidsskr Nor Laegeforen. 2005 Jan 20;125(2):152-4. PubMed PMID: 15665885. *Epub* 2005/01/25. Livet etter akutt hjernehinneblodning. nor.

[30] Kapapa T, Rickels E. Health-related quality of life after subarachnoid hemorrhage. *Neurol. Rehabil.* 2005;11(1):21-8.

In: Spontaneous Subarachnoid Haemorrhage
Editors: Thomas Kapapa and Ralph König

ISBN: 978-1-63485-270-8

Chapter 21

EXPERIMENTAL MODELS FOR THE STUDY OF SUBARACHNOID HAEMORRHAGE

Nicole A. Terpolilli
Department of Neurosurgery, Ludwig-Maximilians University of Munich, Munich, Germany

ABSTRACT

Various animal models have been developed in order to study the pathophysiology of SAH and to evaluate possible pharmacological treatment strategies. The following chapter discusses the most widely used techniques and animal models.

Keywords: experimental SAH, animal models of SAH, MCA perforation model

Various experimental animal models of subarachnoid haemorrhage have been developed to investigate pathophysiological mechanisms and to trial possible new treatment strategies. The following chapter will explore the most frequently employed techniques. Haemorrhage is most commonly induced either by a single or multiple injection of blood into the subarachnoid space or by puncturing/perforating a vessel in the circle of Willis (CW). In the last 30 years experiments were frequently carried out on primates as their physiology and anatomy is similar to that of humans. This enabled the use of clinical examination methods such as digital subtraction angiography and CT angiography for measuring cerebral blood flow and detecting vasospasm. More recently, rodents are favoured as laboratory animals given the scarce availability of primates; besides animal welfare issues and ethical and financial motives, the mouse model in particular is gaining in importance because it offers the possibility of genetic modification, i. e. the creation of transgenic mice. Furthermore, improved *in vivo* imaging techniques, such as two-photon microscopy or magnetic resonance imaging, provide increasingly accurate insights into the processes of posthemorrhagic microcirculation, even when using small laboratory animals.

INJECTION MODELS

Bagley described an animal model for investigating subarachnoid haemorrhage as early as 1928: autologous venous blood was mixed with cerebrospinal fluid and injected into the cisterna magna of dogs [1], which triggered the typical cardiovascular/systemic consequences of human pathology; in some cases multiple injections were required to achieve this effect. Subsequently, the model was adapted for different species, injection sites and injection techniques. Heparinised or non-heparinised whole blood (autologous or heterologous) or haemolysate is injected. The cisterna magna injection model is used extensively in dogs [2-4], different monkey species [5-8], rats [9-12], and mice [13, 14]. Since in the majority of patients aneurysms, and therefore also the bulk of the haemorrhage, are located in the anterior portion of the circle of Willis, it has been suggested that animal models with injection into the anterior cisterns may be better suited to reproduce the clinical phenotype. While transfrontal or transorbital blood injection into the prechiasmatic cistern in monkeys [15, 16] or dogs [17] produced inconsistent results with regard to the development of vasospasm and neurological damage, the model of prechiasmatic blood injection in rats [18, 19] reliably produces subarachnoid haemorrhage with corresponding deficits in a minimally-invasive fashion and with negligible operative morbidity; in this frequently used model auto- or heterologous blood is injected stereotactically into the prechiasmatic cistern via a small frontal burrhole.

In summary, injection models are easy to standardise, particularly with regard to haemorrhage volume, technically easy to implement (compared to other techniques) and reliably result in a range of quantifiable secondary SAH complications, such as decreased cerebral blood flow, intracranial hypertension, neuronal damage, and secondary changes at the cellular and microcirculation levels.

However, injection techniques also have distinct disadvantages as not all aspects of the pathophysiology of SAH can be modelled. In particular, the kinetics of stereotactic volume injection, which usually is performed over minutes, do not correspond to those of a ruptured arterial vessel where haemorrhage happens within seconds with high pressure. Accordingly, intracranial pressure in injection models does not follow the same course as ICP in the human pathology, furthermore the decrease of cerebral blood flow after injection is only short-lived [20]. As the initial and sharp ICP peak and/or the consecutive global cerebral ischaemia are decisive factors for early pathophysiological changes (early brain injury, EBI), it is as yet unclear to what extent injection models are suited to investigating acute pathophysiological changes after subarachnoid haemorrhage.

To better adapt the dynamics of injection-induced subarachnoid haemorrhage to the real-life situation, arterio-intrathecal shunt models were developed. Steiner et al. developed a canine model with femoro-intrathecal shunt in 1975 [21, 22] in order to investigate the pathophysiology of acute mortality after subarachnoid haemorrhage. This approach was modified in the rabbit model by Marbacher et al. to create the so-called shunt model [23]: The cisterna magna of rabbits is transcutaneously cannulated and connected to a catheter that has already been placed in the subclavian artery. When this bypass - which is initially closed with a clip - is opened subsequently, blood enters the subarachnoid space proportional to and dependent on the arterial blood pressure. Afterwards, the shunt is sealed. Previous results with this model indicate that the acute phase of subarachnoid haemorrhage, which is characterised by a CPP-independent decrease in cerebral blood flow [24, 25], may be better reproduced than in other injection models [26].

Re-bleedings which frequently occur and may complicate the clinical course are another factor that cannot be modelled using single injection techniques.

As the occurrence of (angiographically detectable) delayed vasospasm is associated with the extent of subarachnoid blood volume, the injection model may be carried out in a staged fashion, injecting twice or multiple times [27-31] thereby significantly increasing the severity of SAH and of all posthaemorrhagic complications. However, even after double blood injection, the acute decrease of cerebral blood flow is much less pronounced than the CBF drop observed in patients and in the perforation models described below [20, 32]. Lastly, vascular injury and/or endothelial damage, important pathophysiological features of aneurysmal subarachnoid haemorrhage, are missing in the injection model.

Circle of Willis: Perforation Models

In order to adequately model vascular injury and the arterial haemorrhage kinetics of subarachnoid haemorrhage in an experimental setup, large animal models were developed from the 1960s onwards; SAH was triggered by direct vascular puncture of the internal carotid artery [ICA, 33-35], middle cerebral artery [MCA, 36], or arteries of the posterior circulation [37-39]. Catheter-assisted [40] or endoscopic [41] procedures without craniotomy have also been described. In 1995, Bederson was the first researcher to describe the filament perforation model in rats [42]; in this non-invasive technique, a monofilament is introduced via the external carotid artery into the internal carotid artery and then advanced intracranially. The circle of Willis is perforated at the MCA bifurcation, the filament is then quickly removed. Over the years, several modifications of the MCA perforation model have been introduced: in order to control the intensity of haemorrhage, the common carotid artery was ligated [43]. However, this reduces global cerebral perfusion and leads to an increase in posthaemorrhagic global cerebral ischaemia. Use of different filament sizes (3-0, 4-0, 5-0) may be more suited to influence haemorrhage volume and, thus, severity [44]; moreover, replacing the polymer filament with Wolfram wire may help to reduce the perioperative complication rate [45]. Important pathophysiological features of SAH are reliably reproduced in the MCA perforation model: a sharp increase in ICP with simultaneous decrease in cerebral perfusion, the Cushing reflex, and numerous secondary complications such as brain oedema formation, (histologically detectable) neuronal damage and neurological deficits; re-bleeding intermittently occurs and can be quantified [46]. In the late 1990s, the endovascular filament perforation technique was first described in mice and thus could also be used in transgenic mouse models [47-49], but the reported mortality and secondary posthaemorrhagic damage showed wide variations. The routine use of laser Doppler flowmetry and intracranial pressure measurement during perforation helps to prove correct SAH induction and thereby enables a high level of standardisation of the method [50, 51]. Combining the perforation mouse model with transgenic alterations and improved *in vivo* imaging techniques such as intravital microscopy led to important insights into the pathophysiology of the early phase after subarachnoid haemorrhage. This early brain injury is characterised by a significant disturbances of the cerebral microcirculation, involving among other things microthrombosis of cerebral vessels [52, 53], microvascular constrictions (so called microvasospasms) [54], and impaired cerebrovascular CO_2 reactivity [55].

The drawbacks of the perforation model are the challenging and complex surgical technique and the inability to fully control the blood volume. However, after an appropriate training phase, perioperative morbidity decreases significantly. By continuously monitoring intracranial pressure and cerebral blood flow during induction of SAH and at different time-points thereafter, standardisation of bleeding intensity can not only be guaranteed, but also documented. A further albeit minor point of criticism in the perforation model is the lack of a "non-haemorrhage" control group: sham operated animals, in which the filament is introduced but the circle of Willis is not punctured, usually are used as controls. Unlike in injection models, where sham-operated animals are injected saline to separate the effect of intracranial volume augmentation from the effect of blood components, these animals do not undergo any physiological changes. However, in summary, the perforation model of subarachnoid haemorrhage is a well-established tool for simulating most facets of SAH pathophysiology and - despite a few limitations and higher (technical and surgical) complexity than other techniques - the only SAH model that simulates mechanical trauma from vascular rupture. Most studies that address the mechanisms of early brain injury [56, 57] use this model.

Other SAH Models

Placement of blood clots onto or around the circle of Willis vessels leads to delayed vasospasm that is clearly detectable on angiography or by Doppler sonography; this technique has been frequently used for chronic SAH studies and drug trials [58-61] However, a craniotomy and invasive operative procedure are needed to position the blood clot, limiting the successful use of this method to larger species such as dogs and monkeys. The costly equipment and surgical expertise needed for large animal experiments, the increasing restrictions placed on primate experiments, and the shift in research focus to early disturbances in the cerebral microcirculation, have severely limited the dissemination of the clot model. Currently, the primate model is used in a few centres to investigate delayed vasospasms [62, 63].

Various studies report the successful and standardisable induction of intracranial aneurysms [64-66]; however, it has not yet been possible to reliably trigger subarachnoid haemorrhage in these models. Further development of this method or its combination with existing perforation techniques may make a model of aneurysmal subarachnoid haemorrhage feasible in the future.

Conclusion

There are a multitude of experimental techniques for inducing subarachnoid haemorrhage. All models have distinct advantages and disadvantages; given the complex human pathology no single model will adequately represent every nuance of the disease. Perforation models are technically complex and more surgically/manually challenging than other techniques, but perforation-induced SAH appears to be most closely related to the kinetics of haemorrhage, vascular trauma in ruptures, elevated ICP, decreased CBF and other secondary posthaemorrhagic processes of human pathophysiology. In transgenic mouse models this method, combined with novel imaging and visualisation techniques, enables examination of all aspects of SAH pathophysiology, particularly in the early phase (<72 hours) after haemorrhage; if necessary, results obtained in the rodent model then can be tested/verified in clinically relevant, large animal models with respect to their suitability for use in SAH therapy.

REFERENCES

[1] Bagley, C. Jr. Blood in the cerebrospinal fluid: Resultant functional and organic alterations in the central nervous system - Part A: Experimental data. *Arch Surg* 1928;17(1):18-38.

[2] Kuwayama A., Zervas N. T., Belson R., Shintani A., Pickren K. A model for experimental cerebral arterial spasm. *Stroke* 1972 Jan;3(1):49-56.

[3] Mizuno T., Hamada J., Kai Y., Todaka T., Morioka M., Ushio Y. Single blood injection into the ventral cisterna magna through a microcatheter for the production of delayed cerebral vasospasm: experimental study in dogs. *AJNR Am J Neuroradiol* 2003 Apr; 24(4):608-12.

[4] Varsos V. G., Liszczak T. M., Han D. H., Kistler J. P., Vielma J., Black P. M. et al. Delayed cerebral vasospasm is not reversible by aminophylline, nifedipine, or papaverine in a "two-hemorrhage" canine model. *J Neurosurg* 1983 Jan;58(1):11-7.

[5] Chow R. W., Newton T. H., Smith M. C., Adams J. E. Cerebral vasospasm induced by subarachnoid blood and serotonin. An angiographic study. *Invest Radiol* 1968 Nov; 3(6):402-7.

[6] Martins A. N., Doyle T. F., Newby N., Kobrine A. I., Ramirez A. The effect of a simulated subarachnoid hemorrhage on cerebral blood flow in the monkey. *Stroke* 1975 Nov;6(6):664-72.

[7] Delgado-Zygmunt T. J., Arbab M. A., Shiokawa Y., Svendgaard N. A. A primate model for acute and late cerebral vasospasm: angiographic findings. *Acta Neurochir* (Wien) 1992;118(3-4):130-6.

[8] von M. C., Chang J. Y., Delgado T., Owman C., Sahlin C., Svendgaard N. A. Ultrastructural cerebrovascular changes in a model of subarachnoid hemorrhage in baboon based on triple cisternal blood injection. *Surg Neurol* 1990 Mar;33(3):195-201.

[9] Delgado T. J., Brismar J., Svendgaard N. A. Subarachnoid haemorrhage in the rat: angiography and fluorescence microscopy of the major cerebral arteries. *Stroke* 1985 Jul;16(4):595-602.

[10] Solomon R. A., Antunes J. L., Chen R. Y., Bland L., Chien S. Decrease in cerebral blood flow in rats after experimental subarachnoid hemorrhage: a new animal model. *Stroke* 1985 Jan;16(1):58-64.

[11] Doczi T., Joo F., Adam G., Bozoky B., Szerdahelyi P. Blood-brain barrier damage during the acute stage of subarachnoid hemorrhage, as exemplified by a new animal model. *Neurosurgery* 1986 Jun;18(6):733-9.

[12] Sobey C. G., Heistad D. D., Faraci F. M. Effect of subarachnoid hemorrhage on dilatation of rat basilar artery *in vivo*. *Am J Physiol* 1996 Jul;271(1 Pt 2):H126-H132.

[13] Lin C. L., Calisaneller T., Ukita N., Dumont A. S., Kassell N. F., Lee K. S. A murine model of subarachnoid hemorrhage-induced cerebral vasospasm. *J Neurosci Methods* 2003 Feb 15;123(1):89-97.

[14] Kamp M. A., Dibue M., Sommer C., Steiger H. J., Schneider T., Hanggi D. Evaluation of a murine single-blood-injection SAH model. *PLoS One* 2014;9(12):e114946.

[15] McIntyre J. W., Miller J. D., Weir B. K. Anaesthesia for cerebral angiography: cardiovascular and cerebrospinal fluid pressure observations in the monkey under pentobarbital-halothane anaesthesia. *Can Anaesth Soc J* 1969 Jul;16(4):309-15.

[16] Weir B., Erasmo R., Miller J., McIntyre J., Secord D., Mielke B. Vasospasm in response to repeated subarachnoid hemorrhages in the monkey. *J Neurosurg* 1970 Oct;33(4):395-406.

[17] Jakubowski J., McCleery W. N., Todd J. H. Proceedings: Acute haemorrhagic cerebral vasospasm in the dog: an experimental model. *Br J Anaesth* 1973 Dec;45(12):1235-6.

[18] Prunell G. F., Mathiesen T., Svendgaard N. A. A new experimental model in rats for study of the pathophysiology of subarachnoid hemorrhage. *Neuroreport* 2002 Dec 20;13(18):2553-6.

[19] Sabri M., Jeon H., Ai J., Tariq A., Shang X., Chen G. et al. Anterior circulation mouse model of subarachnoid hemorrhage. *Brain Res* 2009 Oct 27;1295:179-85.

[20] Prunell G. F., Mathiesen T., Svendgaard N. A. Experimental subarachnoid hemorrhage: cerebral blood flow and brain metabolism during the acute phase in three different models in the rat. *Neurosurgery* 2004 Feb;54(2):426-36.

[21] Steiner L., Lofgren J., Zwetnow N. N. Lethal mechanism in repeated subarachnoid hemorrhage in dogs. *Acta Neurol Scand* 1975 Oct;52(4): 268-93.

[22] Steiner L., Lofgren J., Zwetnow N. N. Characteristics and limits of tolerance in repeated subarachnoid hemorrhage in dogs. *Acta Neurol Scand* 1975 Oct;52(4):241-67.

[23] Marbacher S., Andereggen L., Neuschmelting V., Widmer H. R., von G. M., Takala J. et al. A new rabbit model for the study of early brain injury after subarachnoid hemorrhage. *J Neurosci Methods* 2012 Jul 15;208(2): 138-45.

[24] Schubert G. A., Seiz M., Hegewald A. A., Manville J., Thome C. Hypoperfusion in the acute phase of subarachnoid hemorrhage. *Acta Neurochir Suppl* 2011;110(Pt 1):35-8.

[25] Schubert G. A., Seiz M., Hegewald A. A., Manville J., Thome C. Acute hypoperfusion immediately after subarachnoid hemorrhage: a xenon contrast-enhanced CT study. *J Neurotrauma* 2009 Dec;26(12):2225-31.

[26] Marbacher S., Neuschmelting V., Andereggen L., Widmer H. R., von G. M., Takala J. et al. Early brain injury linearly correlates with reduction in cerebral perfusion pressure during the hyperacute phase of subarachnoid hemorrhage. *Intensive Care Med Exp* 2014 Dec;2(1):30.

[27] Raslan F., Albert-Weissenberger C., Westermaier T., Saker S., Kleinschnitz C., Lee J. Y. A modified double injection model of cisterna magna for the study of delayed cerebral vasospasm following subarachnoid hemorrhage in rats. *Exp Transl Stroke Med* 2012;4(1):23.

[28] Guresir E., Schuss P., Borger V., Vatter H. Rat cisterna magna double-injection model of subarachnoid hemorrhage - background, advantages/limitations, technical

considerations, modifications, and outcome measures. *Acta Neurochir Suppl* 2015;120: 325-9.

[29] Deinsberger W., Vogel J., Kuschinsky W., Auer L. M., Boker D. K. Experimental intracerebral hemorrhage: description of a double injection model in rats. *Neurol Res* 1996 Oct;18(5):475-7.

[30] Spallone A., Pastore F. S. Cerebral vasospasm in a double-injection model in rabbit. *Surg Neurol* 1989 Dec;32(6):408-17.

[31] Kikkawa Y. A rabbit cisterna magna double-injection subarachnoid hemorrhage model. *Acta Neurochir Suppl* 2015;120:331-5.

[32] Lee J. Y., Sagher O., Keep R., Hua Y., Xi G. Comparison of experimental rat models of early brain injury after subarachnoid hemorrhage. *Neurosurgery* 2009 Aug;65(2):331-43.

[33] Simeone F. A., Ryan K. G., Cotter J. R. Prolonged experimental cerebral vasospasm. *J Neurosurg* 1968 Oct;29(4):357-66.

[34] Frazee J. G. A primate model of chronic cerebral vasospasm. *Stroke* 1982 Sep;13(5): 612-4.

[35] Asano T., Sano K. Pathogenetic role of no-reflow phenomenon in experimental subarachnoid hemorrhage in dogs. *J Neurosurg* 1977 Apr; 46(4):454-66.

[36] Clower B. R., Smith R. R., Haining J. L., Lockard J. Constrictive endarteropathy following experimental subarachnoid hemorrhage. *Stroke* 1981 Jul;12(4):501-8.

[37] Barry K. J., Gogjian M. A., Stein B. M. Small animal model for investigation of subarachnoid hemorrhage and cerebral vasospasm. *Stroke* 1979 Sep;10(5):538-41.

[38] Jakubowski J., Bell B. A., Symon L., Zawirski M. B., Francis D. M. A primate model of subarachnoid hemorrhage: change in regional cerebral blood flow, autoregulation carbon dioxide reactivity, and central conduction time. *Stroke* 1982 Sep;13(5):601-11.

[39] Kuyama H., Ladds A., Branston N. M., Nitta M., Symon L. An experimental study of acute subarachnoid haemorrhage in baboons: changes in cerebral blood volume, blood flow, electrical activity and water content. *J Neurol Neurosurg Psychiatry* 1984 Apr; 47(4):354-64.

[40] Masuda T., Sato K., Yamamoto S., Matsuyama N., Shimohama T., Matsunaga A. et al. Sympathetic nervous activity and myocardial damage immediately after subarachnoid hemorrhage in a unique animal model. *Stroke* 2002 Jun;33(6):1671-6.

[41] Ergun R., Fernandez J., Misra M., Dujovny M. Endoscopic technique: a new model of subarachnoid hemorrhage in rats. *Neurol Res* 2001 Sep; 23(6):627-30.

[42] Bederson J. B., Germano I. M., Guarino L. Cortical blood flow and cerebral perfusion pressure in a new noncraniotomy model of subarachnoid hemorrhage in the rat. *Stroke* 1995 Jun;26(6):1086-91.

[43] Veelken J. A., Laing R. J., Jakubowski J. The Sheffield model of subarachnoid hemorrhage in rats. *Stroke* 1995 Jul;26(7):1279-83.

[44] Schwartz A. Y., Masago A., Sehba F. A., Bederson J. B. Experimental models of subarachnoid hemorrhage in the rat: a refinement of the endovascular filament model. *J Neurosci Methods* 2000 Mar 15;96(2): 161-7.

[45] Hollig A., Weinandy A., Nolte K., Clusmann H., Rossaint R., Coburn M. Experimental subarachnoid hemorrhage in rats: comparison of two endovascular perforation techniques with respect to success rate, confounding pathologies and early hippocampal tissue lesion pattern. *PLoS One* 2015;10(4):e0123398.

[46] Hockel K., Scholler K., Trabold R., Nussberger J., Plesnila N. Vasopressin V(1a) receptors mediate posthemorrhagic systemic hypertension thereby determining rebleeding rate and outcome after experimental subarachnoid hemorrhage. *Stroke* 2012 Jan;43(1):227-32.

[47] Kamii H., Kato I., Kinouchi H., Chan P. H., Epstein C. J., Akabane A. et al. Amelioration of vasospasm after subarachnoid hemorrhage in transgenic mice overexpressing CuZn-superoxide dismutase. *Stroke* 1999 Apr;30(4):867-71.

[48] Saito A., Kamii H., Kato I., Takasawa S., Kondo T., Chan P. H. et al. Transgenic CuZn-superoxide dismutase inhibits NO synthase induction in experimental subarachnoid hemorrhage. *Stroke* 2001 Jul;32(7):1652-7.

[49] Parra A., McGirt M. J., Sheng H., Laskowitz D. T., Pearlstein R. D., Warner D. S. Mouse model of subarachnoid hemorrhage associated cerebral vasospasm: methodological analysis. *Neurol Res* 2002 Jul; 24(5):510-6.

[50] Feiler S., Friedrich B., Scholler K., Thal S. C., Plesnila N. Standardized induction of subarachnoid hemorrhage in mice by intracranial pressure monitoring. *J Neurosci Methods* 2010 Jul 15;190(2):164-70.

[51] Scholler K., Feiler S., Anetsberger S., Kim S. W., Plesnila N. Contribution of bradykinin receptors to the development of secondary brain damage after experimental subarachnoid hemorrhage. *Neurosurgery* 2011 Apr;68(4):1118-23.

[52] Sehba F. A., Bederson J. B. Mechanisms of acute brain injury after subarachnoid hemorrhage. *Neurol Res* 2006 Jun;28(4):381-98.

[53] Sehba F. A., Mostafa G., Friedrich V., Jr., Bederson J. B. Acute microvascular platelet aggregation after subarachnoid hemorrhage. *J Neurosurg* 2005 Jun;102(6):1094-100.

[54] Friedrich B., Muller F., Feiler S., Scholler K., Plesnila N. Experimental subarachnoid hemorrhage causes early and long-lasting microarterial constriction and microthrombosis: an *in-vivo* microscopy study. *J Cereb Blood Flow Metab* 2012 Mar; 32(3):447-55.

[55] Friedrich B., Michalik R., Oniszczuk A., Abubaker K., Kozniewska E., Plesnila N. CO2 has no therapeutic effect on early microvasospasm after experimental subarachnoid hemorrhage. *J Cereb Blood Flow Metab* 2014 Aug;34(8):e1-e6.

[56] Sehba F. A., Hou J., Pluta R. M., Zhang J. H. The importance of early brain injury after subarachnoid hemorrhage. *Prog Neurobiol* 2012 Apr; 97(1):14-37.

[57] Sehba F. A., Pluta R. M., Zhang J. H. Metamorphosis of subarachnoid hemorrhage research: from delayed vasospasm to early brain injury. *Mol Neurobiol* 2011 Feb; 43(1):27-40.

[58] Shiokawa K., Kasuya H., Miyajima M., Izawa M., Takakura K. Prophylactic effect of papaverine prolonged-release pellets on cerebral vasospasm in dogs. *Neurosurgery* 1998 Jan;42(1):109-15.

[59] Fathi A. R., Bakhtian K. D., Marbacher S., Fandino J., Pluta R. M. Blood clot placement model of subarachnoid hemorrhage in non-human primates. *Acta Neurochir Suppl* 2015;120:343-6.

[60] Handa Y., Weir B. K., Nosko M., Mosewich R., Tsuji T., Grace M. The effect of timing of clot removal on chronic vasospasm in a primate model. *J Neurosurg* 1987 Oct; 67(4):558-64.

[61] Pluta R. M., Bacher J., Skopets B., Hoffmann V. A non-human primate model of aneurismal subarachnoid hemorrhage (SAH). *Transl Stroke Res* 2014 Dec;5(6):681-91.

[62] Fathi A. R., Pluta R. M., Bakhtian K. D., Qi M., Lonser R. R. Reversal of cerebral vasospasm via intravenous sodium nitrite after subarachnoid hemorrhage in primates. *J Neuro*surg 2011 Dec;115(6):1213-20.

[63] Pluta R. M., Dejam A., Grimes G., Gladwin M. T., Oldfield E. H. Nitrite infusions to prevent delayed cerebral vasospasm in a primate model of subarachnoid hemorrhage. *JAMA* 2005 Mar 23;293(12):1477-84.

[64] van Alphen H. A., Gao Y. Z., Kamphorst W. An acute experimental model of saccular aneurysms in the rat. *Neurol Res* 1990 Dec;12(4):256-9.

[65] Nishikawa M., Smith R. D., Yonekawa Y. Experimental intracranial aneurysms. *Surg Neurol* 1977 Apr;7(4):241-4.

[66] Morimoto M., Miyamoto S., Mizoguchi A., Kume N., Kita T., Hashimoto N. Mouse model of cerebral aneurysm: experimental induction by renal hypertension and local hemodynamic changes. *Stroke* 2002 Jul;33(7):1911-5.

Editors' Contact Information

Dr. Thomas Kapapa, M.D.
Senior Physician, Associate Professor
Department of Neurosurgery, University of Ulm
Albert-Einstein-Allee 23, 89081 Ulm, Germany
Thomas.Kapapa@uniklinik-ulm.de

Prof. Dr. Ralph König, M.D.
Senior Physician, Associate Professor, CEO
Department of Neurosurgery, University of Ulm
Albert-Einstein-Allee 23, 89081 Ulm, Germany
ralph.koenig@uni-ulm.de

INDEX

A

B

C

D

E

I

J

K

L

M

N

O

P

Q

R

S

T

U

V

W

X